Advance praise for *Joy of Backpacking*

"Joy of Backpacking will supply you with everything you need to know to be comfortable, feel safe, and have fun on your next backcountry adventure."

> —Sheri and Randy Propster,
> Appalachian Trail thru-hikers (2168.2 miles, 1999),
> American Discovery Trail (4200 miles, 2006),
> Get Out More '07 Ambassadors

"Like the ideal backpack, the *Joy of Backpacking* holds all the essentials in one efficient package."

> —John Sterling, Executive Director,
> Conservation Alliance

"The *Joy of Backpacking* cuts through the current dogma that says you have to have a Ph.D. in gear and outdoors techniques and encourages you to discover the true joy of backpacking."

> —Scott Williamson,
> backpacking educator
> and nine-time hiker of the Pacific Crest Trail

"Joy of Backpacking reminds me why I began exploring the wilderness many decades ago; backpacking forces you to abandon the hectic pace of the rat race and focus on the true essentials of life."

> —Stuart Bourdon,
> Editor/Associate Publisher,
> *Camping Life Magazine*

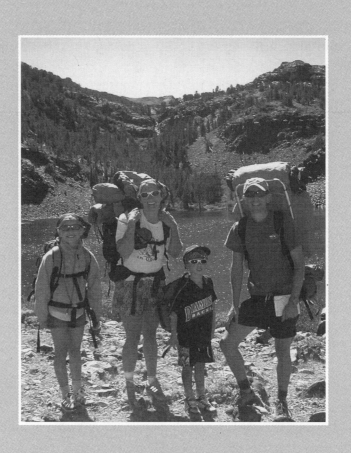

JOY of
BACKPACKING

*Your complete guide
to attaining pure happiness
in the outdoors*

Brian Beffort

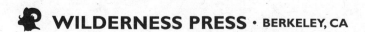

WILDERNESS PRESS · BERKELEY, CA

Joy of Backpacking: Your complete guide to attaining pure happiness in the outdoors

1st EDITION May 2007

Copyright © 2007 by Brian Beffort

Front cover photo copyright © 2007 by Gregg Adams
Back cover photos copyright © 2007 by Brian Beffort, except second from top, by Eva Dienel
Interior photos, except where noted on page vi, by Brian Beffort
Illustrations on page 141 by Paul Purcell
Cover design: Lisa Pletka/Larry B. Van Dyke
Book design: Larry B. Van Dyke
Book editor: Eva Dienel

ISBN: 978-0-89997-405-7
UPC: 7-19609-97405-5

Printed in Canada

♻ Printed on recycled paper (100% post consumer)

Published by: **Wilderness Press**
1200 5th Street
Berkeley, CA 94710
(800) 443-7227; FAX (510) 558-1696
info@wildernesspress.com
www.wildernesspress.com

Visit our website for a complete listing of our books and for ordering information.

Cover photo: Vermilion Cliffs National Monument of the Paria Plateau, Arizona
Frontispiece: The Tresan family, high in the Sierra Nevada

SAFETY NOTICE: Although Wilderness Press and the author have made every attempt to ensure that the information in this book is accurate at press time, they are not responsible for any loss, damage, injury, or inconvenience that may occur to anyone while using this book. You are responsible for your own safety and health while in the wilderness.

Library of Congress Cataloging-in-Publication Data

Beffort, Brian.
   Joy of backpacking : your complete guide to attaining pure happiness in the outdoors / Brian Beffort.—1st ed.
      p. cm.
   Includes bibliographical references and index.
   ISBN 978-0-89997-405-7 (pbk.)
   1. Backpacking. I. Title.
   GV199.6.B45 2007
   796.51—dc22
                              2006103513

PREFACE

I remember my first backpacking trip as though it happened last summer. I was 7 years old, standing knee deep in clear, cold Summit Lake in California's Hoover Wilderness, trying to build up the courage to move deeper into the icy water. I must have been thinking about it for a long time, because while I stood there, a large trout swam slowly out of the depths toward me. I watched as it slid lazily between my legs—its back shimmering in dancing shades of green and red—and back toward the depths. I considered reaching down and trying to grab it, but I was transfixed by my close encounter of the gilled kind.

The whole trip was new and fun—carrying my pack up and over the pass, setting up the tent, climbing trees and rocks, and watching my mom cook dinner over our little green camp stove. But seeing that darn fish was unlike anything I had ever experienced. It gave me a glimpse of the excitement, surprises, lessons, beauty, and joy waiting in wilderness—shining moments of magic and wonder we can rarely predict, which we can witness only by being there. But we can't drive to these experiences. We have to park our cars and travel by other means. Some do it by horse packing; others by canoe, kayak, or raft. I backpack.

Carrying all of your provisions into rugged and inhospitable landscapes can be hard work. It can even be dangerous. But if you plan and prepare well, and make safe decisions while you're out there, you stand a good chance of finding a joy as grand as life itself.

Years of making good and bad decisions while backpacking, of tinkering, fussing, experimenting with systems, and playing with recipes, I've learned to enjoy backpacking in a variety of landscapes and seasons. I wrote this book to offer helpful tips and advice you can use to find the joys of backpacking without having to make too many avoidable mistakes. After all, there's no need to reinvent the wheel ... er, hiking boot.

ACKNOWLEDGMENTS

The information presented here has been gathered from decades of experience, reading, writing, researching, and learning from and with others. My appreciation goes out to all of the following people, and more. First to Mom, for taking me backpacking that first time and getting me hooked. To great outdoor writers, who have helped me learn and explore through words—Edward Abbey, Wallace Stegner, John Muir, Dave Foreman, Doug Peacock, Farley Mowat, Jon Krakauer, and others—as well as outdoor journalists, such as Buck Tilton, Michael Hodgson, Kristen Hostetter, Alan Kesselheim, and others. To the wonderful information and resources in *Backpacker* and *Outside* magazines, as well as the excellent resources contained in the many websites listed throughout this book.

To John Hiatt, Kurt Kuznicki, Blake Tresan, Pete Dronkers, Brian Murdock, James Sippel, Robert Lyon, Sarah Perrault, Craig Deutsche, Darlene and Joey Kitterman, and others for their advice and recommendations. I appreciate Roslyn Bullas, Mary Chambers, James Dziezynski, Barbara Egbert, Scott Graham, Mathew Grimm, Kurt Kuznicki, Laurie Ann March, John Vonhof, and Michelle Waitzman for contributing their "My System" expertise into these pages. Thank you, Kurt, Brian, Blake, James, and others, for contributing your photographs to this project. Thanks to the fine crew at Wilderness Press for working with me. And finally, thank you, Laura and Logan, for patiently enduring the writing of this book. Thank you all! Now, let's go backpacking!

PHOTO CREDITS

Thanks to the following for the use of their photos in this book:

Adventure Medical Kits: Photos on page 230
Howard Booth: Photo on page 16
Laura Brigham: Photos on pages 36, 146, 147, 148, 149, 150, 151, and 162
Roslyn Bullas: Photos on pages 6, 80, 95 (lower right), 105, 112, 115, 124, 143, 183, 187, 190, and 243
Eva Dienel: Photos on pages 57, 156, 159, and 244
Pete Dronkers: Photos on pages 1 and 2
Barbara Egbert: Photo on page 28
Exped: Photos on page 83
Terry Ferg: Photo on page 250
Scott Graham: Photo on page 56

Mathew Grimm: Photos on pages 58, 72, 75, 188, 207, and 220
MSR: Photos on pages 79 (lower right), 86, 87, 90, 91, 92, 93 (upper left), and 95 (upper left)
Kurt Kuznicki: Photos on pages 20, 40, 170, 196, and 217
Montrail: Photo on page 65
Brian Murdock: Photos on pages xii, 15, and 164 (upper left)
Outdoor Research: Photo on page 79 (upper left)
Petzl: Photo on page 64
Adam Richardson: Photos on pages 17, 23, and 104
Scott Sady: Photo on page 10
Scarpa: Photo on page 67 (upper left)
Laura Shauger: Photo on page 74
Ellie and James Sippel: Photos on pages 25, 27, 29, 30, 32 (lower right), 37, 100, 174, 180, and 238
Scott Smith: Photo on page 249
Therm-a-Rest: Photos on page 55
Blake Tresan: Photos on pages ii, 3, 32 (upper left), and 164 (lower right)

CONTENTS

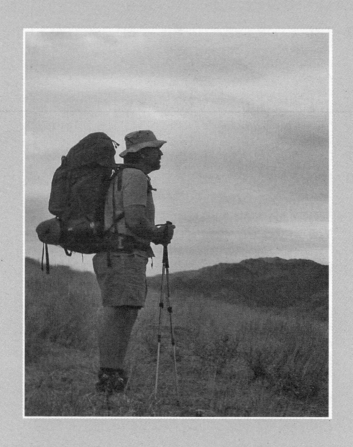

INTRODUCTION

Why go backpacking? Why carry that heavy load into the wilderness, where you'll be exposed to the elements, bugs, and animals with no shower and no real bed to speak of? Millions of people love backpacking, and there are many reasons why. For most people, the joys of backpacking lie somewhere in the list below.

Ten Reasons
Why Backpacking Is Great

Explore the world's most beautiful places. Backpacking can take you to many of the world's most beautiful places, which simply aren't accessible any other way—places such as the twisting inner corridors of the Grand Canyon, the forests of the Appalachian Trail, the high peaks of the Rocky Mountains, the even higher peaks of the Himalaya, and a million other beautiful places.

Get in shape. No matter how you do it, backpacking is great exercise. Huffing your way along a trail is great for the legs, heart, lungs, and upper body (especially if you use trekking poles). Honest physical labor in clean mountain air can do much to undo the damage caused by stress, high blood pressure, and obesity.

Relax. Daily, deadline-driven, and success-oriented lifestyles have a way of winding people up into balls of stress. Although phone

Your joy is waiting for you in the wild.

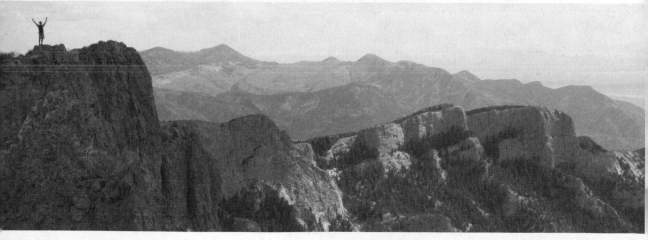

calls, faxes, televisions, commercials, traffic, deadlines, bills, and long to-do lists play important roles in most people's lives, once you hit the trailhead, you'll be able to leave those distractions behind. As walking guru Robert Sweetgall said: "We live in a fast-paced society. Walking slows us down." It's a chance to slow life down to walking speed and take a few deep breaths in solitude.

Focus on what's most important. Spending a few days on the trail can help you forget about the minutiae of your life at home. Concerns will shrink to the essentials: food, shelter, weather, and safety. With these addressed, you can focus on enjoying the scenery, breathing clean air, feeling the sun and wind against your skin, feeling your body work, and letting other matters fall away—at least for a few days. This helps priorities at home adjust

themselves as well; what's most important when you return from backpacking may not be what topped your priority list when you left.

If you are facing a great decision in life, or if you are filled with confusion, stress or angst, hit the trail for a few days. As my friend Sarah told me while backpacking once, "Things tend to get less complicated when you're on the trail."

Get to know the real world. Most of us live our days immersed in a world entirely constructed by humans—from asphalt and air conditioning, to fast-food, fluorescent lighting, office cubicles, and television. Watch or listen to enough media, and you'll start to believe that everything you could ever need or want is a product you must buy. In our daily lives, few of us ever come in contact with the natural world, and we're missing out on so many wonderful

When was the last time you surrounded yourself with true solitude?

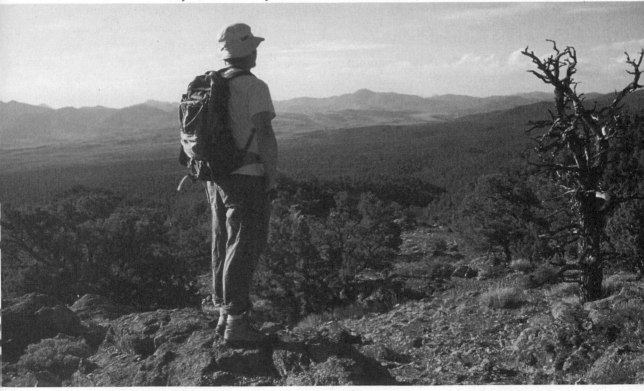

experiences. When was the last time you actually touched bare earth? Lay back and watch the clouds drift across the sky or the stars sparkle against a sharp, black night? Jumped into a clear, cold swimming hole in the mountains on a hot day? Or watched a spectacular sunset fade into the deep blue of twilight? Backpacking allows us to spend time with the natural world—the world that was here before humans built civilization, and the world that will endure long after civilization has crumbled.

Challenge your brain. Although anyone can throw some food and gear into a backpack and head into the wilderness, learning backcountry skills will make it safer and more enjoyable. Planning your trip, packing your gear, anticipating weather and your own body's reactions to hiking, using a map and compass (and GPS, if you choose), and traveling through the wilderness safely and happily without disturbing the natural elements and rhythms of your destination—all of these things will challenge your mind, making it sharper. You'll also learn that persistence and hard work can take you to wonderful places. Not only will these skills make your next backpacking trip even better, they'll give you confidence to meet the tests of daily life.

Get to know yourself. Separating ourselves from the distractions of daily life—from phone calls, faxes, traffic, appointments, and our many other habits and "addictions"—requires us to break free from normal mental and physical patterns. It allows us to see a different side of ourselves, as we react to the beauty and challenges along the trail. This self-knowledge can serve us well as we face the grind of life back home.

Raise happier, healthier, smarter children. Kids love backpacking. It gives them a chance to be kids—to explore, play, push their bodies and their brains, discover the world and learn in ways they can't do at home. Numerous studies show that contact with nature reduces

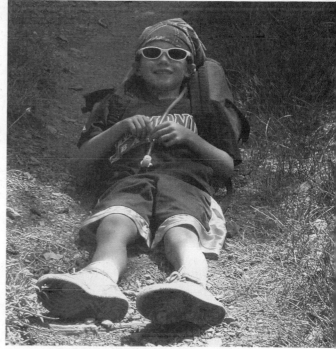
Some days are faster than others.

the risk of developing Attention Deficit Hyperactivity Disorder (ADHD), and it eases the symptoms of those who have been diagnosed with the disorder. Autistic kids have shown similar responses to nature. Wilderness therapy programs have been successful in helping children cope with mental, behavioral, drug, and alcohol problems. No child is too young to backpack (although there are definite challenges to backpacking with infants and toddlers; read more about backpacking with kids beginning on page 24).

Find god. Jesus found his inspiration in the wilderness. Moses found his on a mountain. Buddhists consider mountains sacred homes of the gods, as do many indigenous peoples around the world. Whatever god, goddess, force, higher power, or creator you worship, backpacking can be a deeply spiritual journey because it puts you in direct contact with creation itself. If you do not believe in a divine intelligence, backpacking will put you in the midst of our infinitely complex, integrated, and organized universe. As John Muir said, "The clearest path to the universe is through a forest wilderness." However you define the power behind creation, creation itself is powerful and inspiring to explore.

Enjoy your return home. Whether your backpacking trip is fun or miserable, you'll gain a greater appreciation for pizza, cold fizzy drinks, hot showers, evenings in front of the television, clean sheets, and cozy beds after you've spent a few days in the woods.

Ultimately, what people find while backpacking is a sense of joy. But as you can see from this list, joy can come in different ways. It might come after a day of rain, when you watch the sun dip below the clouds for three minutes of glorious sunset before it sinks below the horizon; when you reach the top of the ridge to

Enjoying the view is a great way to catch your breath.

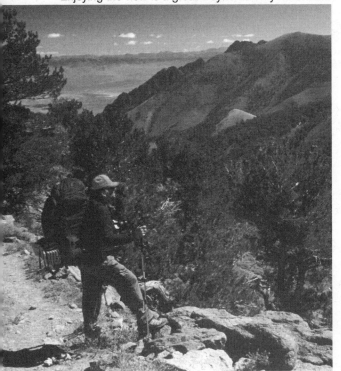

find a view on the other side that stretches over miles of canyons, peaks, and sky; or when you complete a difficult weekend of hiking and say to yourself, "Gee, maybe I'm not in such bad shape after all."

The joy of backpacking is different for every person, and it's different on every trip. It might be the joy of feeling the grass on your bare feet and the sun on your face as you read your favorite book by a shimmering lake; it might be the joy of knowing you have the skills and equipment to survive in the most inhospitable of environments; it might be the joy of watching your child intent in quiet discovery with a rock, bird, or insect; it might be the joy of a cold drink, hot shower, and soft mattress after a voyage into the wild.

Your own joy is waiting for you somewhere out there.

How This Book Will Help

No matter how you cut it, backpacking takes work. Even if you've been backpacking for 20 years, you still need to remember long lists of items to pack, you need to keep up on the ever-changing technology of gear, and you can always find ways to improve your backpacking system. This book is designed to help you work smarter, not harder; to maximize the pleasure and minimize the discomfort of backpacking by showing you how to plan well, pack enough (but not too much), and sharpen your backcountry skills—regardless of whether you're a veteran or a beginner. The better you do these things, the easier your trip will be, and the more fun you'll have on the trail.

You can read books about backpacking until the cows come home (where have those darn cows been all this time?), but the most important thing is to hit the trail. This book is designed to help you prepare for the trip, bring the right gear and food, get fit for the trail, and then travel and camp safely without destroying the places you visit. Included in these pages is everything you'll need to know to get started on the trail, plus suggestions to fine-tune your gear and techniques that most veteran backpackers will appreciate, too. Because backpacking is ultimately about developing a system that works best for you, I've included tips throughout the book from backpacking experts who share their particular systems. You may just find a few new tricks to test on your next trip—or you may be inspired to develop some of your own. I also include suggestions for further reading if you'd like to research particular topics in more detail.

The book is organized into the following general sections:

Planning Your Trip: This section covers how to decide which type of trip is best for you, how to decide where to go and whom to go with, and special considerations for backpacking with kids and with dogs.

Backpacking Gear: This covers all the equipment you will need for backpacking, what to look for in specific types of equipment, and how to care for, clean, and repair your gear.

Food and Water: All you need to know about nutrition, water, food, menu planning, and cooking in the backcountry.

Preparing for the Trail: Essential backcountry skills, such as wilderness navigation, useful knots to use, and how to ford streams safely.

Joy on the Trail: This section covers everything to do with hiking and camping, from finding your pace to knowing when to rest, from setting up camp to keeping yourself clean and your kitchen sanitary, and from breaking camp to going home without a serious case of missing-the-backcountry blues.

Safety and Comfort in the Backcountry: Weather and weather preparedness, wild creatures and poisonous plants, and first aid.

Advanced Backcountry Skills and Travel: There's more to backcountry travel than simple backpacking. This section introduces advanced wilderness skills, such as long-distance or through-hiking, cross-country travel, international trekking, backpacking in extreme conditions or locations, and other types of backcountry travel.

There are as many different ways to backpack as there are people, destinations, and pieces of equipment. The best measure of success is your own happiness. If you're enjoying yourself while hiking through the wilderness while carrying everything you need and want, you're doing something right. And if you're like everyone else who has ever backpacked, you will make mistakes and have moments that are hard to call joyous. Learn from these, fine tune, then do it again. Over time, you will learn by experience and create wonderful memories along the way. Life is a journey. You have to do something with your time on this beautiful Earth … might as well go backpacking.

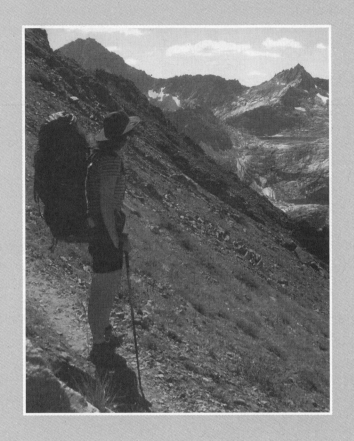

PART I
PLANNING YOUR TRIP

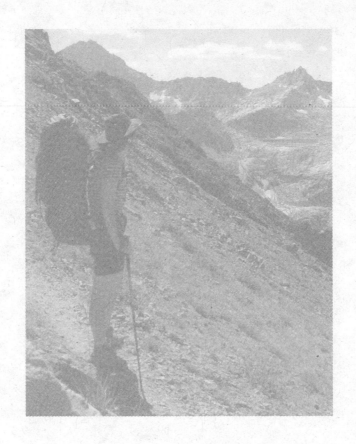

1 CHOOSING A TRIP

Every general knows most battles are won in the planning. Every architect knows the best buildings come from quality blueprints. The same is true for backpacking, and good planning begins with selecting the best trip for you.

As you can see from the top-10 list in the introduction, there are many reasons people go backpacking. The best way to enjoy backpacking is to choose a trip that corresponds with your personal style, and with what you're hoping to experience or accomplish during your trip.

Finding a Trip that Suits You

The first thing you need to do to find a trip that works for you is to consider some questions and cautions:

What kind of trip do you want? Are you hoping to climb high mountains? Sit and read by a peaceful lake? Are you planning to spend time catching up with great friends? Do you need physical exercise to reverse all that desk-jockeying you do from 9 to 5? Or do you just need to get away from it all and think about things for a few days?

Strive to keep your trip simple. Carry only what you need (and a few luxuries, perhaps). Avoid too many logistics and too many miles driving to the trailhead, especially if it's just for the weekend. The more hassles you have to endure to go backpacking, the less you'll enjoy the experience. And if you're not enjoying it, why do it?

Where do you want to backpack? Is there a particular place that attracts you? The top of Mt. Whitney, the Appalachian Trail, or the Grand Canyon, for example? Be careful how you answer this question, as many destinations (such as the ones above) might require a level of fitness you're not ready for, which brings us to the next point.

Know your limits. Some wonderful backpacking destinations are physically demanding. For example, hiking to the Colorado River from the rim of the Grand Canyon (and back) entails an overall elevation change of at least 10,000 vertical feet, which can be hard on the ankles, knees, muscles, lungs, and heart; then there's the possibility of extreme heat, brutal sun, scant water, flash floods, rattlesnakes, scorpions, and other hazards. None of these should scare you away from the Grand Canyon (I consider it a "life list" destination, and hiking the inner canyon is much better than standing on the rim and looking in). But it is important to understand that each destination comes with its own unique set of weather, wildlife, terrain, and other challenges you'll need to address in order to enjoy the trip.

If you're dreaming of a winter assault on Mt. Everest, but you've never backpacked overnight, it's a good idea to start smaller—with

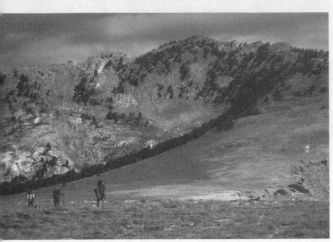
Where in the world do you want to hike?

an overnight to a local state park or national forest in summer. Once you've developed experience and skills at this level, set your sights on the next step en route to your dream trip. Remember, life is a journey, not a destination. Goals are good things to have, and backpacking is a great way to enjoy each step on the path to achieving them.

How far should you hike? If you're a novice backpacker or in poor shape, plan to hike no more than 5 miles each day over easy to moderate trails. If you're fitter, you can set more aggressive goals. (For more on getting fit for the trail, see pages 145 to 151.)

Another question: How far *can* you hike? For your backpacking trip to be successful and enjoyable, plan distances that you can actually accomplish. It's common for people to overestimate the distance they can hike when planning a trip. For moderate, multiday journeys, plan to hike 5 to 7 miles per day—less if you're not fit, your pack is heavy, the trail is steep, you're at high elevation, or you're traveling cross-country. Fit hikers with lightweight gear can cover 10 to 15 miles in a day, as long as the terrain isn't too difficult. On longer trips, give yourself a rest day every few days; your body will appreciate the time to recover.

Find the right balance of gear, fitness, trail, and ambition, and you can cover thousands of miles in a summer. To learn more about through-hiking great distances, such as on the Appalachian Trail, the Pacific Crest Trail, the Continental Divide Trail, and others, see page 17.

Deciding When to Go

When you choose to hike can be as important as where. Weather, trail conditions, and crowds play major roles in whether you will enjoy your trip. Every season offers its own unique beauty and challenges. Summer in northern latitudes is the most popular season for backpacking because that's when the weather is gentlest, the days are longest, and the streams and lakes are warmest. But it's also when crowds, insects and dangerous wildlife encounters are at their worst.

High mountain trails in the northern hemisphere don't often clear of snow until late June or July, depending on the snow pack and latitude. Hike before then in a wet year, and you'll need to be prepared to travel and camp on snow (and don't forget that at high elevations, snow and rain can happen any day of the year). In lower elevations in summer, heat, humidity, and insects can be your biggest challenges.

Call rangers or other local experts to learn how best to avoid or manage these trials where you plan to hike. Learn more about backcountry weather and insects in chapters 23

WILDERNESS WISDOM

Joyous backpackers are happy, safe, and comfortable amid nature's beauty. With proper planning, preparation, and a level head, you can become a joyous backpacker, too.

and 24, respectively. If the weather doesn't get you, the crowds just might. The most popular trails in the most popular destinations are getting increasingly crowded.

Many of the most popular destinations now require a permit; some management agencies prevent overcrowding by restricting the number of people entering the area each day. If you're hoping to avoid those crowds, plan your trip for midweek or off-season, and avoid popular spots on holiday weekends. Call rangers in the area to confirm whether permits are required.

Off-season can be especially rewarding, but you'll face a greater risk of uncomfortable weather or other challenges—which is why it's off-season. For most North American mountain trails, high season lasts from Memorial Day through Labor Day. In hot climates, fall, winter, and spring can be more popular. Call local experts to get their advice on when to plan your trip, and what you should plan to encounter when you do go.

Backpacking is a great way to spend time with friends.

Choosing Your Route

There are three ways to plan your backpacking route: **Point-to-point** trips start at one trailhead and end at another. This is the format of the Appalachian Trail, the Continental Divide Trail, the Pacific Crest Trail, and other through-hikes. These hikes are great because you never have to pass through the same country twice. They can be difficult logistically, however, because you will need to arrange transportation to drop you off at the beginning, pick you up at the end, or you'll need to leave one car at one trailhead and another at your end point.

Out-and-back hikes are the most popular routes for backpackers: Hike to your chosen destination, then hike back out on the same trail. **Loops**, as the name suggests, allow you to hike a loop that takes you through beautiful country and right back to your trailhead. Consult your maps, guidebooks, and local experts to see if there's a beautiful loop trip available where you want to hike.

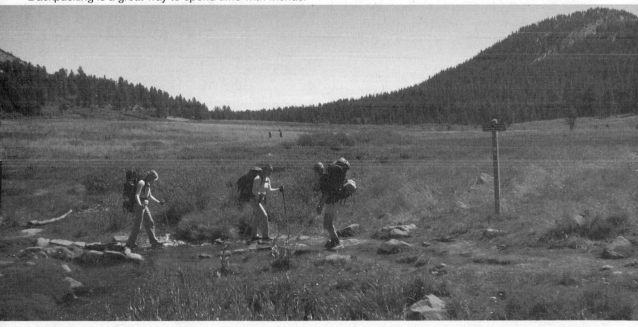

We live in a wide, wild, and wonderful world that would take many lifetimes to explore. Because there are so many beautiful places to backpack, the biggest challenge (at least at this stage) is choosing one trip from the many that are available. Luckily, there is a lot of quality information available about most places you will want to visit. This section will help you find a trip that you will fit your interests and needs.

Researching Your Options

Many sources of information are helpful for researching backpacking destinations. Here are some ideas for finding a great adventure:

Get out the atlas. If you have a map, especially one that shows mountains and canyons, browse it to see if there's a place near you, elsewhere in the country, or anywhere on the planet that you've always wanted to explore. Let your fingers and eyeballs do the walking, and see where they take you. After you find places that intrigue you (sometimes they're indicated by large green blocks on maps), you can do more research in the bookstore or on the internet.

Think about your life list. Are there places you would like to see before you die? There's no time like the present to start checking them off. If those goals are big, start by checking off smaller, more manageable destinations as you build your skills and fitness for the big trip.

Ask people. Friends, associates, family, and neighbors might generate good suggestions of places to explore. The staff at your local outdoor store might also be able to pass on their favorite spots.

Use the internet. If books, friends, and other sources aren't helping you prepare for a backpacking trip, log onto one of the websites listed below. You'll find information on destinations, gear, recipes, and forums where backpackers from around the country and around the world gather to discuss issues and answer questions. You might even be able to return the favor by helping someone else find the information they need.

Hints for internet searches: There are literally billions of web pages out there, with more added every day. To find the information

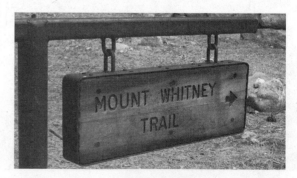

you seek, use as few words as possible, be as specific as possible. Choose search words that refer precisely to what you're seeking, and avoid common words like "and" and "the." If you're searching for a specific place with a compound name, such as Grand Canyon or Appalachian Trail, it's helpful to put the full name in quotes—"Grand Canyon" or "Appalachian Trail"—to help weed out every other canyon and trail website out there.

Some of my favorite sites include:

➤ **www.thebackpacker.com**: The "Trails and Places" section of this site is a great place to read trail reviews and discover new places to explore.

➤ **www.backpacker.com**: The website for *Backpacker* magazine has a destinations section, with trail descriptions and a "Destination of the Month."

➤ **gorp.away.com**: The section called "Destination Guides" will help you discover hikes around the world, and their "National Parks" guide will help you research backpacking options at your favorite National Park.

➤ **www.trails.com**: This subscription site has an extensive database of trail descriptions and maps from published guidebooks, as well as sections dedicated to some of North America's most popular backpacking destinations.

➤ **www.en.wikipedia.org/wiki/Backpacking_(wilderness)**: This open-source encyclopedia, written by people from around the world, offers a good introductory discussion of many issues related to backpacking.

➤ **www.google.com**: Simply type in a destination or activity that interests you—Arches National Park, Virginia trails, hiking California, or Montana backpacking, for example. Pros: Once you hit enter, you'll find yourself rewarded with a wealth of websites on the key words you typed in. Cons: You might just get too much information, which you will then have to narrow down. You might also have to

Questions to Ask About Your Destination

Once you've chosen a destination, you'll need answers to the following questions in order to plan appropriately:

➤ Do you need a permit? Some popular trails and wilderness areas require permits and advanced reservations. If you're planning a trip to one of the most popular destinations, such as Mt. Whitney in California, you may need to apply for a permit several months in advance. Call your local rangers for details.

➤ Is water available? Where? How much will you need to carry? Will you have to treat it?

➤ Is wildlife a concern? Will you need to take special precautions, such as hanging food to keep it away from bears and/or rodents?

➤ Are there restrictions on where you can camp?

➤ Are fires allowed?

➤ What season offers the best weather?

➤ What kind of weather can you expect when you hike?

➤ What season has the best/worst crowds?

➤ Are the bugs bad? Can you time your trip to avoid them?

➤ Will you need any special equipment?

➤ What is the best clothing and footwear for this climate?

➤ Are there sensitive plants, animals, or areas you should avoid?

➤ Ask your local ranger for other advice you didn't cover with your questions.

sift through paid sites by people and companies trying to sell you stuff. Remember, you don't have to buy anything, especially at this early stage.

➤ **www.recreation.gov:** This is a clearinghouse of information about many recreational opportunities on state and federal lands near you. Although it doesn't offer many of the details you will need to plan your trip, it does provide contact information for the management agency responsible for the destination, which should be able to provide you with the information you seek.

Browse the bookstore. There are a lot of great guidebooks to wonderful places, and a stroll through the travel section of your favorite bookstore will provide ample rewards. If you don't find what you want at your favorite bookstore, or if you don't yet know what book you want, try the internet again: Amazon.com is the world's biggest bookstore. You can search for books by any subject (such as Arizona backpacking, or Grand Canyon) to find the books to guide you. Many books on Amazon have been reviewed by readers, so you get to gauge whether the books have worked for other people.

Hit the newsstand. Magazines like *Backpacker* (www.backpacker.com), *Outside* (outside.away.com), *National Geographic Adventure* (www.nationalgeographic.com/adventure), and other travel magazines regularly feature stories on exceptional hiking trails and destinations. Many of the stories in these magazines are also available at the magazines' websites.

Visit local outdoor retailer stores. Many stores that sell backpacking equipment specialize in getting people outdoors. They also have employees who love to explore and who might have good suggestions.

Join a club. Numerous organizations have local chapters that offer organized hikes with experienced leaders. Contact these organizations to find out about local trips and trails. They also have regular meetings where you can see slide shows, hear tales about others' adventures, or meet people who can offer ideas, advice, and companionship on your next backpacking trip. You might have to join the organization to attend their outings, but it's a small price to pay to gain access to their experience and companionship. Here are a few national organizations with local chapters:

➤ **Sierra Club:** www.sierraclub.org; 415-977-5500. America's largest conservation organization has chapters across the country that offer hikes and other opportunities to meet and explore with other outdoor enthusiasts.

➤ **American Hiking Society:** www.americanhiking.org; 301-565-6704. This club serves as the national voice for America's hikers and works to promote and protect America's hiking opportunities for you and future generations. Their website offers a database of local hiking clubs, and the "Trail Finder" lets you download (for a price) chapters from guidebooks in particular areas.

A good regional guidebook can help you plan a wonderful backpacking trip.

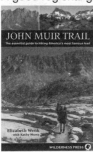
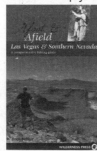
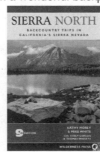
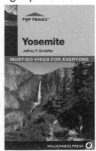
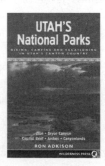

➤ **Audubon Society:** www.audubon.org; 212-979-3000. Dedicated to protecting birds, other wildlife, and their habitat, this organization has regional chapters across the country.

➤ **Appalachian Mountain Club:** www. outdoors.org; 617-523-0636. Dedicated to the protection, enjoyment, and wise use of America's northeast outdoors, this organization has 12 chapters offering hikes and volunteer opportunities.

➤ **Desert Survivors:** www.desert-survivors.org. Dedicated to protecting and exploring the West's desert landscapes, this organization sponsors trips that will help you nurture the desert rat inside you.

➤ **www.hikingandbackpacking.com** has an extensive list of hiking clubs in most states across the country.

Places to Hike on Public Lands

America's public lands (managed by federal, state, and county agencies) belong to all citizens and offer a wealth of outdoor recreation activities. They are also some of the only lands expansive enough to accommodate days of exploration by foot.

National Parks

It's hard to pick more beautiful destinations than America's national parks—Yosemite, Yellowstone, Zion, Great Smoky, Canyonlands, Glacier, Grand Canyon, Rocky Mountain—the list is a long one. The National Park System includes more than 300 protected places in the US, including not just national parks, but also national seashores, national monuments, national lakeshores, national scenic trails, and national recreation areas. Although some national parks are too small or inappropriate for backpacking (historic sites, battlefields, or the White House, for example), many others are perfect for exploring on foot.

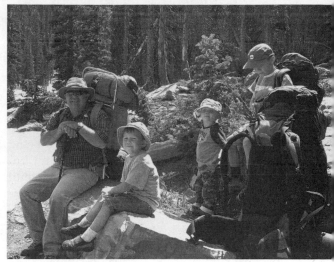

A great family weekend!

Although national parks are beautiful, solitude can be difficult to find, as parks' most popular trails can be crowded; advance reservations and/or permits may be required. Check with specific parks for details and learn more at the following websites:

www.nps.gov: The National Park Service website as a wealth of information, with individual websites for each national park. However, sometimes the information is poorly organized, and you might need to call the individual park in question to get the information you seek.

www.npca.org: The National Park Conservation Association is a nonprofit organization dedicated to keeping the parks funded and managed properly for future generations. Their website has a great park finder section. You can also call them at 800-628-7275.

Wilderness Areas

In 1964, Congress passed the Wilderness Act to preserve shining examples of our national landscape heritage. These areas represent some of our country's wildest and most beautiful landscapes, where man is a visitor who does not remain. In early 2007, there were

702 wilderness areas, covering more than 107 million acres in 44 states. These places are managed by the National Park Service, the US Forest Service, the US Fish & Wildlife Service, and the Bureau of Land Management (see the pages that follow for more on these agencies).

There are also hundreds of wilderness study areas (WSAs), identified by land management agencies (mostly the BLM) as being worthy of wilderness designation. Only Congress can designate a wilderness area, but until it does, agencies manage these areas to preserve their wild and scenic character. Many of these beautiful areas fly under the radar of public awareness, making them great destinations for backpacking. You can learn more about WSAs under the BLM information on page 18.

Because permanent human structures are prohibited in them, wilderness areas are great if you're hoping to leave civilization behind (hard to do in some national parks!).

Many, if not all, make great backpacking destinations, although your experience will depend on where you go, your expectations, and how well you prepare for local conditions. Popular wilderness areas in national parks have trails, signs, designated campsites, and permit systems to manage the large crowds. Other wilderness areas have no trails, few visitors, and no signs to guide you. Ask the land-management agency responsible for the area you're interested in about requirements or restrictions.

A great place to begin your research on wilderness areas is at www.wilderness.net. Its "Search Maps" section will help you narrow down your search and find a wilderness area that suits you, or you can browse a list of all wilderness areas. It also provides contact information for the local land-management agency responsible for the area. Officials there will be able to help you plan your trip.

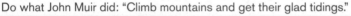
Do what John Muir did: "Climb mountains and get their glad tidings."

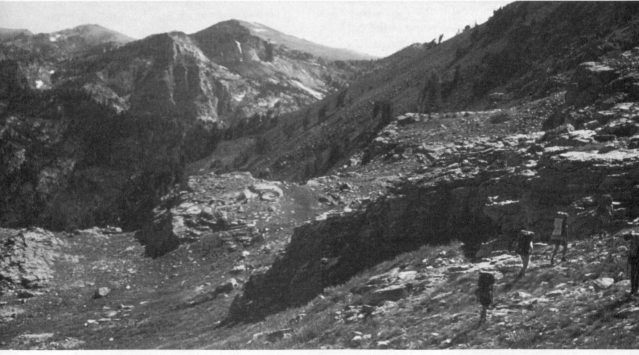

Local wilderness organizations in each state have staff members who know their state well, and these individuals might be able to guide you to destinations suited to your desires and needs. An internet search of "wilderness" and the name of the state you're interested in should lead you to an organization that can guide you.

National Trails

The US has great national trails that offer world-class hikes through amazing country. Some of them are long, but you don't have to do the whole thing; you can always hike just part of it, do pieces over time, or get hooked and end up doing the whole thing. Here are a few of the most popular:

Appalachian Trail. This classic 2160-mile footpath crosses 14 states between Katahdin, Maine, and Springer Mountain, Georgia. To find out more, visit www.nps.gov/appa, www.appalachiantrail.org, and www.fred.net/kathy/at.html.

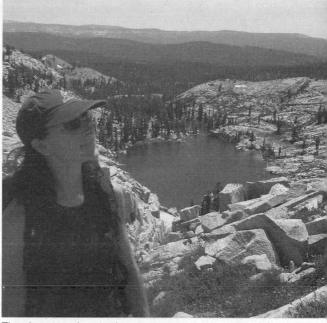
The views can be worth every step.

North Country Trail. This 4400-mile path links communities, forests, and prairies across seven northern states. Although only about half of the trail is complete or non-motorized, what is complete passes through some amazing country—seashores, forests, and wilderness. Find out more by contacting the North Country Trail Association at www.northcountrytrail.org or 866-445-3628.

Continental Divide Trail. This 3100-mile trail spans the Continental Divide between Mexico and Canada through New Mexico, Colorado, Wyoming, Idaho, and Montana. About 30 percent of the trail remains incomplete. Find out more at www.cdtrail.org and www.cdtsociety.org.

Pacific Crest Trail. The 2650-mile, non-motorized Pacific Crest Trail runs along the crest of the Sierra Nevada and Cascade mountains between Mexico and Canada, through California, Oregon, and Washington. Learn more at www.pcta.org or www.pcthiker.org.

John Muir Trail. This 211-mile section of the Pacific Crest Trail runs through Yosemite, Kings Canyon, and Sequoia national parks to Mt. Whitney, the highest peak in the Lower 48. It passes through some of the most beautiful mountain scenery on Earth. Find out more at the Pacific Crest Trail links above.

Tahoe Rim Trail. This 165-mile trail circumnavigates the Lake Tahoe watershed in California and Nevada. Learn more at www.tahoerimtrail.org.

The Desert Trail. Less of a trail and more of a general route, the Desert Trail travels between Mexico and Canada through the deserts of California, Nevada, Oregon, Idaho, and Montana. This adventure is not built for novices—only experienced, prepared, and sunbaked desert rats need apply. For more information, check out www.thedeserttrail.org.

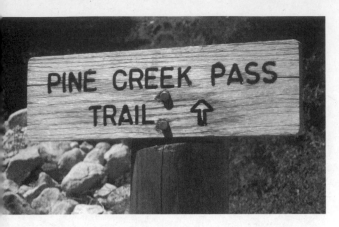

If you choose to tackle one of these wonderful trails, you're on your way to becoming a through-hiker. Congratulations! There are many worse things to be in this world.

National Forests and Grasslands

Managing nearly 200 million acres of land, the Forest Service offers some incredible landscapes to explore. Look on the website www.fs.fed.us for the "find a forest or grassland" page, which will quickly lead you to a national forest worth exploring. A call to local rangers will help you discover hiking trails in their district.

BLM Lands

The BLM manages 261 million acres of your public lands, mostly in the 12 western states. The most beautiful and exciting places in these lands lie within the BLM's National Landscape Conservation System, which includes national monuments, wilderness areas, wilderness study areas, designated wild and scenic rivers, and national scenic and historic trails. Learn more at www.blm.gov/nlcs.

State Parks

Although many state parks won't do for longer backpacking trips, some are ideal for weekend getaways, and there's sure to be one near you. Unfortunately, there is no single clearinghouse for information about state parks nationwide. The easiest thing to do is type "state parks" (include the quotes) with the name of your favorite state into an internet search engine and follow the links. You can also call your favorite state capital and ask to be connected to their state parks division.

Wildlife Refuges

The US Fish & Wildlife Service manages 545 wildlife refuges in all 50 states. They range in size from the Arctic National Wildlife Refuge in Alaska (19.2 million acres) to many small refuges that cover only a few small acres. Whether refuges are appropriate for backpacking depends on their size and particular management plans (some refuges are closed to the public to protect sensitive species). Log onto www.fws.gov/refuges/ to find a refuge that interests you. Then contact officials at that particular refuge to see if backpacking is appropriate there.

3 BACKPACKING WITH OTHERS

For some, few things are more enjoyable than sharing the adventure of wilderness with good friends—indeed, an adventure in the wilderness can transform mere acquaintances into the closest friends. Other people prefer to hike alone. However you wish to travel—alone, with others, or with your dog—understand that each has certain advantages and challenges, and each requires proper planning. However you wish to travel, this section will help you plan appropriately.

Choosing Your Partners

It's safest to hike with other people because multiple heads are better than one when figuring out which way to go, and so you can help each other if you get lost or injured. If you choose your partners well, hiking with others can be very enjoyable. Of course, your safety and enjoyment depends on whom you choose. Here are some things to think about when considering others to be your hiking partners:

Are they experienced? Do they have outdoor experience that will help guide you through the wilderness, or will they be depending on you to guide the party through tough times? If that's the case, are you prepared? Read more about skills required for leading backpacking trips in the Wilderness Leadership section that follows.

What are their expectations? If you're planning to eat nothing but peanut butter while setting record time running from peak to peak, but your partners are planning to photograph wildflowers and cook lavish meals, you're on a beeline toward conflict. Avoid conflict by choosing different partners, or adjusting your itinerary to accommodate both party's interests.

What's their pace? Few people hike at the same pace. You might discover this early in your backpacking trip, when your partner is either far ahead or far behind you on the trail. This is fine, as long as you adapt, communicate, and plan well about when and where to reconnect along the way. Whatever you do, don't lose your hiking partner.

A couple good friends can make a great trip.

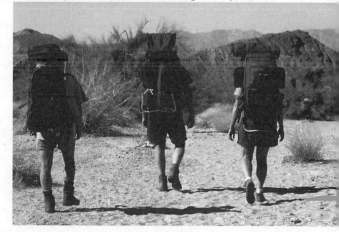

Wilderness Leadership

It's hard to predict everything the wilderness is going to throw at you—weather, animals, challenging terrain, medical emergencies, and personality conflicts. The decisions made by the group in challenging situations can be vital to success and survival in the wilderness. A good leader is someone who can guide a group toward good decisions in challenging situations.

Leadership is a skill, just like reading a map, tying a half-hitch, or splinting a broken wrist. However, it's often neglected entirely when preparing for backcountry excursions. You don't have to be a macho stud-muffin who knows how to do everything to be a good leader. You just need to be someone who can organize the group to reach a common goal successfully—someone who can step up and take responsibility to get the job done, or inspire others to overcome a challenge.

When groups are working together smoothly as a team, there may be no clear leader; everyone brings different strengths—one

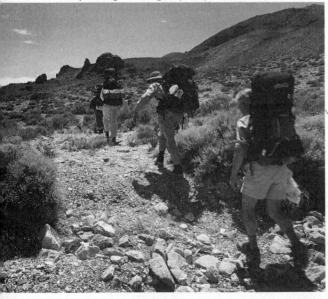

Backpacking with a group requires teamwork.

person's a better cook, another is great at reading maps, a third is adept at resolving conflicts. But when things aren't working smoothly, or during a crisis, someone needs to step back to assess the group's immediate needs (for food, rest, shelter, or first aid) and to anticipate weather and other natural threats. The next step is to come up with a workable plan and help organize the group to accomplish it.

Some leaders are born great, others achieve greatness through study and practice, and some are thrust into the role by crisis. You might not be the official trip leader, but when suddenly the leader gets knocked unconscious or panics, you might be the coolest head remaining in the group, and you will need to step up and chart the group's course to safety.

If you're not a natural-born leader, the following thoughts will help you improve your leadership skills. You never know when you might need them:

Plan ahead and prepare. Think ahead and prepare for dangerous situations you might encounter during your trip (the infamous "what if…" scenario). Aim to prevent problems instead of having to react to them. Do this by researching your trip well, packing the right equipment, then keeping an eye on both natural conditions and the condition of your group.

Compensate for your weaknesses. You don't have to be able to do everything. If you're petite, make sure you bring a friendly ape along who can do the heavy work; if you're not great at first aid or map and compass skills, bring someone along who is.

Respect others. Gain the respect of everyone in the group by respecting who they are, their limitations, and their internal strength (even if they don't see it for themselves). If someone is unable to cross a creek, for example, listen to their fears. Remember when you were in a similar situation, then explain to them exactly how you're going to help them succeed.

Be patient and reassuring. They just might find the strength.

Be yourself. There are many effective leadership styles. Trying to be someone you're not will undermine the trust others put in you. You don't have to know all the answers.

Keep a cool head. When challenging situations arise, the group needs someone who can assess and plan without panicking.

Push the pause button. When faced with a stressful situation, take a deep breath and center yourself. A clear, calm mind is necessary to weigh options, come up with a good plan, and inspire the group to succeed.

Be a role model. If you want others to be on time, be early. Deal with aggressive people by becoming their friend, finding common ground, then building on it. Be in a good mood without faking it. Help others who need it. Share your food.

Be optimistic and supportive. No matter how dire your situation, hope is the most essential thing people need to find their inner strength to prevail. If you honestly believe that your group will overcome this challenge, and if you believe in others, your confidence in them will affect how well they do.

Know when to follow. If someone else has a good plan, the best strategy might be to pitch in and follow her lead as a fellow team member working toward a common goal.

Keep a good sense of humor. A few jokes can do more to ease tension and raise moral than an hour of lectures, warnings, and criticism.

Keep people busy. During emergencies or other stressful situations, people who are not occupied by important tasks can get caught up in obsessive or panicky thought patterns; their panic increases, optimism decreases, and the situation gets worse from there. You can direct people away from panic by giving them something to do. If someone in your party is becoming unstable, assign them a duty to keep their brain focused on something other than the difficult circumstances. If someone gets hurt, allowing them to help themselves—by holding a bandage or cleaning a wound—will help calm them down and focus their attention away from their pain and on a solution. It might be good to assign someone else to keep an eye on them to make sure everyone keeps their cool.

If you're a good leader, your party has a better chance of surviving the curve balls nature and circumstance throw at you on the trail. If you're an exceptional leader, the members of your party will be more confident, more knowledgeable, and happier because of it.

Hiking Alone

It can be difficult to hike with others; finding partners and getting everyone's schedules, hiking speeds, and expectations to correspond can be tiresome and frustrating. Sometimes it's easier to go alone.

One of the first pieces of advice many give to staying found is, "Don't hike alone." Despite the wisdom of this advice, many explorers (myself included) head into the wild alone on a regular basis. Maybe we can't find partners. Or maybe we don't want to, wishing for some time alone to enjoy the wonderful outdoors face to face.

If you're fit and your outdoor skills are strong, backpacking alone might be a reasonable option. But no matter how strong, smart, or capable you are, the risks are greater when you hike alone. If you get lost or injured while hiking alone, you're on your own; there's no one to help. If you plan to hike alone, minimize your risk by following these tips:

Always leave your plans. Leave an itinerary of your trip (where you're going, the route you plan to take, and when you'll be back) with a responsible party at home. Have them call for search and rescue if you're not in contact with them by a specified time (leave generous leeway to allow for distractions and other delays). Don't forget to contact them when you return. Leave the same itinerary on your dashboard, so officials at the trailhead know when to start worrying about you.

Stick to your itinerary. If you decide to change your travel plans, then get lost or injured after changing plans, search parties will be looking somewhere else for you—where you originally told them to look. This rule changes when you encounter a dangerous obstacle, a risky climb, or dangerous river ford, for example. It's better to change your plans or find a detour when facing a dangerous situation and there is no one to help you if you get in trouble.

Be especially cautious. Always make mistakes from which you can walk away. When I hike alone, I am more cautious than I would be with a partner because I know consequences will be more severe if something happens to me out there.

There's joy in them thar hills!

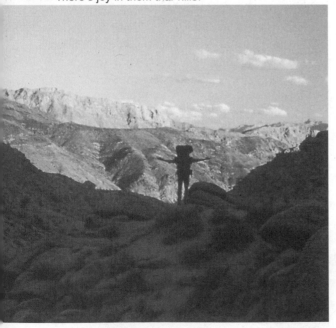

Hiking with Dogs

Fido, Zack, Oscar, Scout, and other fluffy friends can be great companions on the trail, and they can bring immense joy (and security) to your hiking trip. But they require special preparation and attention to keep them safe, and to prevent them from harassing wildlife and other people.

First, you need to find out if dogs are allowed where you're hoping to hike. In general, dogs are allowed in national forests and BLM lands, unless otherwise posted; dogs are discouraged in wilderness areas; and dogs are forbidden on trails in national parks. Nonetheless, always check with officials at your chosen destination to make sure.

Next, you need to make sure your four-legged friend does not harass other people or local wildlife. Despite the fact that they're descendants of wolves, dogs are not part of the natural environment (no matter how convincing their howl is). Wherever you hike with your dog, keep her on a leash or under strict voice control to prevent her from harassing wildlife, other people, or farm animals (every state allows ranchers to shoot dogs that chase cattle). Either pick up dog poop or remove it from the trail and bury it appropriately. At night, bring your dog into your tent with you to keep her warm. This keeps her from bothering smaller wildlife, and it protects her from being eaten by larger wildlife.

Have your four-legged friend carry her own food and equipment (and maybe a few of your things—she'll never know) with special dog packs. Unless your dog is a malamute or other strong working dog, keep pack contents to 25 percent of your dog's weight, and make sure you practice this on your dog at home. There's nothing worse than getting to the trail to find out gear doesn't fit, malfunctions, or is rejected outright by your pooch.

Wrap dog food and other vulnerable dog pack contents securely in plastic bags if your dog likes to lie down in puddles and creeks. If bears, rodents, or other animals are a concern, store all dog food safely with the rest of your food and other tasty or good-smelling supplies. (See pages 178 and 179 for suggestions on proper food storage.) You might also consider buying specialized collapsible dog dishes that are available for their food and water (though Frisbees and old plastic containers work just as well, and they're more affordable).

Finally, keep your pup safe and healthy during your adventure. Be especially cautious during your journey to the trailhead in hot weather. Do not leave your dog in the car parked in the sun on a hot day—the temperature in closed cars can climb quickly to a fatal 150°F in just a few minutes in summer.

Talk to your vet about protecting your dog from heartworm, Lyme disease, and other insect-borne diseases. Frontline and other prophylactic medications can keep bad bugs away from the outset.

Your dog's paws might be sensitive to the hard, hot, and/or sharp ground (how would you feel hiking barefoot on that trail?). If your dog hikes as little as you do, her feet might be as sensitive as yours. Take her on short practice hikes over rough terrain, so her paws have a chance to build calluses.

Booties, dog packs, and other specialized dog equipment are available from the manufacturers below. If you buy anything, make sure to try it at home first to ensure that the fit is right and that you dog is comfortable using it.

➤ Ruffwear: www.ruffwear.com; 888-783-3932.

➤ Wolf Packs: www.wolfpacks.com; 541-482-7669.

➤ Mountain Smith: www.mountain-smith.com; 800-551-5889.

➤ Kelty: www.kelty.com; 800-423-2320.

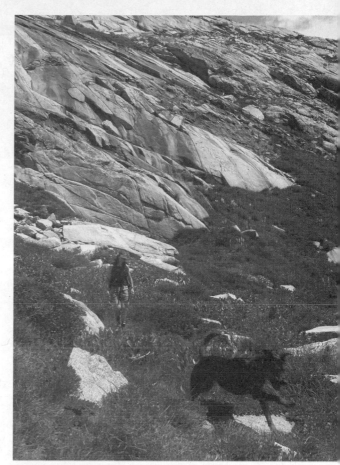

Dogs love hiking!

➤ Granite Gear: www.granitegear.com; 218-834-6157.

In addition to the items in your standard first aid kit, bring the following things to help treat your dog:

➤ Dog brush to clean all the foxtails, sticks, and other things that get stuck in fur.

➤ Styptic powder to help stop bleeds.

➤ An old sock to place over bandages on cut paws (the booties mentioned above work well, too).

➤ Pedialyte powder to add to water to replace electrolytes on hot days.

➤ Towel or extra cloth to clean muddy paws before inviting your dog into your tent.

4 BACKPACKING WITH KIDS

Taking kids backpacking is great for lots of reasons, but the biggest one is obvious—it's fun! Kids love it—climbing trees and rocks, splashing in water, exploring new places, watching the stars, sleeping in tents, and waking up in beautiful, new, and exciting places. If your number one priority is to have fun outdoors with your kids, you have a great chance at success.

The outdoors is also a wonderful classroom. It challenges children's curiosity in ways most books, lectures, and classrooms can't. In the wild, they can learn about the world and how they fit in it, while gaining outdoor skills that will serve them in the future. Some of the best skills they'll learn—confidence and safety-consciousness—will come as they challenge themselves and learn both skills and limits.

For kids, part of the challenge of backpacking is physical. In this age of obesity, getting kids off the couch so they can hike and explore will help them grow up healthier and more active, so backpacking is not only good for their bodies now, it may help them set healthy patterns for life.

Their minds and spirits will benefit as well. Researchers have discovered that outdoor activities in natural settings lead to a great reduction of Attention-Deficit Hyperactivity Disorder (ADHD) symptoms. Other studies show that kids are better able to concentrate on tasks in green surroundings. The success of many wilderness therapy programs shows that nature gives people the perspective to sort out problems and figure out who they are and how they fit into the world. It will also challenge their creativity in ways Nintendo and PlayStation will never do.

This is not to say that backpacking with kids is always easy. It can also be a hassle. There's more gear for you to carry (kids can't carry everything they need), kids (younger ones at least) require a lot of attention and supervision, and there are risks and dangers from which you will need to protect them. But even during the trying times, you will be spending quality time with your children and creating memories everyone in the family will cherish. Ultimately, the benefits far outweigh the risks and challenges.

This chapter covers a few kid-specific ideas to make your trips with them more successful. You'll find more detail about nutrition, clothing, gear, making camp, trail etiquette, wildlife encounters, backcountry threats, and first aid elsewhere in this book.

When to Start

Only you know when your own kids will be ready to start backpacking. Parents have been having, traveling with, and raising children outdoors as long as we've been walking this Earth. Today, intrepid modern parents take children into the wild as soon as Mom recovers from giving birth and is ready to hit the trail. When you start depends on your comfort with outdoor skills and kid management. This discussion will help give you confidence to hit the trail with your tots sooner rather than later.

In some ways, infants are the easiest kids to take into the backcountry. Compared with the 6-year-old who insists on being carried after the first mile, infants are lightweight. They also tend to stay where you put them, and, as long as they're comfortable, they're easily entertained by looking around, watching you, or playing with whatever new object you put in front of them. However, they can't communicate well, so it's up to you to anticipate and accommodate their needs so they remain comfortable, happy, and safe.

Often, one person carries the kid, and hopefully a few other items, while the other serves as the family pack mule—carrying everything else.

Older, crawling infants can be a challenge because of their constant contact with the ground and their need to stick everything in their mouths, including dirt, rocks, and bugs. (My son, Logan, didn't seem to mind when he ate that spider—luckily it wasn't venomous! His mom, on the other hand, freaked out.) Part of the solution is to find a clean campsite, such as on bare rock or deep grass, or to keep your infant in the tent when you're not holding her (tents make great playpens).

Contrary to their little brothers, toddlers are often the most difficult kids to take backpacking. They're able to move, and they're curious about the world. But they are also ignorant about potential dangers, not able to rationalize or comprehend rules, and maybe a little headstrong about following the rules they do understand. They also seem to have their own opinions about which way to hike ("No, Son, we're going this way!"). As I write this, Logan is two-and-a-half. He loves backpacking, and we love taking him, but he needs constant supervision, which requires at least two adults—one to set up camp, cook, etc., and the other to supervise him. Our trips are enjoyable, but busy and exhausting.

Children older than toddlers should be ready to hit the trail after a few practice hikes, and after you arm them with the skills, activities, and equipment discussed later in this chapter.

The kids go hiking one by one, hurrah!

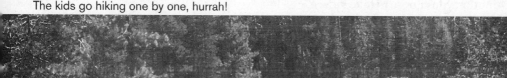

Dealing with Diapers

No matter how you cut it, diapers are a challenge to backpacking with small children. As at home, there are two ways you can deal with the challenge:

Disposable diapers are convenient, but they add up quickly to a smelly, heavy burden in the backcountry. With this option, three days of old diapers can quickly outweigh everything else in your pack, and the smell after a couple warm days could knock you off your feet. Keeping your trip to one to two nights will allow you to enjoy camping without being overwhelmed by the accumulated dirty diapers.

Cloth diapers are a more reasonable (but still messy and inconvenient) option. Two days' worth of diapers (plus a few extra, just in case) should be sufficient, leaving you with enough to use while you wash and dry the dirty ones.

When changing diapers, dispose of the poop by burying it at least 100 big steps from camp and water sources. Leave disposable diapers in the sun (downwind from you) to dry out as much moisture as possible. Pack dirty diapers in a well-sealed plastic bag for transportation back to a proper garbage can (disposable), or until you can wash them (cloth).

You'll need the following supplies for successful changing: diaper covers, wipes, a well-sealing plastic bag or nylon tote to carry soiled diapers, a small bottle of hand sanitizer to use after changing and washing diapers, and a small bottle of tea-tree oil to combat the smell of diapers in the bag. Desitin, or other diaper-rash ointment is also a good thing to have along.

To wash cloth diapers properly, you'll need the following: a bucket or tub, Dr. Bronner's or other biodegradable soap, clothespins and/or a laundry line to hang diapers to dry (preferably in the sun, which will help sterilize the diapers). Also make sure you have enough diapers to get you through that rainy day when you planned to wash and sun-dry your diapers.

Wet diapers are heavier than dry diapers; if you must continue hiking, try to do so with dry diapers, not wet ones.

Where to Take Kids Backpacking

The destination you choose to take kids backpacking will help determine how much everyone enjoys the trip. Adults love hiking—getting outdoors, using their legs and lungs, and enjoying the beauty of nature. Kids just want to play. If you're an avid hiker, disregard your gotta-get-there, destination-oriented attitude. It's not about getting there; it's about enjoying the outdoors right now. Infants and toddlers are perfectly happy with the sticks, pine cones, rocks, and bugs right in front of them. Older children don't want to trudge hours through the heat before the fun starts. In other words, immediate or real-soon gratification is key for younger children; for older kids, the reward must equal or exceed the misery you put them through on the hike getting there.

Choose fun destinations that aren't far from the trailhead. Kids don't care about views, solitude, or exercise. Water is always a hit; you're sure to please kids by camping near rivers, lakes, and streams. Other playgrounds, such as rocks, trees, and other fun places to climb, play, and explore are also sure to please.

When choosing a destination, consider how far your kids will be able to hike (or how far you will be able to carry them, if it comes to that). You understand your kids best, but in general, infants can "hike" as far as you're willing to carry them; toddlers can hike up to a mile or 2, less if they haven't hiked before;

beginning hikers aged 4 to 6 can hike 2 to 3 miles; pre-teens and teens who are beginning hikers will be willing to tolerate your idea of fun for 3 to 5 miles. After that, you might have a mutiny on your hands.

These are general guidelines. When in doubt, plan shorter hikes until you understand your kids. Bring plenty of patience, and forget any expectations of when you'll get there. Try hiking no more than two to three hours in a day. After all, getting to camp is less fun than playing once you're there. After your kids learn how much fun backpacking is on shorter trips, they'll be willing and eager to hike to that really awesome lake that's a *little* farther away than the one on the last trip.

Kid-Friendly Clothing and Equipment

As with adults, kids need clothing and equipment that is comfortable and works well. Unfortunately, they don't always know how to evaluate comfort or function, and they often can't communicate clearly when there are problems. In other words, it's your job as the adult to be mindful of, and anticipate, their comfort and needs.

Footwear

As with adults, happy feet make happy hikers, and painful shoes can stop your kids' expedition in its tracks. Comfort is key when choosing shoes for your kids on the trail. Traction is important, too, if difficult terrain or climbing are on the agenda. Support isn't as important, because kids are light, and they shouldn't be carrying much weight. As they grow bigger and carry more, they'll need more supportive footwear. Pack water shoes or rain boots if they'll be playing in water, in order to keep the hiking shoes dry (hiking in wet shoes is a sure path to blisters).

Clothing

As with adults, dressing kids in several thin layers is better than fewer thick layers; it's easier this way to adapt to changing weather and activity levels by adding or shedding layers. Synthetic fabrics, silk, and wool are preferable over cotton, which is great in warm weather but stays cold when it gets wet. Bright colors are a hit. Kids like them better, and parents have an easier time keeping an eye on kids wearing yellows or reds than forest greens or browns. If you really want to keep an eye on your kids, go to a hunting store and equip them with blaze-orange clothes designed to keep people from being mistaken for game during hunting season. Boy! That stuff sure pops from the surroundings at a distance. Quality kids clothing is available at a variety of department stores and outdoor outfitters.

He'll always remember these times.

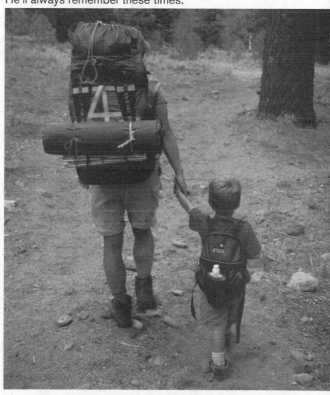

Backpacks

For lighter loads and smaller kids, fanny packs, or kid-sized daypacks should be sufficient. For heavier loads and bigger kids, several kid-sized backpacks, complete with hip belts and suspension systems, are available from manufacturers like REI, Kelty, and North Face.

Because kids don't have hips on which a pack can rest, it's important to fit their backpacks correctly; as with adults, make sure the hip belt rests on the top of the pelvic bones on each side of the waist, which are higher on the torso than the hips (close to belly-button level). If the pack isn't settled correctly on these pel-vic crests, the pack's weight will naturally drop lower, transferring the weight painfully to the shoulders, resulting in an achy (and probably whiny) hiker and less fun for everyone.

Sleeping Bags

Infants and toddlers can share your bag, especially if you're a couple with two bags zipped together. A bag expander provides even more room (see the chapter on sleeping bags, beginning on page 81, for details). My little guy is an active sleeper to say the least; he tosses, turns, and squirms out of the bag quickly. Knowing this, we dress him in a warm, full-body, fleece sleep suit and bring an extra blanket to cover him during his travels.

MY SYSTEM

Backpackin' Baby

Our daughter, Mary, began riding in a baby backpack at about six months. We knew we'd be using it a lot, so we bought a top-of-the-line model (Tough Traveler's "Stallion"), which included a green nylon hood with a clear plastic windshield and open sides. We then modified it for comfort and safety on backpacking trips.

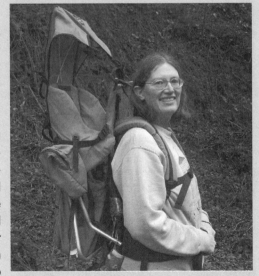

Mary frequently fell asleep in the backpack, and her head would rub on the rough-textured nylon, resulting in a slight rash, so we tore up an old flannel nightgown and used it to cover the parts where she rested her head. Receiving blankets or old crib sheets were attached with diaper pins for a movable sun screen. And for rainy or cold weather, we created a two-part cover with waterproof, ripstop nylon, which we bought at an outdoor recreation store. We made patterns for the top half and the bottom half out of an old sheet before cutting up the nylon. A little simple sewing completed each half, and we used Velcro strips to hold the top and bottom together.

When I carried Mary on hikes, I also carried a little rearview mirror in my pocket, the kind you can buy in automotive stores. That way, I could check on her without disturbing her if she was drifting off to sleep. The backpack came with a stand, so that if I did take off the pack with her asleep, I could prop it up next to where I was sitting and she could just continue her nap.

—**Barbara Egbert**, author, *Zero Days* (Wilderness Press), an account of her journey with her 10-year-old daughter and her husband on the Pacific Crest Trail

North Face, REI, Kelty, and Big Agnes make kids sleeping bags for older kids and juniors.

Tents

Kids love tents! Who wouldn't? They're beautifully constructed forts that make camping an adventure. Choose a self-standing tent for easiest setup. This type of tent will also allow you to set it up in your house, which is a good way to get kids used to sleeping in it, and it makes a great fort inside on rainy days.

Regarding the color of your tent, you have two options: Leave No Trace principles recommend subdued, earth-tone colors to make your camp less obtrusive to other campers and wildlife. However, these colors also make it more difficult for your kids to see your camp from a distance, which makes it easier for them to get lost. A bright rainfly will provide a beacon for your kids, so they can easily locate your camp from a distance (you can also use bright fabrics to signal for help in emergencies). Having said this, it's not often you get to choose the color of your tent or rain-fly; if you find the tent you like, you're usually stuck with that manufacturer's seasonal colors and style.

Home away from home

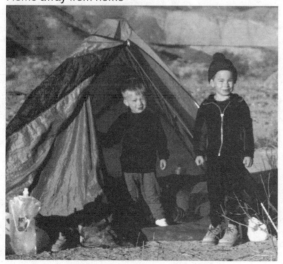

How Much Kids Can Carry

Every kid is different, but here are some general guidelines that should work until you figure out what works best for your kids:

➤ Have kids 10 and younger carry their age in pounds—some snacks, water, a favorite toy and/or a jacket, plus a few more clothes for kids on the older end of this range.

➤ Pre-teens and young adolescents can carry up to 20 percent of their weight—water, snacks, and all of their clothes.

➤ Older teens, like adults, can carry up to 25 percent of their own weight—all their stuff and maybe a communal item or two, such as the stove, fuel, or tent.

Again, these are general guidelines. When in doubt, have kids carry less until you're confident they can go the distance comfortably with more.

While kids are carrying less, you in turn are the pack mule, carrying everything else and possibly exceeding the "25 percent of your weight" rule. Make sure you have a pack with a quality suspension system that supports your burden well, transfers the weight to your hips, and is comfortable all the while. Also keep in mind that if your kids tire on the trail, you'll need extra room in or straps on your pack to relieve them of some of their burden.

Other Necessities

➤ Each kid should have her own **whistle** (on a string around her neck) for emergencies only, a compass (even if she doesn't know how to read it, it makes her feel grown up and outdoorsy), water, and snacks.

➤ **Flashlight or headlamp:** Kids love them, they help kids see at night, and they help you keep track of your kids. Increase their visibility by clipping a small, blinking LED bike light to their jacket or clothes. Glow sticks are also fun for nighttime play and visibility.

➤ One or two favorite **toys and/or books**. Trucks, dolls, or action figures are great because they allow your kids to interact with their surroundings. Just make sure you keep track of their belongings; toys with multiple small pieces may not be the best choices for the trail.

➤ **Bibs:** You can substitute a dish towel held in place with a binder clip or clothes pin—more coverage and more uses.

➤ A **bell** tied to your tent's zipper to alert you if your curious child decides to get out and explore while you're still asleep.

➤ A **positive and supportive attitude** at all times.

Rules for Successful Backpacking with Kids

Once again, kids love being outdoors, but many things can disrupt their fun out there. As the leader of the expedition, your job is to manage their moods and events proactively to keep them happy, to anticipate threats to the fun, and to take the necessary steps to prevent these threats from ruining everything.

Keep them well-fed. Kids have smaller bodies and faster metabolisms than adults. Their blood sugar and energy levels can fluctuate quickly, so frequent snacking is better than three larger meals. Kids are also easily distracted by sweet treats. Use this to your advantage: When they're complaining, when they seem listless, or when they need a morale boost, pull out your secret stash of their favorite treats. You'll be surprised how quickly their outlooks change and energy levels return. There's nothing wrong with plying them with treats (include some healthy ones, if you can) and keeping them snacking all the way down the trail. Think of ways you can use treats to motivate them ("Kids, there's more chocolate waiting at the lake!"). This strategy also works on lackluster adults.

Bring fun food. Choose comfort foods and fun foods that your kids like at home, be it mac 'n' cheese, mashed potatoes, tomato soup, oatmeal, fun nutrition bars, or pancakes. If you can balance the fun with good nutrition, the kids will have better energy, more stable moods, and big smiles on their faces. A variety of treats to choose from is better than one big bag of gorp. Always remember to wash or sanitize hands before meals.

Make sure they drink lots of water. Water is the most important part of nutrition, especially in the heat, cold, or when they're really active. Luckily, water bottles and hydration packs are fun.

Keep them warm and dry. The quickest way to get miserable kids (or adults) is to get them cold and wet. Let them splash in the lake on a warm day, but when the fun is over or temperatures drop, make sure everyone changes quickly into warm, dry clothes. Wet clothes, especially cotton, are a fast lane to hypothermia, a potentially life-threatening condition when the body can no longer warm itself, threatening the bodily functions that support life.

Dry kids are happy kids, and ponchos are fun.

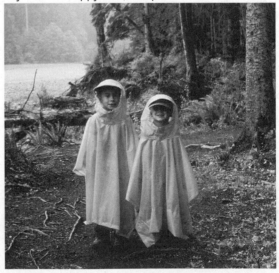

Rules for the Trail

Before you hit the trail, explain the following rules to your kids:

➤ **Stay within sight (younger kids), or within voice range (older kids).**

➤ **Stay on the trail.** Don't cut switchbacks, and always stop and wait for others at forks in the trail, at significant passes or bends, or whenever they're not sure.

➤ **Don't mess with snakes or other animals.** Respect them from a distance. Feeding or annoying them can lead to bites and disease.

➤ **No throwing or rolling rocks toward other people, or where you can't see.**

➤ **Avoid poisonous plants.** Teach them to recognize poison oak or poison ivy. With plants, berries, mushrooms, and other plants that look like they might be edible, use the following rule: "Don't eat anything in the wild unless Mom or Dad says it's OK, even if it looks just like something we eat at home."

➤ **No littering.** Explain why it's important to leave the wilderness cleaner than they found it. Make Leave No Trace a game—when it's time to leave, see if they can make it seem as though you never camped there at all.

➤ **Have a buddy system.** In a group, have kids be responsible for each other.

➤ **If kids get lost, teach them to find a tree or large rock, stay by it, and keep warm.** Wandering, lost people create moving targets, which are harder for searchers to find. At home, we tell kids not to talk to strangers. But all strangers are friends to a lost child. Teach them that a lot of people will be looking for them if they get lost. If they hear voices or noises, blow their whistle or yell out!

Help avoid losing your kids by having a pop quiz from time to time: When hiking along the trail, or exploring from camp, stop and ask them where the car is, where camp is, and what they would do if they got lost right now. Place an identification card in their packs or clothes, so rescuers will know the pertinent details and contact information.

Hiking in the rain can be good fun—it brings out worms, bugs, other wildlife, not to mention great puddles. The challenge is to encourage splashy fun while keeping junior dry. The following system will keep kids dry for hours: synthetic long underwear, fleece tops and bottoms, with rain suit or poncho (nylon is more durable than plastic) and rain boots over all. Add fleece hat or balaclava and waterproof mittens for colder weather.

If someone gets soaked and cold by surprise, change her into dry clothes quickly, then offer a cup of hot chocolate or other sweet treat to warm her back up.

Have them help. Kids want to feel important and grown up. They will be more committed to making your backpacking trip successful if they feel invested in it. Make them partners in the planning. Have them help choose the destination, do advance research, plan and assemble the gear, choose the meals, shop for supplies, and pack everything for travel. If they're able, have them carry important items everyone will need at camp.

Make each kid "in charge" of important duties, such as choosing the campsite, gathering firewood, getting water, helping prepare meals, and making sure that camp is cleaner when you leave than it was when you arrived.

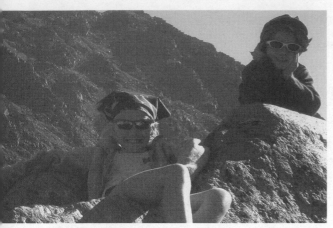
Backpacking makes kids cool!

Every child should have a duty. When hiking, perhaps Sophie can be in charge of making sure everyone has sunscreen or other sun protection, Keeler can be master of insect repellent, and Kaelin can be navigator. If Jimmy's dragging behind, bring him up to the front and ask him to help you lead and make sure everyone stays on the trail. Each of these assignments gives you the opportunity to teach them outdoor skills: Sophie can learn about UV radiation, Keeler about mosquitoes, Kaelin how to use a map and compass (highlight your route on the map, so they can follow it easily), and Jimmy can learn how to recognize trail markers and set a pace everyone can keep. Yes, this all takes time, but remember, it's not about getting there; it's about spending quality time with kids and teaching them skills they'll need to grow into capable, confident, wonderful people.

Having them help is effective because it shows them you respect and trust them enough to make mature decisions. Sometimes this is accomplished simply by encouraging and motivating them to work together toward a common goal, like getting to camp in time to set up and play the rest of the afternoon. In emergency situations, both kids and adults cope better when they have duties to perform; it distracts them with important tasks, so they won't dwell on dire circumstances. This strategy can prevent panic. Assigning duties is helpful on both good days and bad.

Bring a friend. Kids aren't as excited about quality family time as you might be. Years later, they'll cherish the time they spent with you, but now they'd really like to bring their favorite friend. Great idea! They'll help entertain each other, and they'll keep you challenged and entertained along the way. It also gives you the opportunity to enforce the "always stay with your buddy" rule. If they're old enough to let fun overshadow fear, give them their own tent to sleep in. They'll have a blast, but it might take them a while to get to sleep at night.

This rule works for adults, too. Having someone else along means another person to help carry stuff (don't use the word Sherpa when inviting them, though), to help keep an eye on the kids, and to share great times outdoors.

When in doubt, play. When backpacking with your kids, balance the need to get

What I did for my summer vacation…

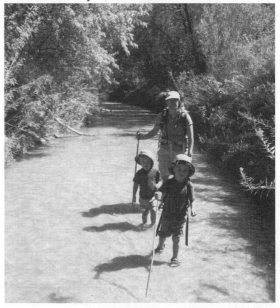

there with the desire to have fun. If moods are faltering because "my pack's too heavy, the trail's too long, it's too hot, my feet hurt, I'm hungry, or Tommy keeps throwing things at me," it's time to change the subject and get their minds off misery. Find a comfortable place to stop, take off packs, and find the "funnest" thing you can—bring out some treats, explore off-trail to check out the cool ferns and moss, turn over rocks to look for bugs, find faces in the trees and rocks, or challenge everyone to a game of Rockhead (see games and activities described later in this chapter). Once morale is high again, hiking can continue.

Follow the pack. When hiking with a group of kids, take up the rear. It's easy to lose stragglers who sit down to rest or wander off another way without telling anyone. You might also be able to raise the spirits and quicken the pace of the child who's feeling last and least.

Play, then chores. When you get to camp, let the kids play or rest for a few minutes before setting up camp. This contradicts advice given for adult hikers elsewhere in this book, but kids can be awfully excited about that really cool lake you chose as your destination. You'll find they're more enthusiastic about chores if they get to revel in their excitement for a little while after your arrival.

Keep a positive attitude. If you're relaxed and enthusiastic about being in nature, kids will be, too. There's no need to share your worries about the weather, getting to the camp on time, or other concerns. Simply take necessary steps to manage situations and avoid risks with a cheerful tone and a smile. A positive attitude is perhaps the most important thing you can bring with you into the wild. The more dire conditions become, the more important this is.

Keep them safe. Kids are even less aware of imminent threats than most adults, so it's your responsibility to keep a watchful eye out for the common threats, so you can take preventative action to avoid them.

MY SYSTEM

How to Keep Me Entertained

To entertain a child on the trail, one of the best things to do is just let them entertain themselves. But just in case, try taking along these items, which will make a foolproof and completely wireless bunch of toys in the wilderness:

A **stuffed animal** is great. It provides a wonderful, comforting cuddle for a homesick youngster. But also, it can be played with like a doll or action figure. You can dress it up with a costume made with a bandanna held in place with hair bands or a couple hair clips. You can also encourage a child to make her own doll, with a pine cone for a head and twigs with large leaves for a skirt.

Percussion instruments are easy to find along the trail. Twigs can be used as drum sticks and tent stakes can become a xylophone. I enjoyed making a giant rattle with empty water jugs tied together with a string, and banged with a stick.

Once, a friend and I entertained ourselves for an entire evening, while the adult filtered water, by creating a city with a palace, king, queen, and several families, just using **acorns and a few rocks**. And try bringing along **paper and a pencil** for a child who likes to write or draw.

A final word of advice: Don't get upset if your child plays in the dirt. She's going to get dirty anyway, and playing in the dirt is fun!

—**Mary Chambers** completed the Tahoe Rim Trail at ages 7 and 9, and successfully hiked the Pacific Crest Trail at age 10.

Avoid blisters. Happy feet are essential to happy kids. Early on the hike, ask kids frequently about painful hotspots or rubbing in their shoes. If so, apply duct tape or moleskin to the area to prevent blisters.

Stay out of the sun. Make sure everyone is wearing protection from sun—long pants and sleeves, wide-brimmed hats, and

First Aid for Kids

In addition to your standard first aid kit (see details on pages 254–255), bring the following items to treat kids:

➤ Children's Tylenol: Don't give kids aspirin; it may lead to a rare condition called Reye's Syndrome.

➤ Children's Liquid Benadryl for allergic reactions. Dose is 1 teaspoon per 25 pounds (maximum 4 teaspoons) every six to eight hours.

➤ Extra Band-Aids: Choose fun ones with colorful characters; they won't admit it, but adults like these, too.

➤ Aloe vera gel for sunburns and other irritations.

➤ Digital thermometer.

➤ Irrigation syringe to wash mud from eyes and dirt from wounds, if necessary.

A note on altitude sickness: Infants and toddlers are more sensitive to altitude than larger people. At high elevations, they may experience difficulty breathing, dizziness, vomiting, headaches, and other discomfort. If you live at sea level, reactions to altitude can occur as low as 5000 feet, especially with physical activity. Be particularly alert to this at higher elevations. Luckily, the cure is easy: Head back down to lower elevations. The more quickly you descend, the sooner your sick kid will feel better.

sunglasses. Apply sunscreen liberally to face, hands, and other exposed skin.

Watch out for insect bites. In this age of West Nile Virus, encephalitis, Lyme disease, and other insect-borne diseases, be proactive in preventing insect bites by having kids wear long sleeves and pants and mosquito netting over their heads if the bugs are thick. Use caution when applying insect repellents containing deet to children. The American Academy of Pediatrics recommends not using deet on children under two months, and they recommend using lowest deet concentration that is effective for time spent outdoors (deet effectiveness does not improve above concentration of 30 percent); there have been reports of side effects. Apply insect repellent to clothes first, and to skin only if necessary.

Keep your kids warm and dry. It's much easier to stay warm than to warm back up after being cold or hypothermic.

Make sure kids drink a lot of water. Give them their own water bottles, and flavor the water with Gatorade or other sweet drink mixes to encourage lots of chugging, especially on hot days when there's a higher risk of dehydration.

Steer clear of potential accidents. Some terrain is more dangerous than others. Decide where to draw the line with clear don't-go-there rules without being too paranoid or quashing their opportunity to grow and explore. If your trail will take you and your toddler past cliffs or other dangers, try a Harness Buddy, a monkey- or doggie-safety harness with leash that also functions as a small backpack. Check them out at www.safetyforbabies.com.

Avoid dangerous animal encounters. Yes, animals are cute, but close encounters can be dangerous. Do not let kids feed or approach any animal. Always keep predators in mind. We forget this when we live in safe neighborhoods and cities, but we are all part of the food chain.

In the wilderness, and along the edges—where civilization meets wild country—there is always a risk of attack by mountain lions, bears, or coyotes. This risk is extremely rare, but each year it happens to an unlucky few. Kids are particularly soft, pink, and helpless—attractive as easy meals. Don't ever forget this. How far away would a mother deer or rabbit let her baby stray? Be cautious of stragglers who drop too far behind the rest of the group. For more on animals, see the chapter on wildlife that begins on page 211.

Keep immunizations current. Before you leave, make sure everyone's up to date on their shots.

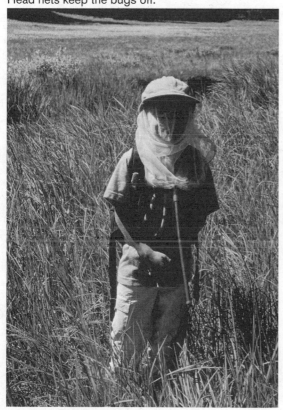

Head nets keep the bugs off.

Games and Activities for Camp and Trail

When boredom or bad weather set in, it's a good idea to have a supply of games and activities to get you through those final miles on the trail or that day in the tent while you wait for the rain stop. Here are a few ideas:

Cards. Compact and lightweight, cards are can help long, rainy days pass. Make sure you can remember the rules to a few key games, such as Spades, Crazy 8s, and Poker.

Hacky Sack/foot bag. These lightweight bean bags offer hours of fun for coordinated folks who still have energy to lift their legs after long days of hiking.

Stories. Reading from a collection of Native American myths from the region where you hike is a great way to add cultural color to your experience and often a moral dimension that leads to further discussion. With older kids, ghost stories might be a good idea, but younger kids (and some adults) can become terrified when dark settles in, ruining all the fun. Ghost stories can intensify the terror. Not being scared of the dark is a lot more fun.

Learn the ropes. Bring a lightweight knot book along (see bibliography on page 260 and sample knots on page 140) and practice useful knots.

Word, memory, and trivia games. Twenty Questions and other favorites like I Spy can lead to hours of fun along the trail or in camp.

Nature guides. Kids will love learning about wildlife, flowers, trees, and rocks.

Star guides. My favorite is the Miller Planisphere, available online and at many outdoors stores (make sure you buy the right one for your latitude).

Frisbee. This makes a great plate, too!

Animal watching. The best times to spot animals are at dawn and dusk. Find a spot by a meadow or near a water hole, then

Fishing with Your Kids

Fishing with your kids is a great way to create wonderful memories for everyone. It's also a great opportunity for them to learn about fish, and it's a great way for you to teach them water safety.

No sophisticated equipment is necessary, just a simple pole, hook and bobber, and appropriate bait (or lure—check with local experts before you go). Fishing licenses are available at almost any bait and tackle store or outdoor supply store on the way to the trailhead.

Depending on local regulations or etiquette, decide whether you'll be eating your fish or simply enjoying catch-and-release. Either way, you'll never forget the look on your kids' faces when they hook their first fish, and they'll never forget the wonderful times you spent teaching them to fish.

After you have inspected your critters, simply let them go. I found mine at www.sciencekit.com.

Take a closer look. Binoculars, magnifying lenses, and bug boxes allow for a closer look at the flora and fauna you'll encounter in the wild.

Rockhead. Thank you, Blake, for teaching me one of my favorite games ever. It's a wonderful challenge for balance and hand-eye coordination. You can play anywhere there are rocks, and the rules are simple:

One person starts with a base rock about the size of your head, give or take (smaller base rocks lead to shorter games, as only so many rocks will fit on top). Players takes turns placing their rocks anywhere on the base rock, or on other rocks that have been added. All rocks must be at least the size of your thumb

How high can it go?

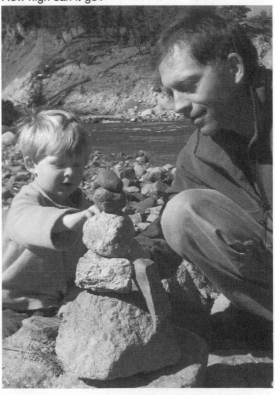

sit quietly and wait. Have everyone sit for 10 minutes and move nothing but their eyes. For greater fun, space everyone apart so they can't see each other. After a few minutes of stillness, birds and animals will begin to appear. Motion and noise are what keep them away. When you sit quietly, they'll forget about you and go on about their business, with luck, giving you a good view.

Animal tracks. Even with your best efforts, animals can be shy and hard to see. Their tracks, however, can tell you when they passed through. Tracks are easiest to find first thing in the morning, especially near water holes. A small plaster-cast kit from your local arts-and-crafts store can help you preserve beautiful tracks for good stories, memories, and study after you get home.

Bug boxes. These plastic containers, with breathing holes and a magnifying lens in the lid, are harmless for the bugs and great for getting close-up peeks at local creepy-crawlies.

above the knuckle, and if you touch a rock, you must use it. Play ends when someone makes the pile collapse.

Watch as you collectively build large, beautiful sculptures. Or it just might be so beautiful, you'll want to leave it as temporary art to admire.

Geocaching/orienteering. A fun way to teach kids map and compass skills is to reward them for learning. While they're asleep or distracted elsewhere, have one adult hide a secret treasure of toys somewhere within a mile of camp. Mark the spot carefully on a map (7.5-minute maps, also called 1:24,000 maps, are best). Then teach the kids the map and compass skills necessary to help them find the treasure where X marks the spot. In case your own skills are rusty, check out the chapter on wilderness navigation that begins on page 127.

Doctor. This is another great way to teach valuable outdoor skills. Go through your first aid kit, and teach the kids how each thing works. Then you can take turns healing each other—stopping a practice bleed or splinting a sprained ankle. This is also a great time to teach the difference between medicine and candy.

Sound exploring. Sit in the tent or outside and close your eyes. How many sounds can you identify? How many different birds are singing? Can you tell the difference between wind and a stream? What else can you hear?

Who lives here? Talk about different animals, where they live, what they eat, and how they survive. Good nature guides, such

Childhood couldn't be better.

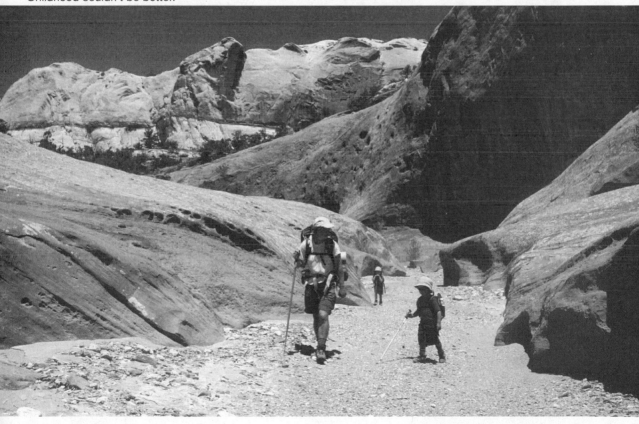

Learn More about Backpacking with Kids

- *365 Outdoor Activities You Can Do with Your Child*, by Steve and Ruth Bennett, Bob Adams, Inc., 1993
- *Camping with Kids: The Complete Guide to Car, Tent, and RV Camping*, by Goldie Gendler Silverman, Wilderness Press, 2006
- *Extreme Kids: How to Connect with Your Children Through Today's Extreme (and Not So Extreme) Outdoor Sports*, by Scott Graham, Wilderness Press, 2005
- *Kids in the Wild: A Family Guide to Outdoor Recreation*, by Cindy Ross and Todd Gladfelter, The Mountaineers Books, 1995
- *Last Child in the Woods: Saving our Children from Nature Deficit Disorder*, by Richard Louv, Algonquin Books, 2005
- *Sharing Nature with Children*, by Joseph Cornell, Dawn Publications, 1998

as Audubon's series on birds, mammals, or insects, or their field guides to regions, are helpful if you're not sure.

Animal and bird calls. Try to copy the animal and bird sounds you hear. If songbirds are present, you might be able to call them by repeating, "Psh, psh, psh…" For some reason, it makes them curious. When it works, it's amazing to watch as they gather and flutter around.

Boat races in the creek. Make your own boats out of sticks and leaves.

Write letters. Bring some postcards or note cards and write to your friends and family back home. Better yet, have your kids draw a picture of a scene from your trip and make their own postcard.

Books. Sometimes there's nothing better than reading a favorite book in the tent while it's raining. If it leads to a nap, even better.

Wilderness stewards. Kids love doing good. Spend some time picking up litter, cleaning up camp, or covering up switchbacks along the trail. While you're doing it, explain to them why this is important.

Practice in the backyard, so you'll be ready for the wilderness.

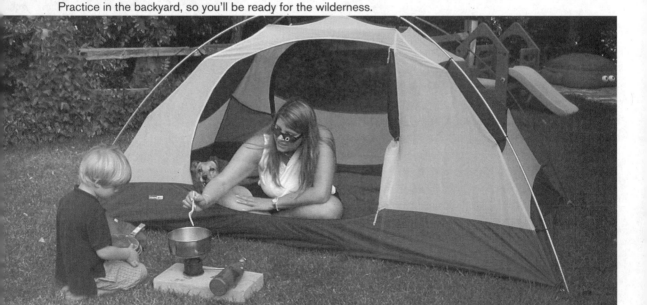

Create a journal, CD, or blog about your trip. Have the kids take pictures and notes in a journal, then create a blog or multimedia CD on the computer once you get home.

Take Baby Steps

Before you launch an expedition into the wild with your children, practice first. Camp out in your backyard—pitch the tent, roll out the sleeping bags, cook backpacking food with a camp stove, and get them used to the equipment and habits of the big outdoors.

Next step, take them car camping. There are thousands of wonderful campgrounds across the country where you can practice using all of your equipment, camp outdoors, and take dayhikes. Car camping might be the easiest and most convenient option for families with diaper-age children, and it allows you to bring more equipment to make the trip comfortable and enjoyable.

After each trip, while it's still fresh in your memory, discuss what worked well and what didn't. Make a list of things you wish you had brought. Cross off things you brought that you wish you hadn't. Next time, you'll be that much more experienced and better prepared.

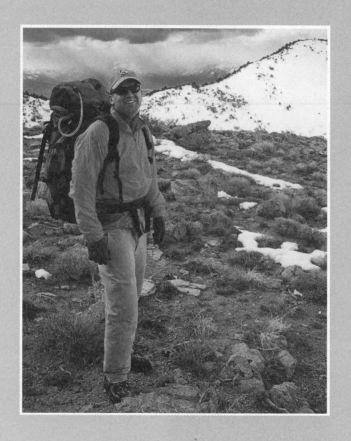

PART II
BACKPACKING GEAR

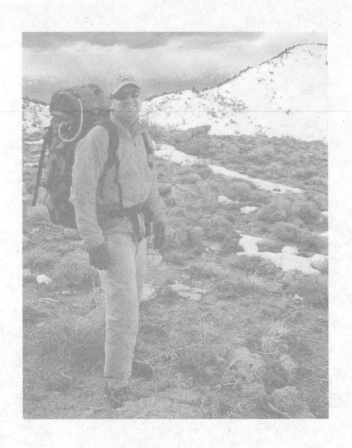

Humans are fragile; we don't have fur to protect us from the cold, nor do we have hooves or claws to help us scale mountains or ward off attack. Yet we can thrive in a rugged wilderness of storms, mountains, and myriad other dangers thanks to our mental savvy and the equipment we bring with us.

The single most important item to bring backpacking is your brain. Don't leave it at home (you'd be surprised how many people do this). No piece of equipment can replace proper planning, careful observation, common sense, respect for fellow hikers and wildlife, and a calm, reasoned response to emergencies. But the brain is just the beginning. The gear you choose to wear and carry while backpacking helps determine your level of comfort in the wild and your ability to deal with a variety of conditions. In extreme situations, the right equipment can tip the balance between life and death.

Choosing the Right Equipment

Your equipment should be comfortable and reliable, and it should function well in a variety of conditions. Choosing the right equipment depends on accurately anticipating the conditions you'll face on the trail, including unexpected emergencies (mosquitoes, rain, a twisted ankle), and then bringing enough gear to meet your needs, but not too much that it weighs you down.

This isn't always easy. Shopping for outdoor gear can be frustrating and confusing. Whether you're in the market for boots, backpacks, tents, sleeping bags, stoves, or clothing, an overwhelming number of products (backed by boastful marketing claims) waits in every outdoor store, catalog, magazine, and website. Each year, changes in technology, innovation, and style bring more.

Luckily, a lot of good companies, led by passionate, committed people, make high-quality gear for backpacking. Sizes and styles are available to fit most every body and every use. Quality gear often—but not always—costs more. Choose right, and you won't have to buy it again for a long time.

Equipment for Women

As we all know, women's bodies are shaped differently than men's (hallelujah!). They also have different needs—for example, women tend to sleep colder than men and need sleeping bags with extra fluff in the right places to keep them warm on chilly nights. Many manufacturers offer lines of sleeping bags, backpacks, boots, and clothing that are designed to fit the particular shape and needs of female bodies. When shopping for gear, ask your salesperson or search online to see if women's models are available.

The Evolution Continues

Outdoor equipment is proof that evolution and intelligent design can coexist. Each year, innovation in materials and design produces lighter, stronger, more durable, and more efficient equipment. Every once in a while, a true revolution arrives that greatly affects the way you travel in the wilderness. Examples of recent revolutions include polyester fleece, LED lights, and possibly radiant-heat stoves. Although these innovations often begin with the most sophisticated and expensive equipment for elite athletes in extreme conditions, the technology ultimately trickles down to everyday backpackers like you and me.

Because new products are introduced and old ones discontinued each season, most discussions in this book will be about general gear categories and features, rather than particular brands and models. I will mention particular products if they have stood the test of time as leaders in their field, or if I really like them. Unfortunately, I can't mention every good company or piece of equipment. I apologize if I leave out quality gear that deserves mention. Ultimately, the best equipment is what works best for you. Don't let me or anyone else sway you from buying what works best for you.

Not surprisingly, in this age of specialization, there is no perfect equipment for all seasons, regions, conditions, activities, or people. There will always be trade-offs between weight, durability, appropriateness, and cost. It's also important to remember that some things—GPS units, maps, compasses, and even clothing—are only as good as your skill in using them.

Buying quality equipment isn't the challenge; buying too much is. Most people, me included, bring more than they need into the wild. It's also possible to get seduced by really cool gear that you don't need—"Sure, that ice axe is nifty, Jim, but why did you bring it to the Everglades?"

This section will help you narrow down your choices, cut through the marketing hype, and outfit yourself with what you need for your next trip into the wild.

Before You Shop for Gear

Before you head to your local outdoor megastore or friendly neighborhood retailer, take a moment to determine your needs. Where and when will you travel? Will you be backpacking in the Pacific Northwest or the Atlantic Southeast, where rain is common? In the deserts of the Southwest? In the high mountains? In spring, summer, fall, or winter? Through thick forest or open expanse? On a trail or cross-country? At high elevations? How you answer each of these questions will determine what equipment you need. For example, do you need a camp stove that will melt snow quickly at high elevation in a snowstorm, or an easy-to-use stove to make mac 'n' cheese on a pleasant weekend outing in summer? Will you need heavy-duty boots to handle a weeklong, off-trail hike in rough terrain, or something lighter and more comfortable for a weekend jaunt on a gentle trail?

Also think about your budget. Is quality more important, or cost? You could waste time drooling over that $400 jacket, but why do that to yourself? Luckily, good equipment is out there for a lot less. More on this soon.

Once you have a general idea of what you need, start your research. Ask friends and associates about the gear they use, or ask staff at your local outdoor store about the gear they carry and recommend. Reputable stores have well-trained staff to help steer you to the gear you need. No brick-and-mortar store can carry every backpack, boot, or tent that might be right for you. If you're afraid of a smooth salesperson talking you into a purchase before you're ready, then leave your credit card, cash, and checkbook in the car while you're in the store. When in doubt, get a second opinion from a different source.

Some great sources are the gear reviews in outdoor magazines and websites such as *Backpacker*, *Outside*, *Camping Life*, and *National Geographic Adventure*. Each year, *Backpacker* magazine awards its Editors' Choice, Gold, and Green awards (www.backpacker.com/editorschoice); *Outside* magazine awards the Gear of the Year (outside.away.com/outside/gear/index.html).

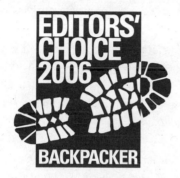

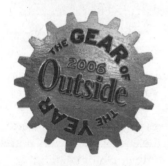

Even when you read the reviews, however, beware of bells and whistles. If you bought into all the marketing claims of gear manufacturers, or every piece of equipment mentioned in this book, you would have so much equipment, you'd never be able to fit it into your pack, let alone lift it and head down the trail. As you're shopping for and evaluating gear, remember the whole point of backpacking is to reduce your material possessions to minimum essentials, and maybe a luxury or two. Cool gadgets are fun, but are they necessary?

Finally, once you've found something that *really* sounds good, try it before you buy it. If you can borrow equipment from a friend or rent it from an outdoor store or outfitter, you can decide if you like it before you commit the big bucks on new gear.

Backpacking on the Cheap

Backpacking doesn't have to be expensive; you don't need to go into debt so you can enjoy a few days on the trail. It's about simplifying your life and reducing your possessions to the most basic of items. It's about getting back to nature, not about shopping.

However, there's also a lot of really cool, sophisticated, high-tech equipment out there that works really well in the backcountry. For this equipment, cost can be a factor. The best, lightest, and most durable equipment often isn't cheap. You can easily spend more than $2000 outfitting yourself with a pack, tent, sleeping bag, stove, clothing, and other gear for the trail. Luckily, once you invest in this gear, which can last for years, the only other expenses you'll face are food, transportation to the trailhead, and the occasional permit at the trailhead.

In this Age of Stuff, you're probably going to end up buying at least some gear for backpacking. Paying more isn't necessary if you're patient and strategic when shopping. Here are a few ideas on how to score the best deals on quality backpacking equipment:

Buy used. You can often find great deals at garage sales, thrift stores, and from classified ads, especially if you're patient. Online, you can find great deals on eBay (www.ebay.com) or Craigslist (www.craigslist.org). Craigslist sites are broken down by city, and there's

Research and Shopping Online

There is a wealth of equipment information online. To find manufacturer websites, type the company name into Google. If there's no store near you, don't be afraid to buy equipment online that must be fitted, such as boots, sleeping bags, and backpacks. But make sure they fit and work correctly before you hit the trail. Just be sure to check their return policy before you buy, so you can send back equipment that doesn't work for you.

The following websites have good information about gear, as well as forums where you can get the advice of other backpackers:

➤ www.backpacking.net: This website for ultralight backpackers offers great advice and suggestions for lightweight gear.

➤ www.trailspace.com: New product reviews, advice for the trail, classifieds, and blogs are all available on this site.

➤ www.backcountrygear.com: This online store has a variety of backcountry gear and some decent sales.

➤ www.backpackinglight.com: This membership site (guests are allowed for some content) has equipment reviews, techniques, forums, trail reports, and equipment for packers looking to shed a few pounds. Subscriptions are required for the most in-depth articles.

➤ www.thebackpacker.com: Designed as a place for beginners to learn about techniques and gear, this site is also a gathering place for more experienced backpackers to share stories and compare notes.

➤ www.backpacker.com: The online companion to *Backpacker* magazine offers everything from feature stories to gear reviews, destination finders, and forums for backpackers to compare notes.

➤ www.en.wikipedia.org/wiki/Backpacking_(wilderness): Written by computer users around the world, this overview on backpacking contains a section discussing the basics of gear.

not an all-Craigslist search engine, but if you go to Google, and type "Craigslist" and whatever you're looking for, you'll get hits for what you want, wherever they are. For example, try "Craigslist backpack" or "Craigslist Arc'teryx backpack" or "Craigslist Optimus stove."

Borrow someone else's equipment. If a friend or relative has some equipment, ask to borrow it. Don't wear out your welcome, though. If you're borrowing a pack for the third or fourth time, it might be time to buy your own.

Wait for end-of-season sales. At the end of each selling season, stores and manufacturers drastically reduce prices to clear stock so they can make room for next season's models. Although you might have to wait for months to put your gear to use, the end of winter is a great time to get great deals on winter clothing. Similarly, the end of summer is a great time to shop for summer clothing and gear.

Settle for less than "best." Top-of-the-line gear is often made for extreme situations that few of us mere mortals will ever encounter. Why pay $400 for a jacket that will protect you from raging blizzards at 20,000 feet on Mt. Everest, when a $50 jacket will work just fine in the summer rain you're more likely to encounter?

Often, second best is good enough. Outdoor specialty retailers are great places to get gear, but you don't have to get all of your gear there. Consider my favorite fleece jacket for backpacking: It cost me $14.99 new at a big-box department store. It's 10 years old, and it still looks good and remains soft and fluffy. I also backpacked every weekend of a summer at the Grand Canyon in a pair of $19.99 hiking boots. Another favorite find is a fleece-lined nylon jacket I bought for $49 at a truck stop. Granted, it's probably not as good at its $180 high-end counterpart, but it has worked well in a variety of challenging conditions.

Unfortunately, there's a price to pay when you buy cheap or used equipment. Second best and used items might work fine, or they might fall apart on you. It can be hard to tell the difference; that's the price of a bargain.

Other Factors to Consider

When buying gear, fit and performance (and cost, of course) are paramount, but there are a few other things to consider before you make your final purchasing decision:

Warranties. Warranties tell you how well manufacturers stand by their gear. If you buy equipment with lifetime warranties, you know the manufacturers are confident in their equipment and value your satisfaction.

If you're not sure about the company's warranty policy for that piece of equipment that just broke, give them a call. Dedicated manufacturers will often replace the product for free; the public-relations value of keeping you satisfied with their service is worth more than telling you "tough luck" and having that reputation spread.

Does it make sense? You shouldn't have to read an instruction manual more than once to put up a tent or operate a stove. It should make sense. Try it before you buy it to see if its design complements the way your mind works. If the "interface" seems complicated, illogical, or unintuitive, find something else that is easy to understand.

Karma. Support companies with good social and environmental ethics. Low prices can often hide the "true" social and environmental costs of making a product, such as dangerous working conditions, sub-living wages for workers, or pollution that results from the manufacturing process.

Luckily, corporate social responsibility is a growing trend in the outdoor industry. Some outdoor companies donate equipment, money, and/or staff time to conserve local landscapes or support local charitable causes. Others are dedicated to making products at a minimal environmental cost. These companies know David Brower was right when he said, "there is no business to be done on a dead planet." Companies may take action on their own, or as a member of a larger alliance, or both. The Conservation Alliance (www.conservation-alliance.com), for example, is a coalition of outdoor industry companies that pool their money to give grants to nonprofit organizations that do good things for the land. Conservation Alliance also lobbies lawmakers to influence laws and policies that affect the land.

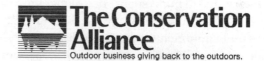
The Conservation Alliance
Outdoor business giving back to the outdoors.

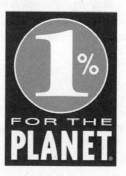
1% FOR THE PLANET

Another group, 1% For The Planet (www.onepercentfortheplanet.org), is an alliance of businesses who donate at least 1 percent of their net proceeds to keeping the planet healthy. It doesn't sound like much, but since 1985, Patagonia alone (a founding member of 1% For The Planet) has donated more than $18 million to good causes.

You can also consider companies that have won *Backpacker* magazine's Green Awards. *Backpacker* regularly honors environmentally groovy products with their Editors' Choice Green Awards.

Buying from these companies rewards them for supporting good causes, and it encourages other companies to invest in a better future. You might pay a few cents more up front, but in the long run, everybody wins with clean air, pure water, livable wages and labor conditions, and landscapes that have been protected for our continuing backpacking pleasure.

There are other ways your gear can help the environment. By bringing appropriate equipment, such as lightweight camp stoves, free-standing tents, and bottles to carry water, you enjoy the freedom to travel lightly on the land and reduce your impact on natural resources. For example, if you're well-prepared and get lost or injured, you won't have to chop down a tree to build shelter or a signal fire.

You might also consider selecting fabrics and equipment with muted earth-tone colors, which will reduce your visual impact on other visitors and on wildlife. A single brightly colored item, however, such as a bright sleeping bag or stuff sack, can come in handy as a signal device in emergencies.

Going Light

Backpacking isn't about stuff; it's about simplifying your life so you can travel through wild landscapes. By definition, backpacking is a lightweight endeavor—reducing your material possessions to only those necessary to survive (hopefully thrive!) in the wilderness. Because you must carry each item, it's important to consider the weight of everything you bring (leave that wonderful cast-iron frying pan at home). There's also a big difference between how much you can carry and how much you'll enjoy carrying it, especially after miles of trail on a hot day. Remember: You will have to carry every gear decision you make.

In the 1990s, backpacker and engineer Ray Jardine grew frustrated with carrying too much weight while through-hiking on the Pacific Crest Trail, Appalachian Trail, Continental Divide Trail, and other epic trails. He fiddled, cut, sewed, thought a bunch, then fiddled some more until he could hike 2000 miles with a pack weighing only 10 pounds, not counting food and water. Jardine's book, *Beyond Backpacking*, has helped backpackers reduce the amount of weight they carry and inspired manufacturers to trim gear weight and design to their barest essentials. The company GoLite was formed to bring many of Jardine's innovations to the market. Many other manufacturers have since developed product lines dedicated to lightweight backpacking.

WILDERNESS WISDOM

Never sacrifice emergency preparedness to save a few ounces of weight. Always make sure you have enough gear to survive emergencies.

There are many advantages to carrying lighter gear: While carrying less weight, you will hike farther, faster, and more easily; you'll enjoy the experience more (because you'll be able to focus on the sights and sounds instead of your aching feet and back); you will be less prone to injury (it's easier to twist your ankle with a 50-pound pack than with a 30-pound pack); and, with less weight to carry, you'll need less support, which means you can use a smaller, lighter backpack and lighter boots, reducing your burden even further.

There are also disadvantages: Lightweight gear often is not as durable as heavier equipment; materials and construction are lighter and less able to withstand abuse. If you try to cram your lightweight backpack with more than it's built to carry, the equipment may fail. If you're planning to go canyoneering, travel off-trail through thick brush, or otherwise be rough-and-tumble with your equipment, you'll want gear that's more durable and up to the challenges you'll encounter—in other words, gear that's heavier. Also, lightweight clothing and sleeping bags might not be as warm as their heavier counterparts. And lightweight clothing, tents, and sleeping bags are also often trimmer in design, which can be constricting. If you need room to move, you'll need roomier, heavier equipment.

Some people have taken lightweight backpacking to extremes. Ultralight packers, also called fastpackers, focus on moving light and fast through the backcountry. This can be a great, adventurous way to travel through the wilderness. However, carrying so little requires strong outdoor skills. Ultralight backpackers have died in the wild because they were not adequately prepared for sudden storms, injuries, and other unanticipated challenges. A little bit of extra weight in clothing, shelter, and food gives you a better margin of error for survival when the going gets tough.

Although weight is always a factor, the function of your gear is most important—a warm sleeping bag on a cold night is more important that a lightweight sleeping bag. Similarly, a tent that can withstand a storm, and a backpack that won't tear apart during your hike, are more important than lighter-weight gear that fails you when you need it most.

My priority is enjoying the outdoors, not shaving another couple ounces off my pack weight or setting a speed record on any given trail. Carrying less helps me enjoy backpacking, but I try not to obsess over it. Consider weight as an important factor when choosing your gear, but take the concept only as far as you're comfortable. There are no rules about this. Your happiness on the trail is the final judge.

WILDERNESS WISDOM

Backpackers discuss and evaluate backpack weight in different ways. The following terms will help clarify discussions you might read online, and they will give you different ways to think about your own equipment:

Base weight: The weight of your pack and everything you carry in it, excluding consumables such as food, water, and fuel.

Total base weight: Base weight, plus weight of gear carried not in the pack, such as clothes, boots, trekking poles, etc.

Total pack weight: Base pack weight, plus food, water, and fuel.

Total weight: The weight of everything you're carrying down the trail—food, water, fuel, pack and everything in it, shoes, trekking poles, and clothing.

Steps to a Lighter Pack

Concentrate on the heaviest items first. Before you cut your toothbrush in half or cut the labels out of your clothing, take a look at your boots, sleeping bag, tent, backpack, stove, and clothing. These are the heaviest items you'll carry; losing significant weight off each of these items can reduce your overall pack weight by 10 to 15 pounds.

Think about systems. Systems are items that work together to meet a variety of conditions. Several lightweight clothing layers that adapt to a variety of conditions are better than a single warm jacket. Instead of bringing a cooking pot and an eating bowl, simply eat right out of the pot. Use that large rain poncho as your ground cloth, or buy a lighter sleeping bag rated to warmer temperatures, and then wear everything you own to bed on chilly nights.

Simply bring less. Always make sure your essential items are in your pack. After that, consider cutting back on the luxuries. Halfway through *War and Peace*? Consider finishing it after you get back home, and instead choose a lightweight collection of poems. Instead of your prized birding binoculars, consider a compact pair that's a fraction of the weight. Better yet, leave the book and binocs at home.

Share. If you're hiking with others, pool your equipment to save weight. One tent and stove is plenty for two to three people; four to six people will do just fine with two stoves. Your entire group needs only one first aid kit, repair kit, and tube of toothpaste.

Be critical—not of your friends, but of your equipment. Lightweight backpacking requires constant critical examination of your gear. Scrutinize every item. Do you really need it? Can you achieve the same results in a different, lighter way?

Other tips on how to shave weight are found throughout the gear and packing for the trail sections.

Resources for Lightweight Backpacking Gear and Wisdom

➤ *Beyond Backpacking: Ray Jardine's Guide to Lightweight Backpacking*, by Ray Jardine, AdventureLore Press 1992

➤ www.backpacking.net

➤ www.backpackinglight.com

Ten Essentials and Other Good Ideas

No matter what equipment you carry into the backcountry, the following items can help you survive most worst-case scenarios that chance, bad luck, or poor planning throw at you. After these essentials, I've added a few items that might not be essential, but they're really good ideas. Details about each item are provided later in the specific gear chapters, where relevant.

Water and extra food. Always carry water, even if water is abundant (what if you get injured and can't get to that nearby water source?). Also carry a filter or water-treatment additive. Throw a couple extra energy bars into your daypack. On longer trips, always bring food for an extra day or two, just in case.

Extra layers for changeable weather. Pack a fleece jacket, hat, and gloves for cold spells, and a shell jacket and pants for wind or rain.

Headlamp or flashlight. It's surprising how often sunsets catch us off guard. I recommend LED headlamps, which are more compact, lighter, and significantly more dependable, durable, and longer-lasting than incandescent lights.

First aid kit. Don't ask whether you or a hiking partner will get hurt, but when. It's also important to know how to use everything in it.

Map and compass. Carry a detailed topographic map in a Ziploc bag. You also need to know how to use it, as well as how to keep from getting lost in the first place, or how to help yourself get found if you do get lost. (Note: A GPS unit is a poor substitute. Read more about this in the section on page 134.)

Emergency whistle, signal mirror, or flare. You can use these items to signal for help. The international distress signal is three long blasts followed by three short ones. Whistles are not toys or conveniences. Use them only in emergencies. Remember the boy who cried wolf?

Fire starter. A lighter or waterproof matches can help you light a fire for warmth or signal others in emergencies. But you might need tinder or another fire starter to get the fire started. Candles are affordable and light-weight, and their drippings or shavings can add quick life to soggy or uncooperative fire-wood. WetFire tinder cubes burn enthusiasti-cally, even when wet. Check them out at your favorite outdoor store.

Sun protection. Glasses with full UV protection, a wide-brimmed hat, sunscreen, and long sleeves and pants can prevent you from getting burned in all seasons. Although

Plan well, and most of your 10 essentials can fit in a small bag.

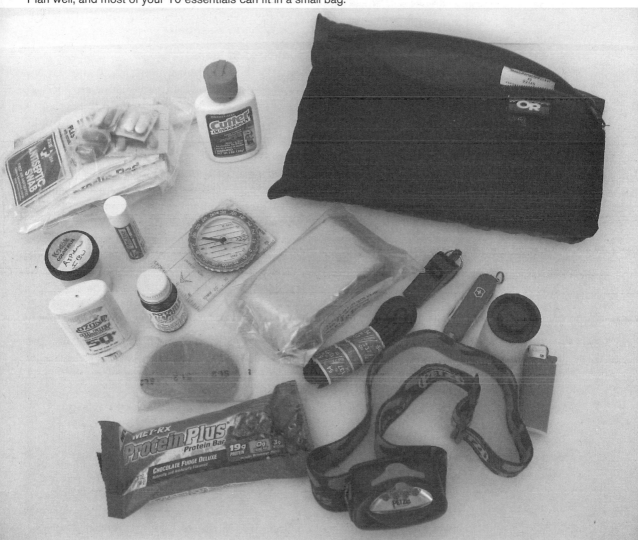

Rescue Beacons

If you're looking for reliable emergency communications, satellite phones or personal locator beacons (PLBs) can be lifesavers. These advancements in technology have saved lives, they are appropriate in some situations, and they are getting more affordable each year.

They have also created controversy. For starters, these high-tech devices create the same false sense of security that cell phones and GPS systems offer. Armed with these devices, too many people head into the wilderness without proper backcountry skills, sound judgment, or proper equipment. They think, "If I get in trouble, I'll just call for help." So what happens when the batteries die, the signal disappears in a forest or canyon, or you drop the device and it breaks?

Instead of relying on technology to get you out of emergencies you create through your own poor planning or bad judgment, concentrate instead on improving your planning, judgment, and other backcountry survival skills. Make sure you have the knowledge, skills, and equipment to handle the weather, terrain, and other challenges you'll encounter in the backcountry. Yes, it's harder, but that's the point. Wilderness travel isn't about convenience; it's about developing backcountry skills and experiencing the adventure and beauty those skills open to you. If you want convenience and comfort, stay home, watch TV, and order pizza.

Search-and-rescue operations cost a lot of money. In some jurisdictions, rescuers charge their "clients" the full cost of search-and-rescue operations, which can easily carry five-figure price tags. Search-and-rescue operations also risk the safety of the rescuers; responding to calls takes them away from quality time with their families and prevents them from responding to people who need help more than you. The choice is yours.

not always essential for survival, sun protection can prevent misery when the sun's rays are relentless.

Emergency blanket. You may need this extra layer of warmth on unexpected overnights on the trail. This is unnecessary if you already have a sleeping bag and tent or bivy.

Knife. For cutting wood, building an emergency lean-to, cutting emergency bandages, and a hundred other uses.

Not every person in your party needs every item (knives, first aid kits, and fire starters, for example), but every group certainly needs the 10 essentials.

Other Good Ideas

The following items might not be essential for survival, but they sure are nice to have in your pack when you need them.

Duct tape. With 1001 uses, this durable tape provides many valuable services on the trail. With it, you can repair torn jackets, boots, tents, and tent poles; secure bandages and splints; tape backpacks, skis, or sticks together to make a litter for evacuating injured people; put some on your foot to prevent blisters; fashion sunglass holders and spoons; repair bindings on snowshoes and skis; lay it across your

Duct tape on your trekking pole—ready to deploy.

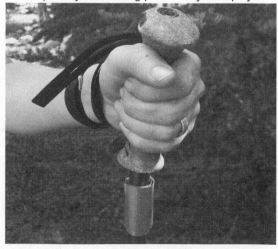

Repair Kit

Duct tape will fix most everything at least long enough to get you back to civilization, but it won't fix everything. Here are a few other repair items to consider bringing:

➤ **Tent pole splint tube:** This hollow aluminum tube fits over tent poles that have split or bent, helping them keep their shape and your tent upright.

➤ **Parachute cord:** A 50- to 100-foot length of this lightweight and durable nylon cord will work for hanging food beyond the reach of bears or rodents; or you can cut shorter lengths to tie items to your pack, replace broken shoe laces, etc.

➤ **Needle and thread:** Make sure you have two sizes of each: small for clothing, large for thicker fabrics. Dental floss also serves as an effective and durable thread. Bring a thimble, or use a hard substitute (a spoon, perhaps?) to protect your fingers while pushing needles through thick material.

➤ **Multitool:** Led by the flagship brand Leatherman, these tools have a variety of blades, screwdrivers, saws, files, scissors, and pliers. There are many styles available (cocktail fork and spreading knife?), so shop around for the one that's right for you. Before you buy, ask yourself if you need everything these tools offer and if the extra weight is worth it.

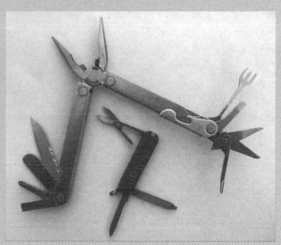

Tools or gadgets. You decide.

➤ **Super Glue:** Small and light, it fixes everything from glasses to cracked water bottles. Place a dab at each end of a rip in fabric to keep it from getting bigger. Super Glue also works to seal small cuts and lacerations, but it stings like a sonuvabitch (Spenco's 2nd Skin is the medical equivalent that stings less). A glue stick (the type used in hot glue guns) is an excellent alternative and fixes many of the same items; simply hold it over a flame and drip your repairs onto any broken item.

➤ **Safety pins:** Pin a few large and small pins to the inside of your first- aid or repair kit bag. Use them to replace lost hinges in your glasses, to affix splints and bandages, to pop blisters (sterilize the pin first over a flame), or to hold torn fabric together.

➤ **Extra batteries:** Make sure you have the right kind to replace batteries in your flashlight or headlamp or other electronic items.

➤ **Extra buckles:** The day your clumsy hiking partner steps on and breaks your hip-belt buckle, you'll be lucky your party has an extra.

➤ **Stove and/or water-purifier repair kit:** These should come with your stove and water filter.

➤ **Inflatable sleeping pad repair kit:** Check with the manufacturer for their recommendations. Different materials require different glue and procedures.

skin, then rip it off to remove cactus spines (and unwanted body hair). Throw a small roll into your pack, or wrap several meters around a water bottle, a trekking pole, or a pencil for easy access.

Straps. A few nylon straps with ladder-lock buckles (the same buckles on the compression straps of your backpack) come in handy when you need to attach things to your pack. They're also good to keep sleeping pads rolled.

Carabiners. A couple of these clips used by rock climbers (I carry one large and one small) are handy for attaching things quickly to your pack, for hanging food bags, or for lowering your pack down cliffs and waterfalls when you need to climb unencumbered.

Bandanna. One of these large, square scarves is as versatile as a multitool—it can serve as a stylish hat, sling, water filter, neck-protecting sun shade from the back of your baseball cap, bandage, strap, face mask for sick people, sun/wind protection, and more.

Plastic bags. Small, produce-style bags over your feet, but under your socks and boots, will work as vapor barriers to lock heat in on cold, wet days. If your boots are already soaked, put a bag over your dry socks to keep your feet drier and warmer. They're also good

for food storage (don't use the same ones you just had on your feet).

Medium-sized bags can carry trash or protect sleeping bags, clothes, and food from rain; small Ziploc bags are great for protecting cameras, GPS units, books, or to pack out your toilet paper or feminine hygiene products. (Note: Ziploc bags are not good for storing powdery or crumby foods; instead, use simpler plastic bags and tie them with a loose knot); and large garbage bags will keep your pack contents drier in rain (line the inside of your pack with one), and they make effective rain vests—simply cut holes for your head and arms. One large bag over each leg will create a quick set of waders for river crossings. For greater reliability, 3-mil (a *mil* equals .001 inch) contractor bags from your local hardware store are more reliable than standard 1-mil lawn bags.

Insect repellent. Depending on when and where you hike, this could be essential. Insect repellents containing deet are most effective. However, reports of side effects are common—rashes, confusion, and seizures.

Avoid the deet controversy by first using repellents made with natural plant extracts, such as lemon grass, citronella, eucalyptus oil, and peppermint. Popular brands include Buzz-Away and Natrapel. If deet becomes necessary, start with repellents containing low concentrations of deet and apply them to your clothes, not your skin; save higher concentrations for when they're absolutely necessary. Avoid high concentrations of deet, direct skin contact, and prolonged use, especially on children.

Long pants and shirts. Tuck your pants into your socks or gaiters. ExOfficio's Buzz Off clothing line is made with Permethrin (an artificial version of natural repellents found in chrysanthemums) incorporated into the fabric.

Subdued colors. Studies have shown insects are attracted to brighter colors. Wear subdued earth tones and keep some distance

Yes, I Can Hear You Now!

Despite the fun of chatting on your cell phone from the top of a remote mountain peak, it's poor etiquette to do so; the whole point of backpacking is to escape civilization and surround yourself with nature. You might not think it's a problem, but people around you are cursing you silently as you're chatting away nearby, even if they're too polite to say so. Talking on your cell phone destroys the solitude for other people. Think about leaving this particular luxury item behind, or keep it turned off.

between you and your friend with the bright, flower-print jacket.

Insect netting. Coghlan's makes mosquito and no-see-um netting that keeps bugs away from your skin. It comes in jackets, pants, and hoods (wear a baseball cap under the hood to keep the mesh away from your face).

Don't Forget Luxury

Although weight is an important factor in planning your trip, so is enjoyment. A strong argument can be made for comfort and good memories. To help you enjoy your trip, bring along a luxury that matters to you. The memories you make will be worth the extra weight. Here are some popular "unnecessary necessities" that can make your backpack a tad heavier, but your trip enormously more pleasurable:

Chocolate. Tired bodies will savor the high sugar and fat content, and its antioxidants actually help your body recover from a difficult day on the trail. In hot weather, store it deep in your pack in a Ziploc bag, and be prepared to eat it with a spoon.

Pillow. It's easy to fold up your fleece jacket and use it as a pillow, but a real pillow will add surprising comfort (and what if you're wearing that fleece to bed?). Therm-a-Rest, REI,

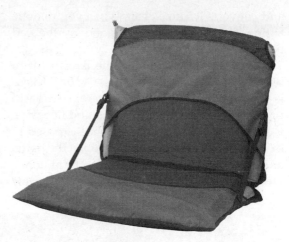
Go ahead, rest your back.

A pillow in the backcountry is the ultimate in luxury.

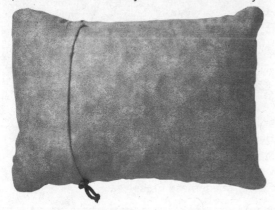

Sea to Summit, and Quixote all make camp pillows. Another approach: Bring a silk pillowcase as a stuff sack, then stuff it with clothes and enjoy a silky-soft night's sleep.

A good book. Nothing beats sitting back and indulging in a good read in your tent on a rainy day, or reading by the side of a lake on a sunny day. Rather than a heavy novel, choose instead a lightweight collection of poems or some musings by John Muir, Emerson, or another great nature thinker. There's also the wonder of learning about the geology, plants, or animals where you're hiking. Ask local sources for their favorite nature guides. For quality, regional guides, check out National Audubon Society's regional Field Guides—relatively compact and lightweight guides to your surroundings in America's Southwest, Southeast, Rocky Mountains, the Mid-Atlantic States, and the Pacific Northwest.

Camp chair. When rocks, logs, and other natural chairs aren't convenient, being able to sit back and enjoy your cup of tea, watch the sunset, or read a book in your tent is a sure way to increase the enjoyment factor of backpacking. Crazy Creek chairs enjoy a devoted following, and the 10.5-ounce Therm-a-Rest Trekker fits over any Therm-a-Rest pad and converts it into a chair. When you're done sitting, simply pop the snaps and lay the pad back out for sleep.

Fine liqueur. Fine wine is difficult to bring on the trail for several reasons: Glass is too heavy; the glass is dangerous to backpacks, tents, and skin if it breaks; and fine wine is good for only a few hours once exposed to oxygen, which means you can't open the bottle and pour the wine into a plastic bottle at home. However, port, sherry, and other sippable snorts offer more punch for the weight, and they carry well in a flask or bike bottle. Caution: Although it makes you feel warm, alcohol contributes to hypothermia. Don't drink much alcohol on super-cold nights.

iPod. Backpacking is supposed to be an escape from civilization, and there are times when electronic escape is a bad idea (such as on the trail, when you need to be paying attention to your surroundings). However, being able to enjoy music or an electronic book can help you

MY SYSTEM

Sweet Seat, Sweet Sleep

In today's lightweight world, it's heresy to admit this, but I'll do so anyway: My wife and I carry Crazy Creek chairs when we backpack.

We get away with doing so by using the chairs as part of our sleeping-pad system. Rather than carry full-length Therm-a-Rest pads, we carry three-quarter-length pads, then use our chairs for the remainder of our pads beneath our feet.

The combination of the shorter pad and Crazy Creek chair is about a pound heavier than a full-length pad alone, but we've found that the benefit of having chairs along while backpacking is worth the added weight. We strap our chairs to the outside of our packs and make use of them every time we take a break.

The chairs also make a nice dry place to stand while changing clothes in camp, they serve as ground-level tables when sorting food and gear, and they work well as a windbreak for the camp stove. Most important, I can report that having a seat with a back rest on the trail and in camp is incredibly satisfying. So satisfying, in fact, that our sons, ages 9 and 12, now elect to carry Crazy Creek chairs as part of their loads on our family backpacking trips as well.

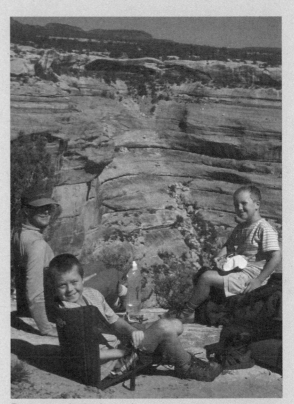
Best seats in the house!

—**Scott Graham**, author, *Extreme Kids: How to Connect with Your Children Through Today's Extreme (and Not So Extreme) Outdoor Sports*, Wilderness Press

endure long storms in your tent and other interminable bouts of nature.

Good food. It's amazing how a long day on the trail can make mediocre, freeze-dried camp food taste like a delicious feast. Imagine what a truly luscious feast would do for the memories and your popularity as a backpacking partner. Once you get used to the challenges and limitations of cooking on the trail, cooking up scrumptious meals in the backcountry isn't too hard. Plan the perfect wilderness feast in the cooking chapter coming up.

Free time. Sometimes the best treat is a little down time. There's no better place to relax than when you're surrounded by the beauty and solitude of wilderness. Instead of cramming your schedule with gotta-get-there, gotta-do-this activities, plan time to settle back and enjoy the beauty of your surroundings. Don't do. Be.

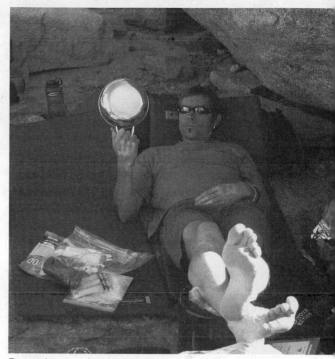

Down time can be the best time.

6 CLOTHING

Your clothes are your first and most important line of defense against the elements. The right clothes will help protect you from the elements while being lightweight, not too bulky, and adaptable to changing conditions. Luckily, we have myriad choices of high-quality, high-tech, and stylish outdoor clothing to fit nearly every body, place, and activity on this planet. Some of this gear is expensive, but not always.

Layering Systems

Grandma was right: Dress in layers. It's a simple concept, and when it's used well, it can make the difference between crisis and comfort in the backcountry. By dressing in several lightweight layers, you can more easily adapt to changeable weather and varying levels of activity. In warm weather, you need little more than lightweight, comfortable clothes, with an extra layer or two for sudden storms and surprise cold fronts.

In cold weather, however, dressing appropriately requires more planning and attention. A thick down jacket is great if you're standing around on a cold day, but if the weather changes, or if you're generating heat and sweat during activity, you'll need a clothing system that can keep you warm while letting your sweat escape and protecting you from wet or windy weather, which is something down can't do. A good layering system allows each piece of clothing to work separately, or in conjunction with other items, to adapt to varying conditions.

How Layering Works

To keep your body warm and comfortable in the backcountry, your clothing needs to perform three functions: transport moisture away from your body, provide insulation (trapped air space) to keep your body warm, and block outside wind and water from getting in to chill you.

A well-designed clothing layer system performs all of these functions and allows you

Layering keeps you dry and warm.

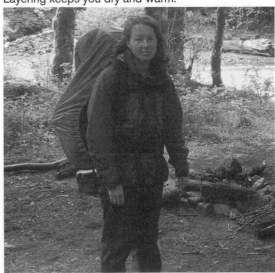

to adapt to changing conditions and activity levels by adding or removing layers as you need. Each of the layers discussed below performs one of these three main functions, yet helps with the other two to keep you warm. Which layers you add or remove depends on which job you need your clothes to do—wick, insulate, or block wind and wet weather.

Base layer. The clothing closest to your skin needs to move moisture away from your skin to keep you dry. Polypropylene, Capilene, and other synthetics, as well as silk and some wool blends, make great base layers because they actively wick moisture away from your skin while providing a certain amount of insulation value. Base layers often come in light, medium, and expedition weights to accommodate different weather conditions and activity levels. Base layers should be comfortably snug (but not constricting) to allow middle and outer layers to fit over them.

Middle layer. This layer provides the fluff, or insulation, by trapping a layer of warm, still air space around your body. It also allows perspiration vapor to pass through toward the outside. Wool and synthetic fleece are best. In warmer temperatures, the middle layer can be thinner or nonexistent. Colder temperatures demand thicker insulating layers, or more of them. Vests, for instance, help keep your core warm without the bulk of a full top. They also make great additional insulation layers on cold days. Fluffier equals warmer.

Shell layer. A good outer shell (usually a windbreaker or rain/snow jacket) should allow the moisture you create as sweat to escape to the outside, while shielding you from heat-stealing wind, rain, and snow. If it's not windy, raining, or snowing, you might not need a shell. If it's really cold, even if it's not windy, a shell can help trap heat close to your body.

Many shell materials these days are waterproof/breathable, such as Gore-Tex, eVent, and other fabrics. These fabrics actually

Dry and Fluffy

Amazingly, dressing with these two words in mind can do wonders to keep you warm in cold weather.

How?

If you get wet in cold weather, you're asking for trouble, because water will steal heat from your body surprisingly quickly, overwhelming your body's ability to warm itself. *Hydrophobic* materials do not like water; they will wick or vent moisture away from your skin (discussed below) and prevent rain and snow from getting in, helping your body keep itself warm. They also dry more quickly than *hydrophilic* (water-loving) materials like cotton. If you get *really* wet, especially in cold weather, change into dry clothes quickly to minimize your chances of getting hypothermia (see page 245 for more on this potentially serious condition).

In addition to staying dry, surrounding yourself with fluff will trap a thick layer of still air around your body, trapping heat close to your body in the same way that insulation in your house keeps the inside warm by trapping dead air in the walls. Moving air carries warmth away from your body through convection, but dead air doesn't move, allowing your body to warm it. The thicker and fluffier that air space is, the warmer you'll be. Synthetic fleece, wool sweaters, and down- or synthetic-filled garments provide the fluff you'll need to stay warm.

have microscopic holes in them that are small enough to allow water vapor (the sweat you're creating inside the shell) to escape, yet too small to let liquid water (outside rain and snow) soak in from the outside. Many shell exteriors are also chemically treated to shed water.

Untreated nylon is a good shell material for dry conditions, because it protects against wind and is breathable if you're working up a sweat. It's also the most affordable shell fabric.

The layering principle works for all clothing, not just your legs and torso. For example, lightweight synthetic glove liners work great on their own when it's cool and crisp, and they add extra warmth to bulkier winter gloves when the going gets downright arctic. Similarly, a thin, lightweight, wind-proof hat can add degrees of warmth to a baseball hat or beanie when temperatures fall or the wind rises, and sock liners can do a lot to keep your feet warmer and drier than just one pair of socks.

Fabrics and Materials

Your favorite T-shirt might seem like a good candidate for your packing list, but think twice. It's fine if it stays dry, or if it gets wet in hot weather, but if it gets wet in cold weather, it can be dangerous; it holds many times its weight in water, and it takes forever to dry. Wet clothes against your skin on a cold day can steal the heat from your body faster than you can say "Jack Frost." And when that happens, you're heading toward hypothermia, a dangerous condition in which your body gets so cold that death is possible. Cotton is also heavier and bulkier than other options; it will fill up and weigh down your pack in no time flat.

For your next backpacking trip, leave your favorite jeans, T-shirt, and sweatshirt at home, or keep them in the car for when you get back to the trailhead. Instead, opt for wool blends, silk, and synthetic materials that are lightweight and hydrophobic (don't soak up so much water). More on these fabrics follows:

Silk. Lightweight and soft against your skin, silk is a warm and effective wicking material. However, it's not as durable as other fabrics, and it might require special care when washing.

Wool. Despite the many advances in synthetic fabric technology, wool remains one of the better fabrics for the outdoors, because it insulates against the cold, wicks moisture, and resists odors. Many people prefer it over newfangled, often expensive synthetic fabrics. However, wool can be heavy, bulky, and itchy. Thin, lightweight merino wool shatters this stereotype with an incredibly soft feel and great insulating and wicking abilities. Wool-synthetic blends are popular in socks, base, and midlayers.

Down. Ounce for ounce, down is the warmest, lightest, most compactable, and most resilient insulator money can buy. It's also more expensive than synthetic competitors, and it requires careful maintenance to keep it performing at peak levels. Here are a few more things you should know about down:

➤ **Fill power:** This is a measure of down's fluffiness (there are different qualities of down), expressed as the number of cubic inches an ounce of down occupies. The higher the fill power, the greater the warmth by weight. You can find clothes and sleeping bags with 400 to 450 fill power (not great), 500 to 600 (better), or 700 to 900 (best).

➤ **Moisture:** Down loses all of its fluff when wet, which makes it useless–and possibly dangerous–because its insulating power depends on its fluff. Many sleeping bag and jacket manufacturers use a waterproof-breathable shell fabric on the outside of down garments and bags to protect the down. A shell bivy sack can protect your sleeping bag from water on the outside, and vapor-barrier liners can prevent moisture from soaking in from your own sweat. But if you're expecting consistently wet conditions, choose a synthetic alternative.

➤ **Cost:** Down costs 30 to 50 percent more than equivalent synthetics, but it should last three to five times longer. If you divide the cost by the years of cozy comfort down provides, it's easy to justify the bargain if you can afford it.

Polyester fleece. Quite possibly the best invention to hit backpacking since the

Waterproof-Breathable Shell Fabrics

Waterproof-breathable might sound like a contradiction, but modern textile technology is pretty amazing. Many shell garments are breathable enough to allow sweat vapor to escape to the outside, but waterproof enough to keep rain and snow from getting in. Textile manufacturers accomplish this in two ways: through waterproof-breathable membranes laminated between the inner and outer layers of a shell garment, and by chemically treating the outer shell fabric.

The most popular waterproof-breathable technology is Gore-Tex. Cooked up in secret laboratories by W.L. Gore & Associates, this expanded polytetrafluoroethylene membrane (known affectionately as PTFE-PU) has 9 billion pores per square inch and is sandwiched between material layers in shell garments. The holes are big enough for water vapor to pass through, but too small for liquid water to penetrate. The result: Rain and snow cannot penetrate from the outside, but sweat vapor can escape to the outside. (Pretty nifty!) All garments with Gore-Tex must also have taped seams to further assure waterproofing.

Gore-Tex is just one recipe among several that have earned the waterproof-breathable accolade. Others include Xalt, WaveTex, H2No, eVent, REI Elements, and Triplepoint. These, too, are proprietary. How well each works depends on which marketing department is talking. Lucky for us, they all work pretty darn well—to a point.

In extreme situations, waterproof-breathable fabrics have their limitations. Extreme humidity can impede the ability of waterproof-breathable fabrics to transport water vapor. If rain is going to be a constant companion on your hike (in the rainy Northwest or Southeast, for example), wear loose-fitting shells with ample vents, combined with an umbrella, if possible, to prevent a steamy terrarium from forming inside your clothes. If you are sweating up a storm, you will need to add and shed layers attentively to walk the fine line between too wet and too cold.

Waterproof-breathable technology also falters when dirt and sweat start clogging the pores, or after years of use, when the technology begins to break down. Old, tired, waterproof-breathable fabrics can be revived by washing them carefully and treating them with specially designed chemical applications. Learn more about these in the chapter on caring for your gear beginning on page 97.

backpack, synthetic fleece is lightweight, soft, fluffy, available in different thicknesses, and it helps keep you warm even when it's wet. It's a perfect insulating layer. Fleece is made from several different recipes, including recycled plastic, and it's available at most outdoor and big-box department stores at affordable prices. Fleece is so common, you probably already own some fleece clothes. If not, make sure to put fleece on your shopping list, and certainly in your backpack the next time you hit the trail.

Other synthetics. Modern textile technology is amazing. Manufacturers are continually coming up with astounding fibers that are lightweight and durable and that provide comfort, insulation, and protection from the elements. Some are designed to resist water, or to let it pass through. A variety of chemical treatments are also applied to achieve a variety of performance results.

There are many synthetic materials to choose from—nylon, polyester, polypropylene, Dacron, Capilene, and DriClime—and each year, manufacturers invent more. Many of these fabrics are trademarks of particular companies, and they may be similar to other fabrics with different names by other manufacturers. Yes, it gets confusing.

Fashion Tips for the Wilderness: Dirt Bags vs. Tech Weenies

Civilized fashion rules don't apply in the wilderness, which is great for those of us who have no fashion sense to begin with. It doesn't matter whether your clothes are the latest style, or even if they match. What matters is that they're comfortable and protect you from sticks, stones, bugs, and weather.

Some of the coolest people in the wilderness are "dirt bags," folks who don't care what their equipment looks like, as long as it works well. Many of their clothes and equipment are downright ratty. But it works, and it's helped them through hundreds, maybe thousands, of nights under the stars.

"Tech weenies" are people with all the latest, expensive, high-tech gadgets but no clue how to use them, or no common sense in the wild. They also have trouble pulling their attention away from their toys long enough to enjoy the wonder of nature.

There are also many things you think you might need in the city, which will work against you in the wilderness. Let comfort and function drive your clothing choices. Leave the following at home:

➤ High heels, pumps, and loafers. Choose instead comfortable shoes with good traction and support.

➤ Cotton, which is heavy, bulky, and soaks up water like a sponge. If it gets wet, dangerous hypothermia becomes a risk.

➤ Perfumes, scented soaps, lotions, and cosmetics. Bears, mosquitoes, and other critters love this stuff. Do you really want to smell that good?

➤ Hair dryers, jewelry, and tight jeans. There are no outlets out there, and the jewelry and tight jeans will only weigh (and slow) you down.

Synthetics are used in all types of garments—wicking, insulating, shell, as well as casual clothing lines. Companies such as REI, ExOfficio, Sportif, and Patagonia (just to name a few) have lines of casual and travel clothing made from fabrics that look and feel a lot like cotton, but are durable, wrinkle- and stain-resistant, and quick-drying. Specialized fabrics are also available to protect against insects and UV radiation. Some technical clothing lines already include locator/beacon technology as well as built-in speakers for your MP3 player. If technology continues to advance at this pace, soon your clothes will be able to massage your back while you hike, and maybe even carry your backpack, too.

Blends. Many socks, shirts, pants, and other clothes are made from a blend of natural and synthetic fibers. There are too many combinations to keep straight, and every manufacturer has its own special recipes and trademarks. One wonderful example of synthetic blends are soft-shell fabrics. These soft, stretchy, flexible, and comfortable combinations of fleece, Lycra, spandex, polyester, and other ingredients that are too hard to pronounce (or type!) insulate you against the cold, breathe, repel weather admirably, and are extremely long-lasting.

Leather. There are several advantages of leather–namely its strength, flexibility, and durability. However, leather is also heavy, does not breathe well, gets soggy and heavy when wet, and dries slowly. If you're not careful when it's wet, it can also dry into new and uncomfortable shapes (common with boots). Although there are still quality, all-leather boots (see more on footwear in the next chapter) available, these days, leather is used less frequently, usually on stress points in shoes, boots, and gloves. Leather shirts, pants, and jackets may be popular in bike gangs and night clubs, but they don't work for backpacking.

Accessories: Sunglasses, Hats, and Headlamps

Although these items are small, each is an important addition to your backcountry toolbox, and each can make a big difference in your comfort and safety while backpacking.

Sunglasses

Sunglasses don't just make you look cool; they also protect you from the sun's dangerous ultraviolet (UV) rays. When shopping for sunglasses, make sure you choose ones that protect against 99 percent of UVA and 95 to 98 percent of UVB. Any less, and dangerous UV rays will affect your eyes, which are worth more than saving a few bucks on glasses. Any glasses worth buying should have a sticker declaring the level of UV protection. On that note, avoid cheap sunglasses. Never mind what ZZ Top says about them—dark lenses that don't provide UV protection can actually be worse than wearing no glasses, because they will cause your pupils to relax and expand, opening your eyes even wider to damaging UV rays.

Choose larger lenses or glasses that fit snugly, so they cover your eyes well. Never mind how cool Keanu Reeves looked in *The Matrix*, larger lenses will provide greater protection against ultraviolet damage creeping in from the sides. They will also help keep out wind-blown debris or dust kicked up on hot, dry trails. When you're working hard in colder weather, you'll need glasses that circulate air well, so they don't fog up.

Quality optic glass provides the clearest view without distortion, but ophthalmologists recommend polycarbonate lenses. Not only does polycarbonate naturally filter UV rays, it's less dangerous because, unlike glass, it doesn't shatter into eye-piercing shards when it breaks.

Consider bringing at least one extra pair of glasses or lenses for your party in case someone loses or breaks theirs. Extra lenses from sunglasses with replaceable lenses work well; with these and a little handy duct-tape craftsmanship, you can quickly fashion an emergency pair of glasses.

After UV protection, the rest is just fashion. But there are a few other things to think about:

➤ Polarized lenses reduce glare from snow and water.

➤ Gray lenses are neutral and sharpen color perception.

➤ Brown and amber lenses enhance contrast, making them good for fog or low-light situations.

For more about sun damage and protection, see page 202.

Hats

Depending on the season, there are three types of hats you will need for backpacking:

Warm hat/beanie. One of these should always be in your pack, unless you're hiking in the hottest of desert summers.

Wide-brim hat. Wide brims protect from brutal sun in any season; if they are waterproof, they work great in rain, too.

Baseball/truckers cap. They don't protect you well against the sun (a hat with 360-degree brim is better), although you can improve sun protection by adding a bandanna,

Umbrellas

In constant downpours and brutal sun, an umbrella might be worth the extra weight. Tie it to your backpack so you can remain drier while hiking hands-free. In rain, you'll be more comfortable in breathable layers; in sun, you'll always have shade. They don't work well in thick forest or wind, though, and your hiking partners might not enjoy those spikes aiming for their eyes.

Lawrence of Arabia-style. You can also keep mosquito netting off your face when sleeping in a bivy sack or wearing a head net, and they help deflect rain and snow from your face when you're hiking in stormy weather.

Light

Lights are important after the sun goes down. Luckily, technology has evolved in beautiful directions in the last decade; light has become cheaper, lighter-weight, more reliable, and more durable.

Incandescent lightbulbs are now going the way of the dinosaurs. Leave your trusty Maglite or other incandescent-bulb flashlight in the closet or your glove compartment, and invest in LED for the backcountry. Light-emitting diodes have numerous advantages over incandescent bulbs: They are many times more efficient (less energy is wasted as heat); they're more durable (no glass to shatter or filament to break); they last longer (burning between 30 and 100 hours on a single set of lithium batteries, which last much longer than alkaline); bulb life is measured in years, not hours as with incandescent bulbs; and they're lighter-weight (smaller bulbs and longer life mean smaller batteries).

For backpacking, I recommend a headlamp over a flashlight. Lightweight and compact, they leave your hands free for more important stuff (like digging through your pack looking for your toothbrush). Just make sure you know where your headlamp is when the sun goes down.

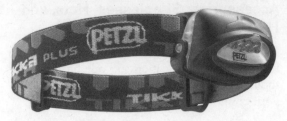

Petzl's Tikka LED headlamp

The smallest LED headlamps are wonderful for reading, tasks around camp, and non-technical travel, but if you're picking your way through a crevasse field on a glacier, or searching for lost people in the woods, make sure you have something more powerful. Several headlamps are available with multiple power options to accommodate your differing needs.

Petzl's Tikka is one of the more popular and reliable LED headlamps. Other companies make quality lights, too, such as Princeton Tec and Black Diamond.

The cheapest lights available are still candles, although they're useless in more than a sigh of weather. A single plumber's candle propped inside your cooking pot (tilted sideways) or in front of your stove's aluminum windscreen creates a romantic ambiance for reading in your tent or moving around camp. Candle shavings or drippings also provide a welcome boost to struggling fires, so throw a candle or two into your pack for emergencies.

7 FOOTWEAR

Warm, dry, comfortable feet are happy feet, and happy feet are essential to happy hikers. This isn't always easy, because there's a lot working against your feet on the trail.

Your feet are a complicated collection of bones, tendons, ligaments, and muscles that receive a lot of abuse while backpacking—not only must they carry you and all your gear along the trail, but they are on the receiving end of hard ground, rocks, sticks, and other obstacles.

For these reasons, don't be miserly when outfitting your feet with the proper boots, socks, and insoles. The footwear you choose for backpacking is the most important gear you will buy. Your boots must be durable and supportive enough to carry you and your gear for miles over rough terrain, and they must be comfortable all the while—a single bad blister can literally cripple you miles from the trailhead. (Read more about preventing and treating blisters on page 165.)

The Best Footwear for Your Hike

To choose the right footwear, first determine your needs. There are big differences among dayhikes, weeklong backpacks, and mountaineering expeditions to the summits of snowy peaks. Hiking and backpacking footwear comes with an assortment of features, falling into several broad categories, depending on the kind of hiking you expect to do. As you move down the list of footwear that follows, weight and cost will increase.

Trail-running shoes. Also called cross-trainers, these shoes are basically street-running shoes on steroids. They're lightweight and flexible, with low tops, sturdy design, and rugged soles, made for moving quickly through challenging terrain. They're great for dayhikes and backpacking with ultralight loads (under 20 pounds). Lightweight-backpacking enthusiasts argue that you don't need any other footwear—if your load is light enough.

However, they don't offer the support necessary to manage heavier loads, and their soles are relatively thin. If you're carrying a heavier pack, if you're hiking cross-country through sharp terrain, or if your ankles need more support, choose heavier shoes or boots. Price range: $50 to $120.

Trail-running shoes might be all you need for light loads.

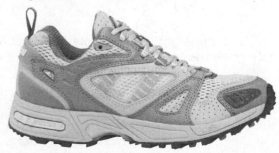

Coordinated Footwear

My preferences in footwear are pretty basic. My trail shoes are by Inov8, a high-quality, lightweight, trail-running shoe with good dirt- and rock-grabbing tread that are quick-draining. For insoles, I toss out the ones that come with the shoes and use the heat-molding Sole Custom Footbeds. They provide inexpensive support specific to my feet. Socks are either Injinji Tetratsoks with their little individual toes, or Smartwool or Teko socks. Honestly, I love socks and always wear moisture-wicking socks with plenty of support and cushioning.

Even more important than my brand choices is the fit—how all these components fit together. I need good toe room and a wide forefoot, with a heel that grips and limits up and down movement. The shoes must be comfortable and "feel" right. They can't have any bothersome seams and must bend in the right places. Support is important for the long days of trail running and hiking. All my footwear choices—shoes, insoles, and socks—must work together to become a system that fits me like a glove.

—**John Vonhof** fast-packed the John Muir Trail in 1987 in 8.5 days, is the author of *Fixing Your Feet: Prevention and Treatment for Athletes* (Wilderness Press 2006, 4th edition), and publishes several newsletters on foot care at www.fixingyourfeet.com.

Lightweight hiking boots. Although heavier than trail-running shoes, these boots are made for lightweight comfort on maintained trails, not for tackling challenging terrain. Usually a combination of nylon and leather uppers glued to a rubber sole, they break in easily, and they cost less than heftier boots. As long as your ankles are strong and your load is less than 30 pounds, these boots will be sufficient for a weekend trip on moderate trails. If you need more support, keep reading. Price range: $50 to $200.

Standard hiking boots. With thick, rugged soles and durable construction, these boots are designed to support you and your full pack over tough terrain for as long as you choose to be out. Made with all leather, or a leather-nylon combination, these boots also have a sturdy sheet of metal or nylon in the sole (called a shank) to make the sole stiffer and more stable. Shanks can be either partial or full-sole, and you'll be able to tell the difference by how flexible the sole is when you walk (you'll want stiffer soles to provide stability and protection on steep or rugged terrain, especially if you're carrying a heavy load). Sides are also thicker to protect you against rocks and other obstacles.

The downsides to these boots are weight and expense. You'll also need to wear them for days or weeks to break them in before they're comfortable. But choose the right pair, and they'll be your trusted companions for many miles and many years on many trails. Price range: $120 to $300.

Mountaineering boots. If you're planning to climb a glacier-covered mountain like Shasta, Rainier, Denali, Aconcagua, or Everest, you'll need a thick, insulated boot to protect you from rocks and cold. These boots come with a stiff sole that has notches designed to fit crampons (the big spiky things mountaineers wear on their feet for traction on ice). These boots better be comfortable the minute you put them on, because they will never give an inch (breaking them in isn't an option—they're designed to be reliably stiff as you kick steps into ice).

If standing atop such lofty summits is your goal, go for it! Life doesn't get much better. But if you're just beginning your foray

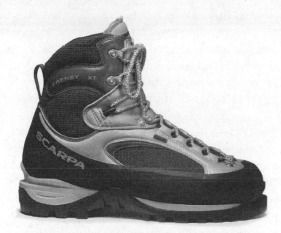

Boot technology has come a long way since the army boots of the 1950s.

into backpacking, please start with shorter and easier trips on lower-elevation trails while you dream and plan for the Big Climb. Price range: $120 to $300.

Regardless of which footwear you use, remember that comfort counts most. Once you choose the footwear most suited to your chosen activity, the best shoe or boot is the one that best fits *your* foot. The most expensive, best-built boot in the world isn't right for you if it's uncomfortable.

Every manufacturer makes boots differently, and one particular manufacturer's mold (called a last) might suit the shape and volume of your feet beautifully, while others might seem closer to Steve Martin's *Cruel Shoes*. Over the years, I have been happiest with boots made by Vasque, Scarpa, and Merrell. For you, other brands might fit better.

If you have an old pair of boots in the closet that you haven't worn in years, take them out and wear them around a bit before you head to the trail. Feet change over time, and your old, trusty boots may no longer fit.

What to Look for in Footwear

Once you have decided on the particular type of hiking footwear that will work for you, there are more factors to consider for the specific boot:

Sole. If you have a heavy pack, if you're a heavy stepper, or if the ground is sharp, you will want a thicker sole to protect you from rocks and other sharp objects on the ground. An aggressive tread will give you traction on uncertain terrain. Heavier boots with stitched soles can be re-treaded, extending the lifespan of your favorite footwear by years. However, stitched soles are becoming rarer as glued soles (which are quicker and cheaper to make) take their place.

Gaiters

Tall, heavyweight gaiters keep rain and snow out of your boots, and keep your ankles and feet warm and dry in wet or extreme weather. They cost between $50 and $100. Lower, lighter-weight gaiters keep rocks and sticks out of your shoes, and foxtails and other seeds out of your socks in dry weather, especially when hiking off-trail. They cost between $20 and $50. And by keeping those plant seeds out of your socks, you can avoid accidentally carrying exotic, invasive plants into new areas where they can colonize and out-compete local species.

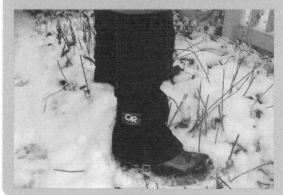

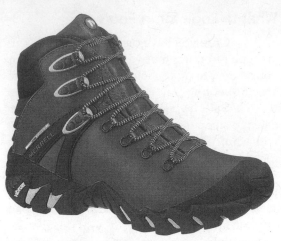

Make sure your nifty new boots are comfy, too.

Padding. Ample padding at the tongue and around the ankles can soften the impact as the boot meets your skin, step after step along the trail. This is especially important with stiff-soled boots.

Flexibility. The more flexible a boot is, the more comfortable it is. However, flexible boots might not provide the ankle support you need to carry you and your gear along the trail.

Support. If you have a heavy pack, weak ankles, or both, you'll need plenty of support. Sturdier, heavier, high-top boots will provide the protection you need. Avoid super-high-top "hunting" boots, as the high tops strain the Achilles tendon.

Protection. Thicker sidewall construction will protect your feet from rocks, sticks, and other hazards on the trail. At the same time, greater protection and support will add stiffness, weight, and cost.

Breathability. This is important in warm weather, and if your feet get wet. Breathable boots help moisture escape, preventing a swamp from forming in your boots, which reduces the risk of blisters, smells better at the end of the day, and is more comfortable while you're hiking.

How to Buy Hiking Boots

The first step in buying boots is to determine why you need them. Do you plan to do mostly dayhikes or longer trips? Over rugged or gentle terrain? Will your pack be heavy or light? How much support do your feet need?

Armed with answers to these questions, head to a quality outdoor gear store. You'll recognize a quality store by its salespeople, who are well-trained in explaining boot construction, quality, and fit. You're going to spend some time in the shop, so don't be afraid to ask for another salesperson or go to another store if your salesperson isn't helping.

The best time to shop for boots is in the afternoon, when your feet are more likely to swell. Wear the socks you plan to hike in when you try boots on. (More on socks in a minute.) As you browse the shelves, look for the lightest boots you can find for what you need, and don't be too picky about size. If you usually wear a size 10 in other shoes, but a size 11 is more comfortable, go with the 11. Every manufacturer's sizes differ from other manufacturers. When you find something comfy, put on both boots to make sure they fit both feet (most people have one foot that's bigger than the other).

> ### WILDERNESS WISDOM
>
> Happy feet make happy campers. Your shoes or boots are the most important gear you will buy for backpacking. The best footwear is comfortable, supports your feet, and prevents blisters.

Now walk around in the store to make sure they're comfortable. Pay attention to where the boots crease against your foot when you step forward. Do they hit your foot in the right places? Walk uphill and down if they have ramps available, and then kick your toes and heels against the floor. Do your heels move easily or rub against the back (they're not

Boots: Does Weight Matter?

Big boots can be fun for stomping around, but they also increase the weight your legs will have to lift with every step. How much unnecessary weight do you really want to drag along the trail? Let's do some basic math to see. Assuming you will take 2640 steps in a mile (each step being about 2 feet long), even a few ounces can make a big difference in how much weight your feet lift while hiking, and how tired your legs will be at the end of the day.

BRAND	WEIGHT PER BOOT/PER STEP	WEIGHT YOU LIFT IN A MILE
"Big Clomper" brand boots	2 lbs.	10,560 lbs.
"Light Stepper" brand boots	1 lb., 5 oz.	6930 lbs.

As you can see, a few ounces of weight can multiply into thousands of pounds in just a mile. What will you lift during a long day? A weekend? The Appalachian Trail? No wonder people's legs get tired with heavy boots.

Boot weight can also affect your overall body mechanics: Some veteran backpackers claim that lifting 1 pound with your feet is the equivalent of carrying 5 pounds on your back. Regardless of whether these numbers are precise, this rule offers a wisdom that's worth heeding: Lighter boots are easier on your body.

Buy the lightest footwear possible without sacrificing protection and support. You'll be less fatigued at the end of the day, and you might still have some spring in your step to keep hiking the next day.

supposed to)? Do you hit your toes when kicking forward (shouldn't happen)? These tests can help you avoid pain miles down the trail. In general, be alert to any slipping, rubbing, tightness, or other discomfort, no matter how minor. A few miles up the trail, minor slipping or discomfort can turn into a major, crippling blister. If you have any concern, get a different size or try another boot.

Ask about the store's take-home policy. Some stores will allow you to return boots if they have only been worn indoors. This will let you wear them around the house or office for a few days to make sure they're comfortable, and return them if they're not. If you step outside, however, they'll know, and you'll have to keep the boots, comfortable or not.

Camp Shoes

A second, lighter pair of shoes is a good idea for river crossings or to wear around camp on longer backpack trips; they bring welcome relief from heavy boots. Lightweight tennis shoes are popular; nylon ones dry faster than cotton. I enjoy my lightweight "aqua socks." Some people enjoy comfortable sandals, although these don't protect feet from insects, cold, or sharp objects. If it's going to be icy cold, consider down booties. Whatever you choose, make sure they fit with the same thick socks you'll wear with your boots. (Another plus to camp shoes: Soft soles are gentler on campsite plants and soils!)

Socks

Although they're not as sexy as jackets, packs, or tents, socks are major players in your comfort and happiness while backpacking: They cushion your feet while you walk; they help keep your feet dry by wicking moisture away from your feet; they prevent blisters by minimizing friction inside your boots; and on cold nights, they help keep your feet toasty. They must also be durable enough to withstand all the impact and friction that occur in your boots while hiking.

For backpacking, thicker socks are better because they add cushion and comfort while hiking. The two-pair system is also popular—a thin polypropylene liner with a thicker sock over that. Whatever you choose, make sure your boots are roomy enough to accommodate your sock system.

Socks are made from a variety of materials, each with its own charms and frustrations. Cotton socks are popular for around town, but cotton is not good for hiking for the same reason it's a poor fabric choice for backcountry attire—it does not wick moisture away from your skin. And when it gets wet, it likes to stay that way. You pay the price with cold, smelly feet and an increased risk of blisters from the wet friction.

Synthetics, on the other hand, include options that are designed to wick moisture from your skin. Unfortunately, some synthetics can leave your feet feeling swampy. There's a diverse and ever-growing world of synthetic materials out there. If you're unsure whether your synthetic socks will work, wear them around for a few days before you hike in them, so you know how they'll perform.

Wool is the tried-and-true classic material for hiking socks; it's warm (sometimes too warm on hot days) and it wicks moisture from your skin excellently. Over time, however, wool loses its flexibility and comfort. Wool comes in a few different varieties: Rag wool is thick and cushiony. For people who are sensitive to wool's scratchy fibers, merino has a well-deserved reputation for being soft; alpaca is even softer.

All this aside, it's difficult to find pure wool socks anymore, although it is commonly blended with synthetics to achieve the maximum benefits of each. Today's high-tech textile manufacturers have combined the best of wool and synthetics into cozy, comfortable socks that keep your feet warm, dry, and protected from blisters. A dose of elastic in the mix improves the socks' ability to fit to the form of your feet.

What to Look for in Socks

Just like boots, there are a number of things to consider when buying socks:

Thickness. Thick cushioning at the heels and balls of the feet will help absorb the pounding your feet will endure over the miles. But the thickness and material you choose may depend on your activity level and the season. Summer dayhikes will call for lighter socks than a long backpack in cold weather.

Fabric density. Thick socks are not necessarily dense socks. Turn your socks inside out and look closely at all the little loops in the fabric. Density of loops (per square inch) is the key to comfort. Big loops might provide cushy comfort while the socks are new, but they'll quickly compress. Tighter, denser loops will provide more reliable comfort in the long run.

Wicking ability. Dry feet are happy feet. Socks need to help transport moisture out of your boots to prevent blisters and that swampy feeling.

Fit. Make sure your socks are snug but not too tight. Your heel should slide snugly into the heel pocket. Baggy socks create ridges and pressure points in boots, which lead to blisters. If you use the dual-sock system, be even more careful about creases in the inner layer.

Trim construction. Lumpy seams and baggy folds can lead to blisters. Look for flat, subtle seams for the best fit.

Ultimately, every foot is different. The best socks are the ones that work best for you. Buy different brands and styles, wear them all, make notes, and then go back to buy your favorites before your next big hike. Socks can be pricey (some cost close to $20 a pair), but this is one place you don't want to skimp. Some of the best hiking socks on the market are made by Smartwool, Thorlo, Teko, Bridgedale, Wigwam, and Fox River. You might wince at the cash register, but you'll be happy you did miles down the trail.

Insoles

You just spent a wad of cash on new hiking boots. Prepare yourself, because you'll need to spend more for quality insoles. The sad truth is that boot manufacturers cut costs by filling their quality boots with flimsy insoles that don't provide the comfort and support you'll need on the trail.

Luckily, insole support and comfort formerly available only by prescription from a podiatrist are now available at many retail stores. Most shoe and outdoor stores sell after-market insoles by manufacturers like Superfeet, Spenco, Shock Doctor, and Dr. Scholl's for $30 to $50. Heel cups on insoles will keep your heels in line and support your arches, improving performance and minimizing pain and fatigue. You can also pay $75 to $150 for insoles custom fit to your feet. Many stores have a custom-fit kiosk available. You can also order ArchCrafters foam molds by mail. Step into the mold, send the impressions back to the factory, and they send back insoles to match those impressions. If you have more serious foot problems, you will need custom orthotics from a podiatrist.

Shock-absorbing insoles are also available at most drug or grocery stores. They don't provide support, but they cushion the blow for heavy steppers.

Although I don't enjoy the extra cost, after-market insoles have made a big difference for me. My feet are noticeably less fatigued after wearing insoles on long hikes.

Your backpack does two things: It holds all your gear, and it provides support to help you carry that gear comfortably and efficiently. Although any pack might do, the right pack can make a big difference in how much you enjoy your trip.

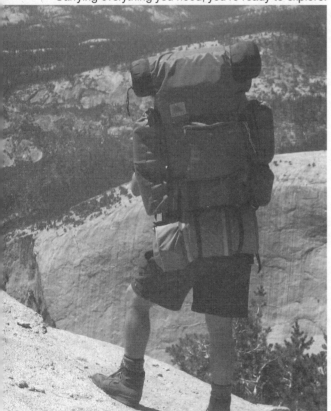

Carrying everything you need, you're ready to explore.

Backpacks have evolved a lot since the steel frame, canvas, and leather packs of the 1950s and '60s. Advances in engineering and materials have produced packs that are lightweight and durable, with suspension systems that transfer the weight to your hips, so you can carry your load with a minimum of discomfort. Today, there are as many different packs available as there are cars on the road.

If you have a light load, you do not need a large pack with a sophisticated frame or harness. In fact, lightweight hiking guru Ray Jardine sewed shoulder straps to a sleeping bag stuff sack, then hit the trail for hundreds and thousands of miles at a time. Then again, his entire load was usually less than 20 pounds.

Heavier loads require more sophisticated suspension and engineering to stabilize the load and transfer the weight to your hips, so you can carry the weight comfortably over long miles.

Finding the Right Pack

The pack that's best for you depends on your size and build, how much gear you need it to carry, and whether you're on gentle trails or rugged backcountry terrain. The quality and weight of the materials and construction, not to mention the engineering of the suspension system, will determine how much you pay; backpacks range in price from $100 to

$500. If you'll be carrying loads greater than 30 pounds, invest in a quality pack. Treat it well, and it will last for decades.

There are literally hundreds of different backpacks available, divided into a few general categories:

Lightweight. Designed for dayhikes and ultralight treks with loads under 20 pounds, these packs don't offer sophisticated suspensions because they don't need them. Lighter materials and construction mean a lighter, leaner load. However, lighter materials and construction are not as durable. If you plan to abuse your equipment (by dragging your pack over rocks on a canyoneering trip, or hiking through thick brush off-trail), make sure it's tough enough to take the abuse.

Internal frame. These packs have a frame; it's just hidden under the pack material. On lightweight packs, it might be no more than a sheet of stiff foam or plastic. Suspension systems on larger packs might be as simple as light aluminum rods, or they might be frames sophisticated enough to make an engineer whistle with respect. Internal-frame packs are designed to keep the weight close to your body, so it can move with you as you twist, bend, and climb over rugged terrain. With no ventilation across the back, these packs can be hot and sweaty in hot weather (although it's never bothered me, and they provide welcome extra warmth on cold days). Packs designed for climbing, mountaineering, and other agility-oriented activities are tall and narrow, giving your arms full range of motion.

External frame. These packs have a large aluminum or plastic frame to support the weight properly and transfer it to your body through your hip belt and shoulder straps. External frames keep the weight farther from your body, which is cooler and sometimes more comfortable. They're great for carrying heavy loads over many miles on stable trails. They're not good if you need balance on rugged terrain.

With the technological advances and popularity of internal-frame packs, external frames are getting rarer. You can still find them in outdoor stores, but they're in the minority.

Within each of these pack types, there are a variety of factors that will help you decide on a specific pack. The first is capacity. Backpacks are categorized by their storage volume, which is usually measured in cubic inches (cu):

➤ 2500 to 3000 cu: Good for dayhikes with a decent amount of gear, or lightweight overnights in warm weather. These packs have minimal, if any, frame or suspension system.

➤ 3000 to 4500 cu: Large enough to hold everything you need for a weekend pack trip—sleeping bag, tent, food, stove, and clothing.

MY SYSTEM

Trekking Poles

For years, I resisted using trekking poles. Now I won't backpack without them, for several reasons: Four legs are better than two—they increase power and speed, help pull me uphill, ease me down with less risk of injury, and they add balance and support on rough or slippery terrain and during river crossings. As a veteran of back surgery, I experience significantly less discomfort with poles after a long hike.

Disadvantages include the expense ($50 to $200 for "real" trekking poles, although an old pair of thrift store ski poles can cost $5); they're awkward when you need your hands for anything else; they add to the amount of gear you'll have to carry and manage; and they click-clack annoyingly over rock.

There's also the time-honored wooden hiking staff—classier than high-tech metal, but also heavier and only half as effective. Learn all you need to know at www.trekkingpoles.com.

–Brian Beffort, author

➤ 4500 to 6000 cu: For several days to a week or more, this is the pack you'll need.

➤ 6000+ cu: Yes, it's true, you're a pack mule. You'll need this pack if you're the designated family Sherpa, if you're going to hike for longer than a week with no resupply, or if you're packing for an expedition in winter. Make sure the suspension is adequate, the hip and shoulder pads are thick and soft, and your back and knees are up to the task.

After capacity, look at the actual size of the backpack. The pack needs to be long enough to fit your back, but not too long. (See the section that follows on fitting your pack.) The materials and construction of a pack also matter. Durable packs will last longer and stand up to more abuse. Thinner materials and lighter-weight straps and stitching can result in a pack that weighs less, but is it ready to handle

"Now, where did I pack my sunglasses?"

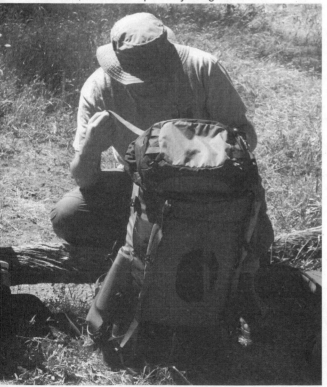

the weight of your gear and activities? With a light load and gentle hiking, a lighter, less durable pack might be just right.

The weight of your empty pack depends on the load it will carry and the abuse you will give it. Lightweight packs for lightweight loads can weigh less than 2 pounds. Sophisticated suspension systems and durable materials mean a heavier pack. Reliable packs for heavy loads and extreme conditions can weigh 7 pounds before you start packing them. Generally, the more you plan to carry, the better the suspension you'll need to transfer the weight properly to your hips, making the load less of a burden over the miles.

Another design feature that's easy to overlook when fitting your pack is the access it provides to gear inside. The design, shape, and placement of pockets can make a big difference in how well you will enjoy your pack. External-frame packs are usually better at providing separate storage areas for different types of gear. Internal-frame packs offer two general ways to access gear: panel- and top-loading. Panel-loading packs have a U-shaped zipper to allow easy access to all of your gear at once. Zippers, however, can leak water, and they tend to blow out if the pack is stuffed with too much heavy gear.

Top-loading packs have only one access hole at the top, through which you can access your gear, which can turn your pack into a gaping black hole that makes gear hard to find or organize. Some models feature an additional zipper near the bottom to access your sleeping bag or tent. These packs stand up to heavier loads and are more weatherproof, but they require good organization on your part. With top-loading packs, I use internal compartmentalization—different colored stuff sacks to keep food, clothes, and other gear organized.

Many packs come with additional straps to carry extra gear (ropes and other hardware for rock climbers, skis and climbing skins for backcountry skiers, crampons and ice axes for mountaineers, etc.). Getting a pack that can carry your favorite toys is a good idea. Just remember that every additional strap, stitch, and pocket means extra weight and added expense. If you don't need it, why carry it?

Those of you hiking in wet conditions will appreciate recent developments in waterproof packs. Made with urethane-treated nylon, these packs are basically dry bags with shoulder straps and hip belts.

Fitting Your Pack

A backpack performs best when it fits your body. It's most important to match the length of your torso with the length of the pack. There can be little correlation between your height and pack size (I'm 6'6" tall, yet I wear a medium-sized pack with some brands). Quality salespeople can help you with this. If you're buying online or from an unprepared sales staff, a friend can help you with this at home:

Use a cloth measuring tape to measure the distance from your seventh cervical vertebra (the prominent bump at the base of your neck) and the imaginary horizontal line between the tops of your pelvic bones on each side of your waist. Although some manufacturers will vary, in general, your torso will fall into one of the following categories (double-check with the manufacturer to be sure):

➤ Small: Less than 18 inches
➤ Medium: 18 to 20 inches
➤ Large: More than 20 inches

Once you buy a pack (and before you hit the trail), adjust the pack to fit you. Depending on the pack's manufacturer and style, the shoulder straps and hip belts might have different settings to allow it to fit your particular size and shape. We'll discuss how to fit and adjust your full pack for the trail later, on page 161.

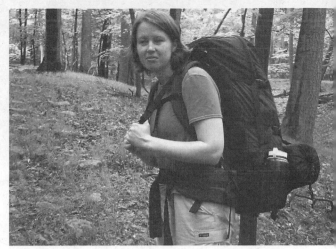
Most of your pack's weight should rest on your hips.

Daypacks and Travel Packs

If you're planning dayhikes during your trip, bring along a lightweight daypack, or buy a larger backpack that has a lid or pocket that detaches and works as a day- or fanny pack. You can save weight by ignoring this advice, emptying your backpack's contents into your tent, and carrying it only with those things you'll need for a dayhike.

Backpacks designed for wilderness travel are not well-designed for taking on and off buses and in and out of airplanes; the straps tend to get caught in airport conveyor belts and other pack-eating machines and protuberances. Travel packs have few external straps and buckles, and their hip belts and shoulder straps tuck or zip neatly away in hidden compartments. Once you arrive, pull out the straps, put on the pack, and set off for adventure.

For more than 10 years, I traveled with an MEC travel pack. It survived falling off the top of an Egyptian bus at 60 miles per hour with no visible damage, then it performed beautifully and comfortably during weeklong backpack trips up Mt. Kenya and into the Japanese Alps. If only every piece of gear were made as well as that pack.

When the weather and insects cooperate, the best shelter in the backcountry is a blanket of stars overhead. Unfortunately, wilderness doesn't always cooperate. There are four common reasons why you will sooner or later need a tent or other shelter while backpacking—protection from wet weather, warmth (even a simple tarp-style shelter without walls is warmer than no shelter), protection from insects and other creepy crawlies, and privacy from other campers. How high these needs rank in your world will determine the type of shelter you should buy.

There are several different types of shelter for the wild. Tents are the most popular, but they are not the only option. What follows is an overview of your choices for protection against the elements.

Finding the Right Tent

Compact, portable, well-designed, and attractive, good tents go up in minutes, and, presto! No matter where you are, you have a cool little shelter to sleep in while you're away from home. Everyone who's ever had a fort or secret hideout as a kid will get to relive the adventure as an adult.

There are many styles of backpacking tents to choose from, ranging from cozy and

With the right shelter, you'll feel at home in the wild.

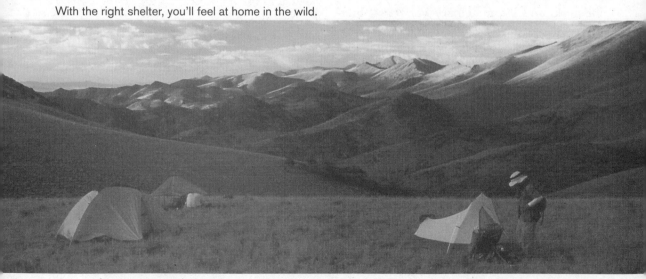

lightweight one-person tents to larger, heavier expedition tents that will shelter four during a high-altitude blizzard.

Although they are the shelters of choice for most backpackers, tents have some disadvantages: They can be stuffy in warm conditions or when filled with smelly, sweaty bodies; they can be heavy; they isolate you from beautiful views and sparkling stars overhead; and they can cost a pretty penny.

What to Look For

As with any gear, you need to determine your needs before you commit to a particular tent. More than anything else, a tent needs to shelter you from the elements—to keep you dry, warm, and protected from insects and other critters. The type of tent you buy depends on your group size and your season of travel. Are you a solo hiker looking for a lightweight tent, or do you want something for two, three, or four people? Are you planning weekend trips in summer, or longer expeditions in harsher seasons and conditions?

Tents are made to provide protection in two-season, three-season, or four-season conditions. Two-season tents are little more than mosquito netting to protect you from bugs and mild summer weather. Most backpacking tents on the market are three-season tents, equipped with optional rain-flies—large sheets of nylon that attach to the outside of your tent and are designed to repel wind, rain, and snow. These can help protect against most storms. Four-season tents are designed to stand up to wind and snow during expeditions in the worst possible conditions. These are understandably heavier and more expensive than two- and three-season tents.

Once you've figured out what type of conditions you need your tent to protect you from, think about size: Usually, you'll spend most of your time outside and use your tent only for sleeping. However, heavy weather

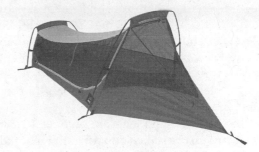

This one-person tent is for light and fast travel.

and persistent insects might drive you in for long stretches of time. Make sure the tent you buy has enough room for you to sleep and perform necessary tasks, such as sitting up and getting dressed, and that it will accommodate a long day of waiting out the weather or bugs without driving you stir crazy. For tall people (over 6′5″), many tents aren't long enough. Before you buy, climb in, lie down, move around, and see if a candidate tent offers enough space. Roomy tents, however, are heavier and often more expensive. Weigh all these factors before you choose.

Regardless of the size, some tents are well-designed and easy to set up—others aren't. Before you buy, practice setting tents up in the store to see if they are easy and make sense. Ask

A three-person, three-season tent

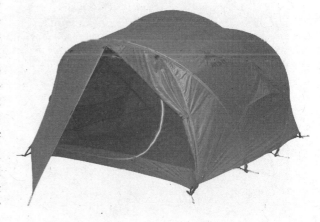

the salesperson to help you, and watch closely. Then practice again at home. You should be able to set your tent up at night in the rain in five minutes, because some dark, stormy night in the future, you just might have to.

Here are some other features to consider before buying:

➤ Self-standing tents are preferable over tents that must be staked down in order to stand up. They're good where the ground is too soft or hard for tent stakes (such as sand, snow, or rock), they cause less impact on the land, and kids will love them set up in the living room.

➤ Vestibules in the rain-fly help protect backpacks and other gear from wet weather.

➤ Ventilation: Doors and/or windows can allow cross-ventilation, which helps minimize stuffiness and condensation.

➤ Convenient pockets and attics inside are great for storing headlamps, bug repellent, toothbrushes, etc.

➤ Multiple doors allow all inhabitants to come and go easily, and they enhance cross-ventilation, which minimizes stuffy air and condensation.

With a quick-pitching tarp, it's easy to snooze.

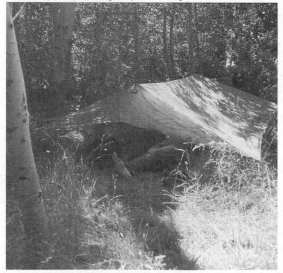

➤ Tent poles with elastic shock cords make assembly quick and convenient. Aluminum poles are lightweight and relatively durable; fiberglass tends to splinter and break; steel is strongest but very heavy.

➤ Pole sleeves vs. clips: Your tent poles will either slip through a sleeve on the outside of the tent to hold it up, or the tent will connect to the poles with clips. After using both for many years, I prefer clips; they're lighter, faster, less frustrating, and they don't rip when the pole develops a hangnail or rough spot.

Tarp-Style Shelters

Tarps pitch like tents, but most have no walls or floor. Shelters have several advantages over tents: Most are lighter weight; they're versatile, allowing a variety of configurations for different settings and conditions; they ventilate well, eliminating stuffiness in warm weather or when filled with smelly hiking partners; and they minimize overnight condensation on sleeping bags and other gear from breath and dew. They're also good to pitch over the kitchen or social area in wet weather. Disadvantages include too much ventilation during heavy weather and easy access for mosquitoes and other creepy crawlies.

Reputable shelter manufacturers include GoLite, MSR, Kelty, Mountain Hardwear, Sierra Designs, Integral Designs, REI, and North Face.

If you own a tent with a rain-fly, you probably already own a shelter. Cleverly designed tents have rain-flies that can set up without the tent. Consider also simple plastic tarps, available at most outdoor and hardware stores. They're affordable and easy to string up between trees or trekking poles, but they're not always lightweight, and they take up more space.

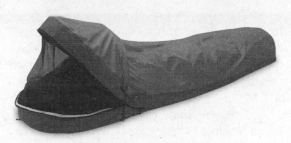

Bivies are lightweight but not roomy.

Bivy Sacks

Few things are nicer than sleeping under a blanket of stars, especially when bugs and weather allow. Bivy sacks, nylon shells that slip over your bag, allow you to leave the tent at home without abandoning all protection against the elements. Because they weigh less than tents and shelters, they're often the choice for minimalist adventurers. They add significant warmth to your bag, and they protect your bag from moisture. For these reasons, a bivy can be a welcome addition, even when you use a tent or shelter. Some bivies are simple nylon sacks that slip over your bag; others, like Black Diamond's award-winning Lightsabre Bivy, create a small tent over your head, complete with poles, netting, and doors. All bivy sacks, however, are snug–a disadvantage if you get claustrophobic, or if you want to do anything else in them other than sleep; there's no room for sitting or changing clothes. A variety of sizes, weights, and designs are available from companies such as Outdoor Research, Black Diamond, Mountain Hardwear, Integral Designs, and Sierra Designs.

Tent and Shelter Accessories

Depending on the conditions and your personal preference, there are some things you might want to add or change about your shelter. For instance, a sheet of plastic or tarp on the ground under your tent or shelter will keep you drier in wet conditions, and it will protect your tent floor from scuffs and dirt, increasing the life of your tent. Many tent manufacturers sell ground cloth "footprints" designed to fit the particular dimensions of your tent. You can also save a lot of money by making your own footprint by cutting one out of tarp. Some ultra-light backpackers scoff at the extra weight ground cloths entail and choose to lay themselves and/or their shelter directly on the ground. It's up to you.

If heavy weather is on its way, you'll need to secure everything you don't want flying away (self-standing tents make great kites!). There are several different types of tent stakes, depending on where you'll be pitching your tent (hard or soft dirt, snow, sand), how much weight you want to carry, and how much you're willing to spend. Many of the styles that follow come in different materials—steel (heavy but durable), plastic (lightweight but not so durable), titanium (very lightweight, very durable,

Tent stakes come in a variety of styles.

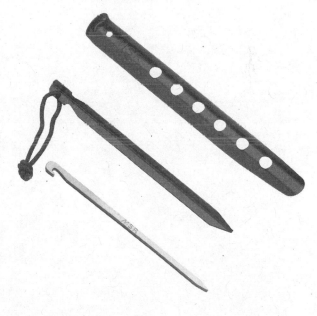

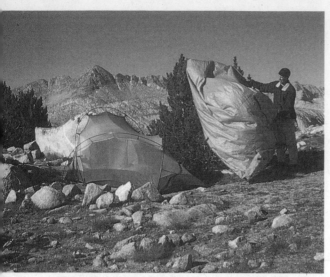

Stake your tent down—don't let it become a kite.

and very expensive!), and aluminum (lightweight, affordable, and moderately durable). Statistics listed below are for basic aluminum. Prices vary by length and manufacturer. For titanium, expect the price to triple:

Shepherd's hook. This is your basic tent stake, which comes standard with most tents. They'll work fine on lawns with no rocks to get in the way or hard weather to pull them out. If you expect worse than favorable conditions, get longer stakes, or a different style. Length: 7.25 inches. Weight: 0.35 ounces. Cost: $0.75.

Power peg. These plastic stakes will take a beating, but they are bulkier and heavier than others in this list. Length: 9 inches. Weight: 1.2 ounces. Cost: $0.75.

Y-pegs. These Y-shaped pegs hold well and don't bend like basic stakes. Length: 7 inches. Weight: 0.6 ounces. Cost: $1.50.

U-shaped pegs. For sand and snow. Length: 9.5 inches. Weight: 0.85 ounces. Cost: $1.75.

Nylon snow and sand anchors. In soft sand or snow, stakes and pegs don't work well. Fill these nylon parachutes with sand or snow, then bury them for greater strength. Weight: 3.7 ounces for a set of four. Cost: $9.75 per set. Thick, plastic grocery bags work well, too (double them up for strength), and they're a lot cheaper.

10 SLEEPING BAGS

It can get darn cold at night in some of the planet's best backpacking destinations. What type of sleeping bag you need depends on how cold and wet it will be where you plan to camp, as well as your particular needs as a sleeper.

The best sleeping bags are those that provide enough fluffy insulation to keep you warm, while being both lightweight and compressible. This is harder than it might seem, because it's one thing to make your bag small and compact enough to fit into your backpack. It's another to pull the bag back out and have it expand back to its full and fluffy glory, time and time again.

Because a cozy night's sleep is essential to enjoying your backpacking trip, it's important to get the right bag for your needs. If you're interested in trimming weight from your backpack, you can shave a couple pounds by buying a lightweight bag. Of course, the warmest, most compressible, and lightweight bags are also the most expensive.

If you have the money, spend more on a lighter, warmer bag. You can shave pounds off your pack weight with the right lightweight bag, and it's easier to unzip your bag to cool off on a warm night than it is to put on more clothes for a shivery night, especially if you're already wearing everything. Warm sleep is worth it.

To buy the sleeping bag that's right for you, pay attention to the discussion on other features later in this chapter.

Temperature Ratings

All manufacturers give their sleeping bags temperature ratings (also called comfort ratings), which indicate the lowest temperature at which the bag will keep you warm. Although reputable manufacturers determine these ratings through rigorous testing, there is

MY SYSTEM

A Perfect Night's Sleeping Bag

I have a lightweight bag rated to 40°F, a fleece sleeping bag liner, and a bivy sack. On warm, summer trips, I use only the liner and bivy. On colder nights, I use my sleeping bag with bivy sack. When it gets frickin' cold, I use them all and wear everything I own to bed. This strategy has allowed me to save money on expensive gear, sleep comfortably in a variety of seasons and weather, and it's kept me warm on nights when temperatures have dropped into the teens. But that's me. What sleeping system will work for you?

—**Brian Beffort**, author

no industry standard for tests or ratings, and competition-driven marketing can push manufacturers to exaggerate their claims. The lesson: Buyer beware—take temperature ratings with a grain of salt. In general, it's a good idea to buy a bag with a rating at least 10 degrees colder than the conditions you expect; if you think it might get down to about 30°F on your upcoming pack trip, buy a sleeping bag rated to 20°F. This will give you some insurance, just in case the temperature drops into the 20s, you're a particularly cold sleeper, or the bag's performance doesn't live up to its rating.

Down vs. Synthetic

The type of fill material you buy—synthetic or down—depends on how cold it will be where you camp, and, perhaps more importantly, how wet it will be. Down is the lightest, warmest, and most compressible material available, but it fails miserably when wet. Some manufacturers help protect down bags with waterproof-breathable shells. However, if moisture will be a persistent factor on your trip, such as in humid or rainy climates, choose synthetic.

Down garments and bags are made with different "fill power" ratings, which reflect the volume (also called loft) of the down used, measured in cubic inches (cu). Fill power ratings range from 500 cu to 900 cu. Higher fill power means more fluff, greater warmth, and a higher price tag.

Synthetic bags are made with Polarguard 3D, Polarguard Delta, Quallofil, PrimaLoft, and other fills. They maintain most of their insulation when wet, dry quickly, and are non-allergenic. They are less expensive than down bags, but they're also heavier and don't last as long because the insulation eventually compresses, leaving you with less fluff to keep you warm.

Other Features

Beyond temperature rating and type of fluff, you'll need to consider a few other features for your perfect backcountry bed.

One is shape. Mummy bags keep you warmer by providing a hood to prevent heat loss. Cinch cords let you close the opening down around your face, reducing heat loss through your head. For backpacking, they are better than rectangular bags with large openings, which let too much heat out on cold nights. If you're claustrophobic, you might need to do some deep-breathing, calming exercises to keep from freaking out. They're also more expensive than other bags.

Obviously, you also want to make sure your bag fits. Larger and taller people need extra room, and many manufacturers make bags

Sharing Your Sleeping Bag

Cozy couples and parents with kids might not need two bags. Save the weight and expense of two sleeping bags with a bag expander. It's a panel made of the same material as your bag, with zippers on both sides that zip into your bag to give you extra girth for multiple bodies. Mountain Hardwear, North Face, and REI all make bag expanders in both down and synthetic. They cost in the neighborhood of $50.

If you're planning a backpacking trip with your favorite snuggle partner, you also have the option of getting bags that can zip together. Intimate couples will enjoy being able to cuddle body heat together on cold nights. Consider buying two bags with opposing zippers (one bag that opens on the right; one that opens on the left), so you can zip them together. Just make sure the zippers match—there are a few different kinds.

in long sizes to accommodate people over 6 feet tall (thanks, guys!). Most manufacturers also have at least one product line with extra girth for larger bodies and active sleepers.

You can also buy women-specific bags. Not only are women shaped differently than men, they tend to sleep colder, too. Most bag manufacturers make women's bags with special designs and extra insulation where it matters for women.

Regardless of whether you're male or female, if you're prone to sleeping cold, consider finding a bag with a draft collar that minimizes heat loss, or draft tubes between you and the zipper that keep warmth in and cold air out.

In checking fit, don't be shy—roll candidate bags out on the showroom floor, climb in, and take them for a spin. Do you have enough space to wiggle around comfortably? Extra space makes your body work harder to heat it. Not enough room, and you'll either feel claustrophobic, or you'll push up against the sides (or the end), which compresses the insulation and keeps you colder. Every body is different. Find the bag that best suits yours.

Lastly, check out the design. Quality bags are designed with overlapping insulation compartments (called baffles), so there's never a gap in insulation. Some zippers zip smoothly; others are hard to get started, and/or they catch easily on the bag's fabric.

Sleeping Pads

It's not enough to have a warm sleeping bag when you plan to put it on the cold, hard ground. You will also need a sleeping pad to soften the bumps and insulate you from the cold. In fact, sleeping bag temperature ratings are determined assuming you have a sleeping pad. Like your sleeping bag and clothing, sleeping pads keep you warm by trapping still

An Ultra-Lightweight Alternative

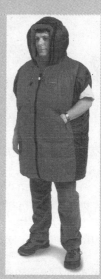

Do you really need both a warm jacket and a sleeping bag? You can shave a few pounds by leaving one at home. The Exped Wallcreeper might be all you need for 30°F nights. It's a jacket/sleeping bag combo available in down or synthetic. It has arm holes, pockets, a hood, and a hole at the feet that tightens with a draw cord. Wear it as a long (or longer) jacket, then pull yourself in, batten the hatches, and you have a sleeping bag. Weight: Less than 2 pounds. Cost: $150 to $200.

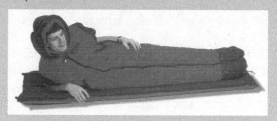

air. How warm the pad keeps you depends on how much air it traps and how little that air circulates.

As with the insulation in your house, the insulating power of sleeping pads is measured by their R-value, which reflects the material's resistance to heat flow through conduction. R-values with sleeping pads range from 1 to 7; the higher the R-value, the warmer the pad. Insulation against heat loss isn't so important if you're camping on a hot summer night; on cold rocks or snow in cold weather, it becomes much more important.

When shopping for sleeping pads, factors to consider include insulation, comfort,

Sleeping Bag Liners

Fleece, cotton, silk, and synthetic liners are available for sleeping bags. They increase your bag's warmth by up to 15 degrees, and they can prolong the bag's life by keeping dirt and body oils from clogging the liner and damaging the insulation. Manufacturers include Sea to Summit, Kelty, Cocoon, and Marmot.

weight, volume (bulkiness), durability, and cost. There are several types of sleeping pads:

Open cell. The same foam used in most car seats, couches, recliners, and generic "foam rubber" mattresses is available in sleeping pads that are comfy, lightweight, and affordable. However, open-cell foam is bulky and absorbs water like a sponge (sponges also happen to be open-cell foam). It also shreds easily. Cost: $10 to $20.

Closed cell. Open-cell foam allows air (and water) to circulate; closed-cell foam does not. Closed-cell pads, made of Ensolite or Foamlite, are good for backpacking because they provide the same insulation at a quarter of the volume of open-cell foam. However, closed-cell pads must be thicker to provide the same comfort. Some manufacturers add ridges or egg-carton-shaped pits to add comfort without extra weight—Therm-a-Rest's Z-Lite and RidgeRest are examples of this. Although more durable than open-cell foam, closed-cell pads also shred easily. They are adaptable because you can cut them into sections to fashion a splint or make a seat, something you can't do with inflatable pads. Usually priced between $20 and $30 each, closed-cell pads are among the more affordable and more popular sleeping pads for backpacking.

Inflatable. Air mattresses are comfortable and can be inexpensive. However, affordable pads are bulky, heavy and easily punctured. They also allow air to circulate, which reduces their insulating value. Cost: $10 to $30.

Self-inflating pads. These have open-cell cores in inflatable nylon shells. However, these tend to be more expensive; the lightest and most durable models can cost well over $100.

No sleeping pad is perfect: Both open- and closed-cell pads can shred, and inflatable pads can puncture easily (although with some, repairs are easy—but not necessarily in the middle of the night after they've popped and deflated). Consider a stuff sack for your pad, so you can minimize damage when it's strapped to the outside of your pack.

I prefer simple, less-expensive, closed-cell pads. I use two because the ground seems to get harder as I get older. I don't like the weight of more affordable self-inflating pads, and I'm afraid of the low durability of the lighter-weight and more expensive self-inflators—more stuff to worry about, and another repair kit to carry for when it pops. But then again, I'm clearly in the minority; self-inflating pads are very popular. Admittedly, sometimes I push my wife off hers in the middle of the night, because it's darn comfy.

If you do use a self-inflating pad, don't forget your repair kit—you'll need it eventually.

Before You Buy a Pad

Determine your needs. Which is more important to you, weight, durability, or comfort? Will you be camping on soft ground or hard? Cold or warm weather?

Try before you buy. Unroll a self-inflating pad on the showroom floor. Check the valve for ease of operation and obvious leaks. At home, over-inflate the pad, close the valve, then check on it the next day for slow leaks. Return it if it has one.

Sleeping pad manufacturers include Therm-a-Rest, REI, Big Agnes, Exped, and Insul Mat.

You can cut weight by buying no more pad than you need. Use a pad long enough to cushion your shoulders and hips but not your legs. Cut non-inflating pads to your preferred length, then use the remainder to carry in your daypack as a seat. Use clothes or your backpack to insulate and pad your legs and feet.

Store your sleeping pads flat, with valves open. Both self-inflating and closed-cell foam pads have memories; roll them up tight, and they'll stay squished up; store them flat, and they'll maintain maximum cush, and they'll keep you comfy longer.

There are numerous types of stoves, dishes, and utensils you can buy for backpacking. There's sure to be something out there to fit your style. Whatever you choose to cook and eat with in the backcountry, make sure that it is, above all, reliable. After all, quality backcountry kitchen gear is as important as, well, eating.

Stoves

One of the great romantic fantasies of camping—cooking over an open fire in the wilderness—is getting rarer in the backcountry for several reasons: Popular backpacking destinations have been picked clean of firewood by previous campers, and there's not much left; some destinations—high elevations above treeline, for example—don't have much wood to begin with; many national parks and forests prohibit campfires to conserve the resource or prevent wildfires in dry seasons; fires are time-consuming, messy, and awkward for cooking; and fires impact the environment by depleting natural biomass (wood) and by scarring the ground with ugly fire rings.

Luckily, high-technology comes to the rescue: A wide variety of dependable, convenient, and lightweight stoves enable backpackers to travel quickly and lightly through the wilderness, without leaving undue impacts, and while eating well. There are several dif-ferent styles of camp stoves from which to choose.

Butane Canister Stoves

Lightweight and convenient, these stoves are great for weekend backpack trips in mild weather—light the match, turn the knob, and presto! You're ready to cook. These stoves screw into disposable isobutane (also called

MSR's Pocket Rocket is great for quick meals in mild conditions.

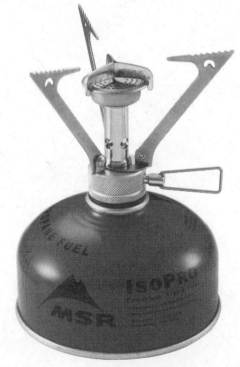

86

liquid propane gas, or LPG) canisters, which are available in several sizes at most outdoor stores. They're also more easily adjustable than most liquid-fuel stoves (discussed next), allowing backcountry chefs to simmer sauces to perfection.

However, they do have several disadvantages: They don't perform well in cold temperatures or at high elevations. It's hard to insulate them well from the wind because the heat can be reflected down to the fuel canister, causing undesired fireworks, so cooking in wind can be a time- and fuel-consuming experience. As fuel bottles empty, pressure drops in the bottle, which decreases efficiency and increases cook time. Many are tall and narrow, so cooking with large, full pots can be precarious (make sure the one you buy has wide supports or a stand to prevent this). The canisters cannot be refilled or recycled, creating a poor environmental legacy in landfills. Not all canisters are alike, which can be frustrating when the canisters on the store shelf don't fit the stove in your hands. Make sure your stove screws properly into a new canister before you get to the trailhead.

Liquid-Fuel Stoves

Stoves with refillable fuel canisters are more dependable in extreme cold and high elevations than butane or liquid-propane canister stoves. The standard fuel for those in North America is white gas, which is available at most outdoor and hardware stores. Some models are little more than glorified blowtorches, designed to melt snow and boil water quickly in extreme conditions, but not to simmer meals. However, recent innovations with these stoves allow more sensitive flame control.

If you're unsure about which fuels will be available (a consideration if traveling overseas), choose a multi-fuel stove that will burn almost anything, including kerosene, gasoline, diesel, alcohol, or jet fuel.

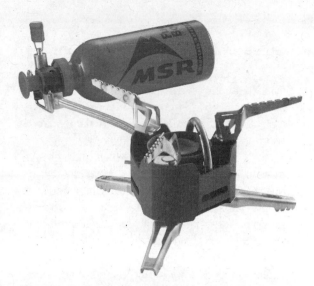

MSR's XGK will burn hot in the most extreme conditions.

The biggest disadvantage to these stoves is inconvenience; they have to be primed with fuel before they're ready to cook (not too hard, really, but they're not as quick-and-easy as butane canister stoves). Fuel assemblies also tend to clog, although manufacturers have found good ways to prevent clogging, such as MSR stoves with "shaker jets."

For liquid fuel, use only bottles that are approved for fuel. Fuel bottles are always metal (plastic can degrade and leak at the lid; glass can break), compatible with your stove, distinctive (so you don't mistake it for your Gatorade bottle), and leak-proof. Always pack your fuel below your food so a fuel leak won't destroy your sustenance.

Solid-Fuel Stoves

Solid-fuel stoves come in two types: simple metal frames that unfold to hold solid fuel cubes (such as Esbit fuel cubes). With these, tablets spit out decent heat for about 10 minutes, making them great for heating up a quick pint or two of water in mild weather.

Stove Evolution and Revolutions

In 1973, Mountain Safety Research (MSR) revolutionized backcountry cooking by separating stoves from their fuel source, allowing campers to shield pots and flames from wind and greatly increase efficiency.

Heat exchangers, which maximize a stove's heat transfer to pots, have greatly increased stove efficiency. Jetboil has become many backpackers' favorite, with its sophisticated heat exchanger built directly into the bottom of a specialized pot.

MSR's Reactor stove combines a heat exchanger with a burner that uses both convective and radiant heat for great heat output, and a pressure regulator that maintains relatively constant pressure over the life of the fuel bottle. MSR claims this combination creates "the fastest-boiling, most fuel-efficient, windproof stove system available."

The stats look promising: The stove boils 22 liters of water per 16-ounce fuel canister, as opposed to 15 liters with other stoves, greatly improving efficiency and reducing fuel weight for long trips. Boil time with a new fuel bottle is three minutes and only about three-and-a-half minutes when the fuel bottle is nearly empty (compared with much longer boil times with old, depressurized fuel canisters on other stoves).

Although the stove looks good on paper, as of this writing, it hadn't been proven on the trail. Does it clog? Will it hold up to backcountry abuse? What other frustrations will users meet while using it? Such questions and the $150 price aside, it looks as though campstove technology is changing, and the potential for radiant heat technology to improve cooking with white gas, kerosene, and other liquid fuels looks promising in the coming years.

There are also stoves that burn sticks, twigs, pinecones, and such. These stoves are great for lightweight trekkers who want to travel far without carrying fuel. You'll have to fidget for consistent flame, and you'll need to go without hot food if fuels are unavailable or wet, or when gathering wood is against the rules.

Solid-fuel stoves are great for single hikers in fair conditions. But if you're planning to prepare meals for several days in the cold and/or at altitude, chose one of the far more reliable stoves described in the previous pages.

Homemade Stoves

A little ingenuity with metals shears can transform an old tuna or soup can into a functional stove that burns alcohol, wood, or other fuels. Check out www.zenstoves.net or the "make your own gear" section of www.backpacking.net.

Fuels

Depending on your stove, you may be able to use one or more of the following fuels:

Kerosene. Kerosene burns hotter than other fuels (boil times are often determined using kerosene), but it can be difficult to light, and it leaves a heck of a lot of soot, which creates a mess and clogs stoves easily. It also creates lethal fumes, so don't ever cook in your tent with it. It's widely available internationally.

White gas. Sold by Coleman and other camp-fuel brand names, this is one of the most common fuels available in the US for refillable-fuel stoves. It lights easily, burns hot and clean, but it isn't available widely internationally.

Butane. Butane lights easily on its own. It's available internationally, but its performance falters significantly in cold temperatures and high altitudes. Note: Knowing this, bring something other than a Bic or other butane-filled lighter to light your liquid-fuel stove above 10,000 feet.

Isobutane and butane-propane blends. These blends improve on butane's performance, but only slightly in the cold and at high elevation. Gaz and other canisters contain a butane-propane blend.

Denatured alcohol. This burns cleanly and quietly and is a popular option for lightweight trekkers. But it doesn't burn as hot as other fuels.

Liquid-propane gas (LPG). LPG offers the best performance of pressurized gas canisters, but the canisters are heavier to accommodate the greater pressure, and international availability is limited.

Questions to Ask When Shopping for Camp Stoves

➤ **What fuel does it use?** Is this fuel commonly available (an important question if you're traveling internationally)? How efficient is the fuel? Is the fuel dirty (do you mind getting soot all over your pots, all over your hands, and all over the inside of your backpack if you're not careful)? Does the fuel work well in cold temperatures or at high elevation?

➤ **Is it reliable?** Some stoves don't light easily or burn reliably. Performance for all stoves will drop significantly in cold temperatures and at high elevations.

➤ **Is it stable?** How stable will it be with a large pot on an uneven surface? Will it tip easily? Hungry, tired campmates don't take kindly to spilled meals.

➤ **How big is the burner?** What are your cooking needs—a small pot for a single hiker, or a big meal for everyone in camp? Note: Several two-burner backpack stoves are available.

➤ **How quickly does it boil water?** The time it takes a stove to boil one liter of water, also called "boil time," is a standard measurement you can use to compare stove efficiency and strength. Remember, however, boil times are determined under ideal conditions in laboratories. How well your stove boils cold water on a cold, windy day at high elevation with a near-empty fuel canister is a different matter. Boil time is also affected by how clean your fuel is, how clean your stove is, how well the flame is protected from the wind, whether your pot is rounded or flat (rounded bottoms absorb heat better), whether your pots are black or not (black absorbs heat better), and let's not forget operator efficiency (do you really know what you're doing?).

➤ **Can it simmer?** Does the stove have adjustments that allow you to cook with low heat as well as high?

➤ **How does it perform in wind?** Are windscreens available to shield the stove from wind?

➤ **How well does it perform at low temperatures and high elevations?**

Before you rush out to buy a stove, ask yourself if you really need one. In cold temperatures, warm meals are not only welcome, they are often necessary. In winter, stoves are necessary to melt water. But for a two-day trip in summer, do you really need one? Not carrying a stove, fuel, and cookware makes pack weight significantly lighter, and it saves time, although menu options are leaner. Some consider traveling without a stove too hardcore. If you need to impress a first-timer, or if you just gotta have some civilized lifestyle on the trail (a nice, cooked meal is important to many people on a deep, emotional level), indulge in a stove and quality menu. If you're hiking lean and fast in summer, consider leaving it behind.

Water Purification

Although many streams and lakes in the backcountry might look pristine and clean, many are not. Microscopic organisms that make you sick, such as giardia, cryptosporidium, and numerous types of amoeba, are relatively common in all but the most remote places on the planet. Because water is essential to life, it's important to take necessary precautions to make your water safe to drink.

Boiling is the most effective method to kill all organisms that can make you sick. All disease-causing organisms are killed by the time water reaches a boil, even at high elevations, where water boils at lower temperatures. If you don't believe me, let it boil for another minute or two, just to be sure. Boiling is fuel-intensive, which presents a weight challenge on longer trips. It's also time consuming, and unpacking pots and stoves every time you need to disinfect water can be inconvenient. Finally, it does nothing to clear up muddy water or remove chemical contaminants.

Perhaps because of these disadvantages, water filters have become standard equipment for many backpackers. They are the quickest route to drinkable water (you can be drinking after only a few minutes of pumping), but they also have several disadvantages: They're heavy (many weigh up to a pound), they're expensive (prices range from $50 to more than $200), they pump slowly and clog easily in murky water (can you clean the filters, or do you need to bring extras?), and no filter can screen out viruses (to be safe, combine filtration with chemical treatment). Water filter manufacturers include Katadyn and MSR.

Chemical treatment (halogenation) is a lightweight, affordable, and effective way to kill bacteria, viruses, and protozoa in backcountry water sources. However, chemical disinfection takes a relatively long time to work (30 minutes to several hours, depending on the factors in the discussion that follows), and they can leave an unpleasant aftertaste in the water.

How well these chemicals work depends on several variables: the concentration of chemical (higher concentrations work quickly, but they pose a higher risk to you, so lower concentrations are recommended), temperature of the water (cold water takes longer), murkiness of the water (murky water takes longer and/or a higher dose of chemical), and time (giardia and cryptosporidium cysts have

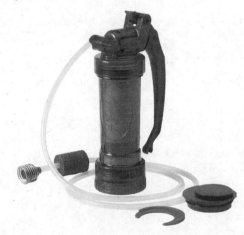

Water filters are standard equipment for many backpackers.

thick shells, and longer contact is necessary to destroy them). Because of the extended time of treatment, it's wise to plan ahead; treat water well before you get thirsty. There are several chemicals used in water disinfection:

Iodine. Iodine is not effective against cryptosporidium cysts. Standard treatment is one small tablet for each quart of water, then let sit for 30 minutes. Increase concentration and time in cold or murky water, and be prepared for an unpleasant aftertaste.

Potable Aqua. Because iodine leaves a less-than-pleasant taste in the water, it's also available with a separate bottle of PA Plus, ascorbic acid (vitamin C) tablets, which neutralize the iodine taste and color. The shelf life of Potable Aqua is four years if unopened; one year if opened. One bottle treats 25 quarts. Cost: $6; $8 with PA Pure.

Polar Pure. This fist-sized glass bottle is filled with iodine crystals. Simply pour water into the Polar Pure bottle, wait one hour, pour water out into the quart of water you're planning to treat (a trap will keep crystals from pouring out), wait another 20 minutes, and you're ready to drink. One bottle treats 2000 quarts. Cost: $10.50.

Chlorine dioxide. This is effective against all organisms, but it can take up to four hours to kill cryptosporidium in cold and murky water. And while iodine leaves an icky taste, chlorine dioxide can actually improve the taste of foul or stagnant water. Both Katadyn and Potable Aqua have individually wrapped 30-tablet packs. Simply drop a tablet in a quart of water, wait four hours to treat cryptosporidium, then drink. One package of 30 tablets treats 30 quarts. Cost: $14.

Cookware and Utensils

The best backpacking cookware is designed simply—lightweight, compact, and efficient—allowing you to prepare meals under changeable backcountry conditions. There are a range of materials and designs from which to choose:

Stainless steel. It's durable enough to endure years of abuse on the trail, and it disperses heat well to minimize scorching, but it's considerably heavier than other options.

Aluminum. Lighter than stainless steel and cheaper than titanium, aluminum is the best value for backpacking. However, it tends to scorch food, so stir frequently or choose pots with a nonstick finish.

Composite. Some manufacturers have combined stainless steel on pot insides (to reduce scorching), with aluminum on the outside (to reduce weight). This combination carries a higher price tag than either material alone.

Cast Iron. Don't even think about it. Despite the beauty of a fine Dutch oven stew, or a brook trout sizzling in a cast-iron pan over an

Stainless steel pots are durable.

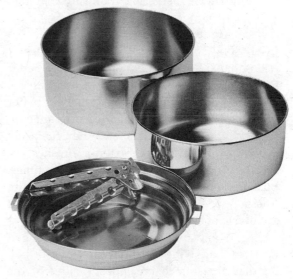

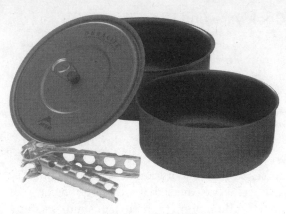

Aluminum pots are light and affordable.

open fire, leave this heavyweight to outfitters, horse packers, and car campers—unless your hiking partner insists and is willing to carry it.

Titanium. If lightweight cookware is a priority and cost is no concern, titanium is for you. Durable and half the weight of stainless steel (but often triple the cost), titanium is the best cookware available for those who want to travel light and fast. Don't turn your attention from stirring for even a minute, though, or your food will burn.

Cookware Features

After considering cookware material, look for design features.

Tight-fitting lids make cooking efficient, and some lids can double as plates or frying pans. Rounded bottom edges are better for even heat distribution and easier cleaning. Likewise, a wide, flat pot absorbs heat better than a tall, narrow one. Rounded rims are easy to grab with pot holders, and they fit nicely against your lips. Black exterior finishes absorb heat quickly and speed up cooking times. Buy blackened pots new, soot them over a fire (messy!), or spray them with black stove paint (available at hardware stores).

Some pots and pans have hinged handles that swing out from the sides, or bail handles that attach on opposite sides of the rim and lift from the top. All handles can get in the way of windscreens and get hot enough to make you scream. Many are also unstable and can spill food easily all over the ground—which will lose you points with cold, hungry campmates. The better bet is to choose instead handle-free pots that you lift with pot grippers or lightweight pliers.

You can avoid scorched food with a nonstick finish, but there are consequences: Such finishes are vulnerable to scratching and flaking off, especially if you scour your pots with sand like I do. The leading nonstick material, Teflon, can release toxic particles and gasses into your food and the air. However, a silicon ceramic alternative is winning rave reviews.

Cookware comes in many sizes, from 8-ounce to 4-liter pots to accommodate your group size and menu plans. Well-designed kits have "nesting" pots that fit nicely inside each other.

To contain your "kitchen," pack your cookware in a stuff sack. This will keep soot and cooking mess from getting everywhere in your pack.

MSR, Snowpeak, Primus, Vargo, Evernew, and Coleman are leaders in quality backpacking cook sets.

Other Kitchen Items

MSR's heat exchanger. If a longer expedition is in your plans, consider bringing MSR's heat exchanger. It increases cooking efficiency by 25 percent, eliminating significant fuel weight and making its $30 price tag and 7 ounces of additional weight worthwhile. Just make sure it's compatible with your pots before investing in this item.

Oven. If your goal is to impress camping partners with fresh-baked bread, lasagna, or soufflé, you'll want to include one of the three following ovens in your pack: Outback Oven, which can bake just about anything, once

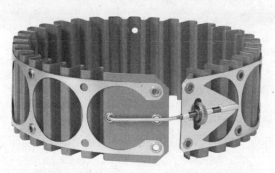
Heat exchangers increase your cooking efficiency.

you practice keeping the heat constant. Hungry testers at *Backpacker* magazine awarded the Outback Oven the Editor's Choice Gold Award in 2001—proof that one way to win acclaim is through tired, hungry tummies. A more affordable alternative oven is the Bakepacker, which uses oven bags (these add hefty pennies to the cost of each meal, and the bags mean more garbage). Although it requires practice to bake well, the most affordable backcountry oven is two pie tins held together clamshell-style with office binder clips, suspended over coals, with coals or a twiggy fire on top (cover the top coals with foil for best results).

Plastic utensils and dishware. When shopping for utensils, bowls, and plates, look for items made from Lexan, a type of plastic that is lightweight and virtually unbreakable. To eat in colorful style, check out Orikaso—lightweight, flat sheets of plastic you can use as cutting boards, then fold into cups and bowls. Old Tupperware-style bowls from your cupboard aren't as elegant, but they are lightweight, durable, and a heck of a lot cheaper. The main disadvantage with plastic is that you can't cook and eat out of the same pots, as you can with metal.

Cup. Everyone needs something to sip, and everyone seems to prefer some types of cups over others. For years, stainless-steel Sierra Club cups were ubiquitous, clanging along the trail, hooked to people's backpacks. Some

people prefer insulated plastic mugs with well sealing lids to prevent spills and keep liquids hot. Despite the cost and weight, I prefer my Nalgene bottle; it doesn't insulate as well, but it makes a great hand warmer or hot water bottle for inside my jacket or sleeping bag; it also seals well for spill-free transportation.

Little bottles. Small bottles are great for carrying spices, sugar, coffee, cocoa, olive oil, and more. Make sure the lids screw on tightly and won't open (pop-top lids are guaranteed to open inside your pack). Hotel shampoo bottles (well-cleaned!) and vitamin bottles are perfect. Film canisters also work well (Kodak canisters are more secure than Fuji canisters; they don't pop open if squeezed). Never mind the rumor about film canisters being toxic; it's a myth. If you don't believe me, call Kodak environmental services at 800-242-2424.

WILDERNESS WISDOM

You know you've chosen your stove, cookware, dishes, and utensils well when they all nestle together into a lightweight, compact package that fits easily into your pack.

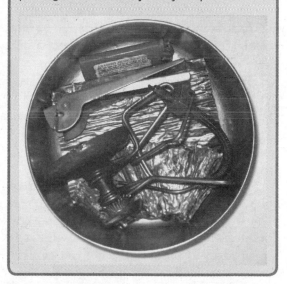

Caring for Your Cookware

If you take care of your camp kitchen, it will likely last a long time—so long you may start to feel nostalgic for past trips when you pull out your favorite pot to make your morning oatmeal. But only if you care for it! Here are some tips:

Nonstick Teflon coatings on pots chip easily. Stir your food with a plastic or wood spoon to avoid scratching it, which ruins the nonstick quality of your pot and makes you ingest toxic Teflon.

Always wash your cookware immediately after meals. Not only is it easier to clean when food is fresh, but you'll be happier facing a clean pot when it's time to cook again. If you don't have a pot scrubber, sand, snow, small, soft, pinecones, sprigs of pine needles, and other natural scrubbers work just fine. To help loosen the gunk, pour some hot water into the pot after you have served the dinners, cover it, and let it soak for a while.

Always wash cookware (and yourself) at least 200 feet from water. Use biodegradable soap (Dr. Bronner's or Campsuds are good ones), and never pour waste water or food waste in water sources or near camp. Take it at least 200 feet upwind from camp (to reduce the chances an animal will be attracted by other smells in camp), and equally far from water, then scatter or bury it there.

Water Bottles

There are many types of bottles and reservoirs you can choose to carry water. Here are a few options, with their pros and cons:

Grocery/convenience-store water or soda bottles. Pros: These are the cheapest and lightest of all options, and they are surprisingly durable. They even come pre-filled with your favorite drink. Cons: They're not good for hot liquids, and small mouth openings make them

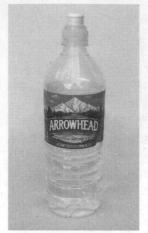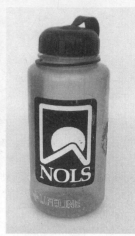

Every water bottle has its pros and cons.

hard to fill and hard to clean (wider-mouthed Gatorade-type bottles are better). Cost: $1 to $2.

Nalgene-type water bottles. Pros: These durable bottles have a wide mouth, which makes filling and cleaning easier. They are also designed to withstand boiling water (they make great hot water bottles for your bag at night). Cons: They're moderately pricey, at $6 to $8 per bottle.

Hydration bladders/reservoirs. Pros: Their easy-to-access tubes make drinking convenient—great for staying well-hydrated while on the go. They are also collapsible, so they're compact when empty. Opt for a reservoir with a wide mouth for easier filling and cleaning. Cons: They're hard to clean and can be hard to fill. They also can puncture easily, and water can freeze in tubes in winter. They're pricey, at $15 to $20.

Dromedary bags. Pros: A Cordura outer shell makes these large bags durable. Plus, they're collapsible, so they're compact when empty. Opt for wide mouth for easy filling. Cons: They are pricey, at $20 to $30, hard to clean, heavier than other options, and opaque, so you can't see the biology experiment breeding inside (then again, do you want to see it?).

Bagging It

One of most indispensable pieces of gear that my husband, Michael, and I add to our packs is about as low-tech as you can get, weighs only a few ounces, and cost us about $5: a 5-gallon plastic bladder encased in a nylon bag with carrying handle. (You could also use a bladder from a wine box, taking care not to puncture it.)

This simple water bag gives us the freedom to dry camp in our favorite Sierra terrain where water might not be close by: off-trail granite shelves with dramatic views. Even when we're near water, we fill up our bag and keep it in camp for convenience. It contains more than enough water for a couple of meals and washing up, and we can even pump clean water from it with a water filter.

We also use it as a shower bag when we need to shampoo or have a serious soap cleanup, well away from creeks and lakes. If we have a layover day and remember to do it, we'll fill it in the morning and let it soak up the sun during the day, bringing the water to near-tepid temperature within a few hours. Then, with one person standing on a higher surface and holding the bag, we give each other showers, thus avoiding the dreaded "legs sticking together in sleeping bag" syndrome. (We used to attach a water nozzle that comes with the bag, but now we don't bother.) A full bag has enough water for a complete shampoo-soap-rinse. Of course, only the first bather gets that warmer water!

—**Roslyn Bullas**, managing editor, Wilderness Press

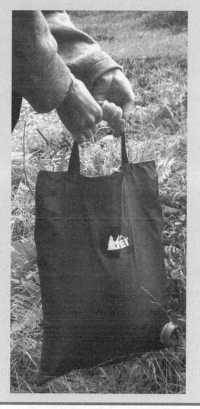

Dromedary bags are flexible and durable.

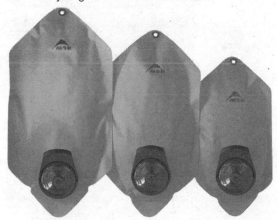

Collapsible water jugs. Pros: These are good for keeping cooking and washing water on hand in camp. Large jugs reduce repeated trips to the water source and are compact when empty. Make your own by using a Mylar or plastic liner from wine in a box (the valve pops off with the blunt end of a knife). Store it in a nylon stuff sack for extra protection. Partially inflated, they also make great pillows! Cons: Emptying the bag of wine the night before you hit the trail leads to a heckuva hangover. Good thing it makes a pillow, so you can sleep it off.

Cleaning Water Bottles

It's no good disinfecting water to drink if your water bottle has a thriving biology experiment living in it. Keeping water bottles clean will help keep you healthy. To do this, take the following steps:

Wash bottles and hydration bags at home with simple dishwashing soap. Use a bottle brush inside to clean well. Clean hydration tubes with a long pipe cleaner, or by pulling through a long piece of string, knotted with cloth to scrub out mildew. Cleaning kits are also available for about $20. Air dry by removing drinking valve and inverting bag over a broomstick or dowel to keep it open. Place in the sun, where UV rays will help sterilize.

Disinfect by filling with water, adding 2 teaspoons of bleach, then letting it sit overnight. Rinse well. Remove odors by filling with water, adding 2 teaspoons of baking soda, then letting it sit over night.

On the trail, wash with biodegradable soaps like Dr. Bronner's or Campsuds, rinse frequently, and air dry. Wash and rinse yourself and all items at least 200 feet from water sources.

Like most equipment, backpacking gear lasts longer and performs more reliably when you take time to get to know it, and when you provide necessary preventative maintenance, such as regular washing and proper storage. Here are a few tips on how to get the most out of your equipment and help it last for years of reliable use on the trail. There is a lot of different equipment out there, and some might require care and storage practices not mentioned in this book. When in doubt, check with your manufacturer for advice on how to get the most out of your gear.

Getting to Know Your Equipment

Now that you have everything you'll need in the backcountry, practice using it at home. Make sure all the parts are there and that everything works properly. Practice assembling, lighting, and cooking with your stove. Set up your tent in the backyard. Then break it down and set it up again. Time yourself. If you can't set it up in five minutes, keep practicing or buy a different tent—you'll be glad you did when you're setting up camp at night in the pouring rain.

Cleaning, Maintenance, and Storage

Your outdoor gear will perform better and last longer if you take proper care of it.

Here are a few specific tips for handling, storing, and washing your gear. When in doubt, call the manufacturer for specific instructions.

Protect from ultraviolet damage. Over time, the sun's rays can damage fabrics in jackets and rain-flies, making them weak and brittle. This happens more quickly at high elevation and high latitudes in summer (in Alaska or New Zealand, for example). Nothing can repair the damage once it's done. The best protection for these fabrics is to avoid prolonged exposure to the sun when possible. Yes, I know, it can be hard to do outdoors.

Care for zippers. Sand, grit, and dirt can impede zipper function. Use water and an old toothbrush to clean them. Keep them zipping smoothly by rubbing them with lip balm, a bar of soap, or candle wax.

Keep gear dry. Mildew smells bad and can break down or clog fibers. It's especially hard on tents and sleeping bag insulation. If possible, dry your gear before packing it for the trail each day, and especially before you put it into storage between trips.

If mildew begins to form on your tent (you can tell by the small, cross-shaped spots on the tent), sponge-wipe the tent with one of the following solutions, then air dry completely before packing it away: a half cup of Lysol to a gallon of hot water, or 1 cup each of lemon juice and salt to a gallon of hot water. This should kill the mildew, but it might not remove the spots. Because mildew can affect the tent's waterproofing, you might need to re-waterproof it with one of the solutions described in the next section.

Keep gear clean. Although technical fabrics can protect you from the harshest weather, they fall easy prey to sweat, dirt, and spilled food and drinks, which can clog waterproof-breathable shell fabrics and reduce the loft of down and synthetic insulating materials.

Unfortunately, washing can break down the waterproofing properties of shell materials. Washing sleeping bags and insulation-filled jackets incorrectly can ruin them. Resist the urge to wash your tents, rain-flies, sleeping bags, down jackets, and outer wear. Try instead to keep them clean, or at least tolerate the dirt, for as long as possible (but please throw that stinky long underwear into the laundry).

When you do wash, be particularly cautious: Liquid detergents and fabric softeners can gum up down, ruining its loft. Even on low heat, dryers can shrink wool, silk, and synthetic fabrics. Spray-on water repellents can ruin waterproof–breathable fabrics by clogging their pores.

For the best results, follow these tips:

➤ Read the label. Manufacturers know best, and they might recommend special treatment that's not mentioned here; as such, their recommendations supercede all information given here. When in doubt, call them.

➤ Spot-clean stains using a toothbrush and the following concoction: one part each of glycerin (available at most drug stores), liquid castile soap (like Dr. Bronner's), and water.

➤ Wash all blended or technical fabrics in cold water.

➤ Avoid hot dryers, which will shrink or melt sensitive fabrics. Air drying is best.

➤ Do not dry clean, use liquid detergent, or use fabric softeners. They leave residues that can clog breathable fabrics and make down clump.

➤ Wash tents by hand using one of the technical washes mentioned below. Set up tents out of direct sunlight to dry them; it will ensure the tent dries completely and will prevent it from shrinking out of shape.

➤ Washing down bags and jackets requires special instructions:

Wash by hand, or in a front-loading washer (the agitators in top-loading washers can tear apart the baffles that compartmentalize the down). Close all zippers before washing. Wash in cold water, using a soap especially formulated for down.

Rinse repeatedly and thoroughly to make sure all soap residue is gone.

Do not wring garment. Instead, gently press the water out, or send the garment through the spin cycle several times to extract as much water as possible.

Dry in a large front-loading dryer set at the lowest heat. Make sure you have plenty of quarters and a good book, because it will take a long time. Ignore the unwise advice about throwing in tennis balls or an old shoe to fluff up the down—they can damage the down, and its own weight will fluff it up well. Make sure bag is completely dry before you pack it away. Otherwise, mildew can build up on the down, affecting its loft.

Waterproofing Fabrics

There are so many technical fabrics and materials on the market, and each needs to be washed and waterproofed in a particular way to maintain peak effectiveness. Eventually, every waterproof fabric will start soaking water in rather than shedding it. When this happens, refresh its waterproofing oomph with the proper solution from Nikwax or Granger's.

Whatever fabric you're washing or waterproofing, both Nikwax and Granger's have a variety of washes and treatments for

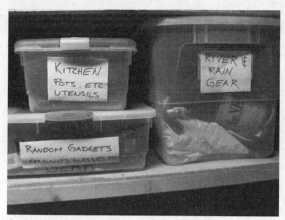
A place for everything

items ranging from Gore-Tex to down, leather, silicone-impregnated nylon, soft-shell fabrics, fleece, and wool—and for boots, clothing, backpacks, and tents. If you're unsure, call the manufacturers for their recommendations.

Stitches in shell materials need special attention to be waterproofed, or they'll leak generously. Waterproof-breathable shells often already have taped or sealed seams (all Gore-Tex garments have taped seams). If yours doesn't, or if it's gotten tired over the years, chemically seal the seams using a product like Seam Grip or Aqua Seal, both of which are available at many outdoor stores. Be aware that seams must be sealed in warm, dry weather, and they must be given time to dry before storage. You're out of luck if you try to seal seams in the rain; it doesn't work.

Storage

When it's time to pack up your gear post-trip or post-season, follow these steps:

➤ Clean and dry everything before storing it.

➤ Store all pieces together. Avoid the frustration of unpacking your stove in the wilderness, only to find you've forgotten your fuel bottle or windscreen, or to realize your tent poles are still in the garage.

➤ Stuff sleeping bags loosely in a large cotton or mesh bag when you're not on the trail, so they will maintain their loft. Do not store your jacket or sleeping bag stuffed tightly in a stuff sack—both down and synthetic fill will compress and lose their fluff.

➤ Store sleeping pads unrolled and flat to keep them thicker and warmer longer.

➤ Use large plastic tubs to store backpacking gear together in one place, so it's easy to gather when it's time to hit the trail again.

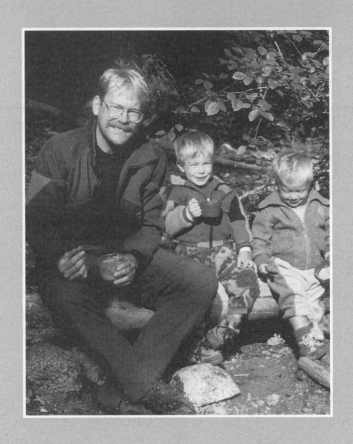

PART III
FOOD AND WATER

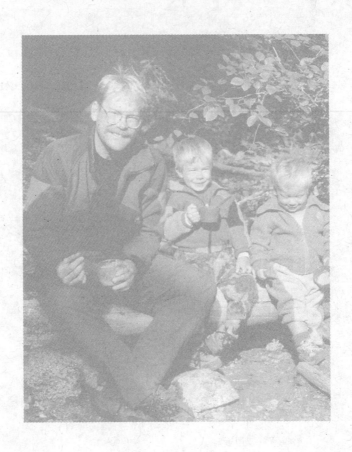

13 NUTRITION FOR THE BACKCOUNTRY

Just as your car needs gas, your body needs fuel to carry you and all your gear through the wilderness. However, eating on the trail isn't like eating at home; there are no refrigerators or fast-food restaurants, and you must choose foods that won't spoil, and that aren't too heavy or too bulky. Beyond these constraints, there aren't many hard-and-fast rules about which foods to bring backpacking or how to prepare them.

Eating on the trail is as simple or as sophisticated as you make it. Some backpackers prefer to bring only the most basic, easy-to-prepare nutrition necessary; others enjoy preparing fine cuisine in the wilderness. With a little planning, you can bring food that is both delicious and nutritious. Your body will appreciate the premium-grade fuel when it's working hard in the wilderness.

Water

Water is your most important nutrient. Good hydration keeps the body's chemical reactions balanced and efficient, it improves circulation and helps keep you warm, it facilitates the transport of nutrition to—and wastes from—our cells, and it helps transport wastes out of your body efficiently through sweat and urine. You might not notice what water does on your insides, but you will notice the improved mental clarity and physical performance that good hydration brings.

A good rule of thumb is to drink two quarts of water a day; if you're working hard, in very hot or very cold weather, or at altitude, you will need four to five quarts a day. The convenience of hydration packs encourages more frequent drinking, as do sweeteners like Gatorade.

Read more about how to stay hydrated and how to ensure safe drinking water later in this book.

Calories

After water, your body needs energy, which is measured in calories. A calorie is simply the amount of energy it takes to raise 1 gram of water 1°C at 1 atmosphere of air pressure (the air pressure found at sea level). A calorie of food provides your body the same amount of energy to maintain metabolism and hike along the trail.

At home, the average woman burns roughly 1600 calories in a given day; a man burns about 2000 calories. On a hard day hiking, plan to double your caloric intake (3500 to 4000 calories); if you're hiking or climbing hard in cold weather, plan to eat 4000 to 5000 calories a day, because in cold weather we burn calories just keeping ourselves warm.

Empty vs. Nutrient-Rich Calories

Although quantity is important when eating on the trail, so is quality. Not all calories are equal. Your body needs more than just energy; it needs nutrition—molecular building blocks to build and heal bones, muscles, and organs; to power your metabolism; and to keep you healthy during your long, illustrious life. Those building blocks come in several different forms: macronutrients (carbohydrates, proteins, and fats) and micronutrients (vitamins and minerals).

Planning Your Daily Caffeine Fix

If you're like me, the morning caffeine fix is more than a wonderful ritual (picture sipping your morning cup of Joy in crisp morning air, with birds singing joyfully nearby, and romantic beams of sunlight dancing at soft angles through the trees), it's also necessary (I just don't move well without it), and both coffee and tea contain antioxidants, which help your body recover from long days on the trail. Luckily, there are numerous options for backpackers to enjoy a daily perk up; they range from gourmet-but-relatively-heavy to lightweight-unromantic-but-effective. Here are some options:

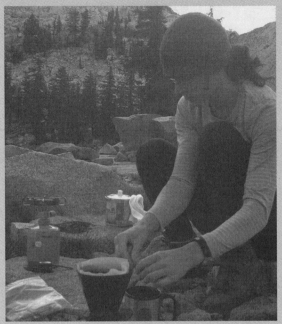

"Please don't talk to me until I've had my coffee."

Cowboy coffee. It's easy: Pour in ground coffee, add hot water, wait a couple minutes, and drink. Adding eggshells or a sprinkle of cold water on top will help the coffee grounds sink to the bottom. You can also filter the coffee before you drink ("Honey, hand me your bandanna, please?").

Tea. Teabags are the lightest and most compact way to enjoy a healing, energizing cup of warmth. Or drop one in your water bottle and hang it on the outside of your pack for sun tea along the trail.

Espresso maker. GSI's stove-top espresso makers come in 1-cup and 4-cup sizes, weigh 7 ounces and 15 ounces respectively, and range in price from $18 to $26. If one of these is in your pack, I'll be your hiking partner any day.

French press. These Lexan versions of fine restaurant coffee makers are relatively heavy and bulky, but they produce a fine cup of Joe. GSI's Java Press comes in 10-ounce and 33-ounce sizes, costs $16 to $20, and weighs less than a pound.

Who needs to cook? If you're traveling fast and light, bring chocolate-covered espresso beans, caffeine gum, or caffeine-enhanced energy goo—not the same ritual as a morning cup, but they'll get you going, fer sure!

Disposing of grounds: Please don't scatter your tea or coffee grounds willy-nilly. Either scatter or bury them well away from camp, or pack them out with the rest of your garbage (let them dry first).

If you're a junk-food junkie, it doesn't really matter what you eat on your weekend backpack trip; you've eaten the same stuff for years, and you feel great, right? For longer trips into the backcountry, consider nutrient-rich foods, because you're going to be pushing your body harder than normal. This doesn't mean you have to leave the cookies at home, but you should eat other things that are good for you while you're on the trail.

Macronutrients

Macronutrients consist of proteins, carbohydrates, and fats. Proteins—and the 22 amino acids they comprise (nine of which the body cannot manufacture)—are essential to the structure and function of all living cells. They are necessary to build, maintain, and repair all tissues in your body (bones, muscles, organs, cells, etc.), they catalyze chemical reactions as enzymes and coordinate bodily functions as hormones, and, as antibodies, they defend you against infection and disease. Good protein sources include meat, fish, beans (especially soy in its many forms—tofu, tempeh, and soy nuts), powdered eggs, and dairy.

Carbohydrates are the primary source of fuel for your body. They come in two forms: simple (sugars) and complex (starches). Sugars are digested easily and provide calories for quick energy. It's always a good idea to have

sweets in your pack for when you need a quick boost. However, calories in sugars are empty; they contain no vitamins or minerals, over-consumption can upset hormone levels, and they're stored as fat if you don't need all that energy—all good reasons to keep their intake moderate.

Starches digest more slowly and provide longer-lasting energy. Fruits, vegetables, and whole grains also contain other essential nutrients. In general, the more colorful your carbohydrates are (leafy greens and berries, for instance), the more protein, fiber, vitamins, minerals, antioxidants, and other good things they contain (dyed foods like candy, cookies, and soda don't count). White carbohydrates, such as pasta, potatoes, flour, and rice, though relatively empty of nutrition, help provide energy for hard-hiking bodies.

These days, many carbs—from snack chips to breakfast cereals—are so overprocessed, there's no significant nutrition left. Wheat, corn, and other grains are stripped of their nutritious hulls, ground into powder, combined with unhealthy fats, sugars, and/or salts, then sold back to us as chips, breakfast cereal, and other snacks. They're scientifically

Goal: Tasty *and* nutritious food.

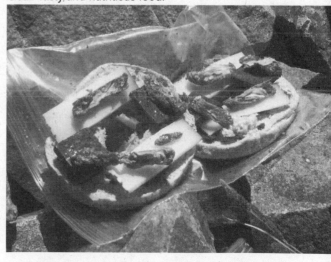

Learning from Fad Diets

If you believe the headlines you read at the supermarket checkout stand, you're certain Elvis is alive and breeding with extraterrestrials. You're probably also confused by the competing claims of various fad diets: Atkins, South Beach, and the Zone, for example, all claim to be the true path to health. Luckily, a closer inspection shows they're not so different. Though they disagree on the details, they all agree on the big picture: Everybody needs a balance of proteins, fats, and carbohydrates; the best nutrition comes from foods that are fresh and unprocessed; variety is the spice of life; and it's better to get micronutrients from your food than from supplements. Interestingly, this is also what sports nutritionists prescribe for world-class athletes—good enough for me.

To follow their advice, strive to eat a balance of carbs, proteins, and fats somewhere between the 40 percent carbs/30 percent protein/30 percent fat ratio recommended by the Zone diet, and the 65-15-20 ratio recommended by many sports nutritionists (the harder your body works, the more carbs you need). Rather than working to get the ratios precise (unless you're hoping to beat Lance Armstrong's record), strive instead to ensure that all of those macronutrients are high quality, from a variety of unprocessed sources, and that all contain ample micronutrients. Choosing organic will help you avoid industrial hormones, antibiotics, pesticides, fertilizers, and other things mother nature didn't intend for your body. You'll also support local, working farmers instead of multinational agribusiness fat cats.

designed to taste great and crunch perfectly. They're marketed to make you want them, but they do your body little or no good at all, because they don't provide nutrition your body needs.

Whole, unprocessed grains, such as whole oats and whole-grain rice, are healthier for you, but they present a challenge for backpacking because they take a long time (and lots of fuel) to cook. A food dehydrator can solve this. Simply cook your rice, oats, or pasta at home, dehydrate it for the trail, then rehydrate it when it's time to eat at camp. Read more about dehydrating food later in this chapter.

Fats have a bad reputation these days because Americans eat far more than they need. That aside, fats are essential to bodily functions: They help build and regulate hormones, they absorb and transport fat-soluble vitamins, and they help the body use carbs and proteins efficiently. When you eat calories your body doesn't need, it stores this excess energy as fat to use later. Stored fat helps cushion bones and organs.

Fats also provide critical energy for life on the trail. Fat contains double the calories as protein and carbohydrates (9 calories per gram, compared with only 4 calories per gram of protein or carbs); those extra calories help fuel hard-working bodies on the trail. They also help keep you warm when it's cold. In winter, bring plenty of high-fat foods, such as precooked sausage and pepperoni, cheese, chocolate, butter, and nut butters to help keep your internal furnace stoked. If you're going to be sleeping in subzero conditions, toss a healthy handful of cheese into your soup for dinner, or a cube of butter into your hot chocolate before climbing into your bag for the night.

Monounsaturated and polyunsaturated fats, found in fish, vegetables, olive oil, and nuts are healthier than saturated or trans fats, which are found in butter, cream, cookies, crackers, and other processed foods.

Micronutrients

Micronutrients are vitamins and minerals. Your body needs vitamins for many essential functions, but it can't make these necessary nutrients for itself. Water-soluble vitamins (the B-complex family and vitamin C) are not stored in the body and must be replaced each day. Fat-soluble vitamins (A, D, E, and K) are stored in fat tissues and in the liver.

Make sure you get enough vitamins while backpacking, particularly on longer trips. Vegetables, fruits, and other fresh foods are the best sources of vitamins. Because fresh fruits and vegetables don't travel well, it might be necessary to bring supplements to make sure your body gets what it needs.

Minerals are the building blocks of molecules, which are in turn the building blocks for proteins, carbs, and fats. They are essential to the millions of vital chemical and molecular processes taking place in your body every second. Americans used to get their minerals from vegetables and meat; now minerals in our soil have been significantly depleted, and most of us (including the animals we eat) have switched to largely processed diets. Ensure your body gets the minerals it needs every day, especially on the trail.

Electrolytes (sodium, potassium, chloride, calcium, magnesium, bicarbonate, phosphate, and sulfate) are minerals that your heart, nerve, and muscle cells need to carry electrical impulses across cell membranes and to other cells. These minerals are lost when you sweat and pee. Drinking a lot of water without replacing electrolytes can upset the body's natural chemistry, a dangerous condition known as hyponatremia.

Good electrolyte sources include salty and spiced foods, such as chips, cured meats, and soups, as well as fruit (dried bananas and apricots are great for the trail), whole grains, legumes, vegetables, and Gatorade or other electrolyte-replacement drinks.

Fiber is another essential nutrient that is available in fruits, vegetables, and grains (especially whole grains). Soluble fiber helps maintain blood-sugar levels and may lower cholesterol; non-soluble fiber may help reduce your chances of colon cancer, and it keeps your bowels moving regularly, which can be a challenge while backpacking.

When your muscles work hard during a difficult hike, or when you're stressed, or exposed to tobacco, alcohol, radiation, or other toxins, your cells produce free radicals—forms of oxygen that are missing electrons; they steal electrons from your cells, which can damage cell structure and the genetic material packed inside. This damage speeds aging and increases your chances of cancer, heart disease, and other diseases.

Fortunately, antioxidants neutralize free radicals, help slow aging, and reduce your risk of disease. Antioxidants include vitamins A, C, and E, as well as compounds found in broccoli, kale, spinach, and other dark green vegetables, citrus fruits, mango, papaya, apricot, strawberries, blueberries, nuts, tea (both black and green), coffee, and cocoa(!).

Recovery Nutrition

World-class athletes and their coaches have learned that eating quality nutrition soon after a workout is essential to help athletes recover quickly from the damage they've just inflicted on themselves. It helps them build muscle, improve conditioning faster, and perform at peak levels more often.

Sports nutritionists often refer to the "golden hour"—that first hour after a hard workout (or hike), when your body is craving the nutrients lost during exercise. This is a good time to drink lots of water, eat simple sugars to help you restore energy levels, and eat carbs, protein, vitamins, and minerals (especially electrolytes) to replace nutrition stores

Freeze-Dried Options

Companies like Mountain House, Alpine Aire, Backpacker's Pantry, and Natural High make cooking in the backcountry easy. Just boil water, reconstitute the foods in their own foil bags, and presto! Beef stroganoff, chicken a la king, and lasagna are ready to eat. These companies spend a lot of time thinking about how to make their food better.

Over the years, quality has improved, and often those eating the food are the winners, but these meals can disappoint. Freeze-dried meals can also be expensive. Also, don't trust their serving size estimates; though packages might say they contain two servings, ravenous teens and anyone who's just hiked 13 miles over a high pass will disagree strongly. Test a meal or two before you stock up for the week.

and repair damage. Some recovery nutrition experts advise avoiding much fat in this golden hour because fat inhibits your ability to absorb electrolytes, carbs, and protein.

Good recovery foods include energy and nutrition bars (more on these later in this chapter), dried fruit (especially apricots, bananas, apples, and berries), grains, and low-fat dairy.

Food Factors: Weight, Durability, Spoilage, Variety, and Simplicity

Enough about nutrition. There are other things to consider when planning your meals for the trail. For one, how much does your food weigh? The longer your trip, the more important this becomes. For a weekend trip, weight isn't a big issue because you're only bringing a couple days' worth. If you don't mind carrying the extra weight, weekend trips and the first couple days of longer trips are good times to indulge in fresh veggies and fruits—heck, even steak and a bottle of wine (pack out the bottle). Eat your heaviest food first to shave pack weight quickly.

Because the majority of food's weight comes from water content, if you're going on a longer trip, you'll need to reduce the weight of your individual portions so you can carry enough to last you for days without spoiling. This narrows your options to dried and/or dehydrated foods.

If you strive to keep food lightweight and compact, it's possible to carry enough to last a week to 10 days. On a moderate trip in warm weather, you will need only 1.5 to 1.75 pounds of dried food per person per day (pppd), which is about 2500 to 3000 calories. In cool weather when you're hiking hard, you'll need to eat about 2 pppd (3500 to 4000 calories). On hard-working trips in cold weather, push your daily intake up toward 2.5 pppd (5000 calories). If you plan to be on the trail much longer than a week, you'll need to resupply (for more on how to do that, turn to page 237).

You should also consider the food's durability. After all, you won't be packing it into a spacious kitchen with cupboards, a pantry, and a refrigerator. Some foods are fragile, such as bananas, eggs, plums, potato chips, fluffy loaves of bread, and other easily broken or bruised foods. If you insist on bringing these, you need to take steps to keep them safe, or be prepared to eat mush and crumbs.

Another aspect of durability is how long it will last on the trail before spoiling. The more water or oil content foods have, the faster they'll spoil. Removing water lightens food weight significantly, and it helps increase the time before spoilage. A variety of dried and dehydrated foods are available at your nearest grocery store. A food dehydrator is a wonderful way to prepare food for the trail (more on this later).

Variety is also important, for both complete nutrition and high morale, especially

MY SYSTEM

The Basics of Variation

By planning my backpacking menu around the following ingredients, I can enjoy a variety of delicious meals while keeping ingredients and planning to a minimum.

For dinners, I bring a few main starches, such as pasta, rice, and instant mash potatoes, and veggies, such as dried tomato powder, dried onions, carrots, peppers, etc. Then I bring a variety of protein sources, such as precooked, dehydrated meats, or cured meats (like sausage or pepperoni). Tofu and textured vegetable protein (TVP) make great alternatives (in fact, the right stock and a half a cup of TVP in any soup or stew can really give them an essential oomph that many people crave but can't put their fingers on). A few different cheeses, such as cheddar, Parmesan, or Asiago, can really make the difference between good and great meals.

In my spice kit, which fits right in my cook set (I keep spices in little plastic bottles), I bring several types of stock: veggie, beef, pork, or chicken. Sometimes, especially when it's cold, I bring margarine or butter in a screw-top container (don't trust Tupperware or other lids that can pop open in your pack) for extra taste and for a source of fat to keep warm. I repackage everything in plastic bags that tie shut. No frigging Ziplocs for food. Don't forget the cooking instructions if you're following a recipe.

Now I have everything I need to enjoy a variety of delicious meals over a week. I don't always have strict recipes. Instead, I simply combine the ingredients above in fresh combinations each night. Here are a few examples:

➤ Peppers, cumin, and dehydrated beans with chicken, beef, or pork (and matching stock), over rice or noodles with cheddar, for Mexican.

➤ Oregano, rosemary, basil, nice andouille sausage, and other herbs over noodles, with Parmesan or Asiago for Italian.

➤ Curry powder with tofu or dehydrated chicken for Indian (add dried coconut milk for Thai!), over rice.

—**Kurt Kuznicki**, just another guy who loves to backpack

Keeping Fresh Food Fresh

In cool to cold weather, you can keep food fresh if you pack it well-insulated from the weather deep in your pack. Freeze meat or fish ahead of time, keep it frozen in a cooler on the drive to the trailhead, then bury it deep in your pack (make sure it's in a plastic bag). It will thaw while you're hiking and be ready to cook that first night.

In warm to hot weather, or if there's any chance food will spoil, err on the side of caution. Avoid bringing fresh fish and/or meat, which can spoil quickly and infect you with botulism, salmonella, E. coli, or other undesirable hiking partners. In warm weather, fresh fruits and vegetables will last for a day, maybe two, if you pack them deep in your backpack, where your clothes and/or sleeping bag can insulate them from the outside heat.

In cool to cold weather, fresh fruits and veggies can last two to three days in your pack. But do you want to carry that much weight for so long?

if you plan to be on the trail for a while. I once ate nothing but energy bars for three days. I realized the error of this decision before the first day was over, but it was too late. Needless to say, the last one didn't taste nearly as good as the first. Challenge yourself to mix up your menu to keep things interesting. Avoid eating the same dinner more than twice in a week. Although it takes more time and effort when planning your trip, you'll appreciate the extra work days later on the trail.

Don't forget to save room for treats! One great advantage to backpacking is that you need to eat a lot to fuel your body for the journey. Leave your strict diet (or best diet intentions) at home. Instead, always make room on your menu, and in your pack, for indulgence.

Scrumptious treats are great for a quick burst of energy and morale on the trail, and nothing produces smiles faster than passing around a decadent chocolate bar, or some Cheez-Its, during a rest stop.

All backpacking meals fall somewhere on the spectrum between quick-and-easy (just tear open the wrapper and start eating) and complicated. ("Honey, keep stirring the alfredo sauce, and don't let it come to a boil. I'll be over here folding egg whites into the soufflé.")

Although fine cuisine is always a pleasure to eat, it can be difficult enough to prepare at home, surrounded by all the ingredients and gadgets you need. On the trail, fine cuisine takes planning and cooperative conditions.

WILDERNESS WISDOM

Regardless of how much you like to cook, make sure you have several easy-to-fix, one-pot meals in your pack. If you're exhausted after a long day, if the mosquitoes won't let you out of the tent, or if the rain is falling sideways as you're trying to light your stove, you'll be very happy with a fast, filling, warming meal.

The simplest hot meals are ready to eat as soon as the water's done boiling, or those that can be made quickly in one pot. Keep a couple extra easy-to-fix meals in your pack as emergency rations, then turn to them when weather or other challenges change your menu plans.

Keep meals that require more than one pot, many steps, or lengthy preparation time, to a minimum, unless you're ready, willing, and able to pull them off with panache.

14 COOKING IN THE BACKCOUNTRY

Eating in the wilderness isn't the same as eating at home for a few reasons: Unless it's downright cold out the whole time, food can spoil quickly, food can be heavy and/or difficult to transport, and you don't have access to the same assortment of pots, pans, and utensils as you might at home. Add to this the challenges of weather, insects, animals, fatigue, and peer pressure from fellow campmates, and it's easy to see why it's necessary to think carefully about what you plan to cook and eat while backpacking. This chapter will help you assemble foods that will travel well, taste great, and suit your particular style for eating in the wild.

Planning Your Menu

To bring the right amount of food, you need to plan your meals carefully. Create a list of every meal and the number of breakfasts, lunches, and dinners. Also make a list of cooking supplies, utensils, and extra spices you'll need for each meal. The shorter your trip, the more freedom you'll have in planning your menu. For one or two nights, you'll be able to carry more fresh foods and kitchen gadgets; for longer trips, you'll rely more on dried foods that are compact, lightweight, easy to prepare, and won't spoil.

The following options will help you decide what kind of food to bring and how much fuel to bring for your stove (or whether to bring a stove at all), depending on how much you want to cook:

Cook once a day. Enjoy granola, fruit, and energy bars for breakfast, get your caffeine from chocolate-covered espresso beans, enjoy pita with cheese, hummus, or cured meats with trail mix for lunch, and save the cooking hassle and fuel weight for dinner.

Cook twice a day. Hot cereal, pancakes, and coffee, tea, or cocoa make a great start for your day. Bring snack and lunch items, such as cheeses, jerky, and dried fruit that don't need cooking, then cozy around the stove at night for dinner.

Cook three times a day. In cold weather, you'll need to cook morning, noon, and night to melt snow for water and to prepare hot (high fat!) meals to get warmth coursing through your body.

> ## WILDERNESS WISDOM
>
> Appetites often drop for the first couple days in the mountains, but they'll kick in after a few days. Decrease ration size a bit in the beginning, and increase it by the third day of your trip.

Don't cook. On short trips in summer or fall, consider leaving the stove at home and

Useful Kitchen Tools

If you plan to backpack regularly, you may want to invest in some of the following home kitchen items, which can help you prepare good meals and snacks for the backcountry:

➤ Dehydrator: Your universe of trail cuisine will expand deliciously if you invest in one of these; they're available for as little as $50. You'll be able to prepare a wide variety of dried vegetables, fruits, soups, sauces, even rice and pasta, and dehydrate them for the trails. Just make sure to start dehydrating your meals days in advance of driving to the trailhead; it takes a goodly amount of time. Note: Stoves set to low can also dehydrate food, but I have found that they don't work as well, and I'm nervous leaving the oven on all night.

➤ Food processor or blender: When drying sauces, it's important to get the sauce smooth first. Food processors also help chop fruits and vegetables if you're preparing a lot of food for a lengthy backpacking trip.

➤ Kitchen scale: If you're planning a long trip with a group, a scale that measures ounces (or grams if you're using the more-reasonable-but-hard-for-Americans-to-learn metric system) accurately will help portion out your portions well.

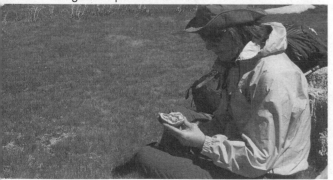

Bagels are perfect trail food.

compensate with a healthy variety of tasty snacks that don't need cooking, such as grains, cheese, powdered hummus, dried fruits and veggies, cured meats, and nutrition bars. You'll save significant weight without a stove, fuel, and pots, not to mention cooking time and hassle. Do not attempt this if you're going to face freezing temperatures; you'll need that stove to melt water or just stay warm. It takes a Spartan attitude to pull this off; if you or someone in your party needs a semblance of modern convenience and comfort, abandon this plan for the heavier and more comforting cooking option.

As you're planning your meals, ask your hiking partners about their needs and likes. On the trail is the wrong time to learn about food dislikes or allergies. And remember that despite the best-laid plans, meals can, and eventually will, go terribly wrong. Nearly every veteran backpacker has a story about that horrible meal in the backcountry. In my book, anything that turns into a good story is all part of the adventure, although some stories are better to hear than tell (or taste).

Recipe Ideas

There's a whole lot of delicious dining taking place on backcountry trails around the world. Listed below are a few of my favorite dishes. Many more can be found by reading the books listed at the end of this section.

Breakfast

Mountain Muesli

Not only does muesli offer the nutritional benefits of whole oats, barley, nuts, fruits, and seeds, you can eat it raw on warm summer days or pour hot milk over it for a quick, hot breakfast that sticks to your ribs in winter. Like granola or gorp, muesli is a generic term; a variety of packaged mueslis are available at most grocery stores, or you can mix your own. I usually start with packaged muesli and add a half cup each of the following for extra nutritional boost: coconut, flax seeds, wheat germ, sunflower seeds, sesame seeds, raisins, and other dried fruit. For extra sweetness, add sugar before you eat on the trail.

Sierra Scramble

Eating powdered eggs isn't quite the same as eating freshly cracked eggs, but they'll be a welcome treat on a chilly mountain morning. At home, package the following ingredients in separate plastic bags:

- One bag with powdered eggs (or egg whites): ½ cup powder per person
- Another bag with ½ cup each of dried onion, mushroom, bell pepper, or jalapenos. Add to bag 1 teaspoon garlic powder.
- 2 tablespoons powdered milk (keep this with the rest of your milk stash until you're ready to cook)

In camp, pour dried vegetables into a bowl several minutes before you start to cook. Add enough water to cover the veggies; let them rehydrate for 10 minutes before cooking. Next, add an equal amount of warm water to your powdered egg mixture (it's a good idea to start with a little less—you can always add more water, but you can't add less). Stir eggs into the water with a fork until the lumps are gone (a small whisk will make up for its extra weight if you're planning to cook eggs in the backcountry regularly). Then scramble in a pan with oil or butter. Top off with grated cheese and/or hot sauce.

Snacks and Lunch

Tofu Jerky

Even my hardcore carnivore friends ask for more when I break this out on the trail. It's a great vegetarian alternative to beef or turkey jerky. You can make it with any marinade that doesn't include oil. Good marinade recipes are available online; store-bought ones, such as teriyaki or barbecue, work fine, too. Here's my favorite recipe:

Note: It takes a couple days to make this recipe—one night to marinade, and one full day to dry, so give yourself time.

Slice a 1-pound block of firm or extra-firm tofu into quarter-inch-thick slices (equal widths are important, so they all dry to the same texture). Lay slices on a towel, then cover with another towel for 15 to 30 minutes to soak out the water. Marinade in your favorite sauce or one of the following recipes for several hours (overnight is best), stirring occasionally to ensure even coverage (these same marinades will work great on beef or venison).

Original Jerky Marinade

- ½ cup soy sauce
- ½ cup Worcestershire sauce
- 1-2 cloves garlic, pressed or minced (more if you really like garlic)
- 2 tablespoons brown sugar or molasses (more to taste)
- Tabasco sauce or cayenne pepper to taste (if you like heat)
- Salt and pepper to taste
- ½ cup orange juice for a nice tangy-sweet touch (optional)

Sweet 'n' Sour Jerky Marinade

- ¼ cup soy sauce
- ¾ cup pineapple juice
- ½ cup balsamic vinegar
- 1-2 garlic cloves, pressed or minced (more to taste)
- ½ cup brown sugar or molasses
- 1 tablespoon minced fresh ginger
- Salt to taste

Arrange the slices in your dehydrator, and dehydrate for eight to 12 hours. Check after eight hours. Time it right, and you'll get a texture very close to that of beef jerky; dehydrate too long, and it becomes dry, brittle, and less enjoyable. Note that the jerky will continue to dry and harden a bit after you take it out of the dehydrator.

Accessorizing Meals

Who ever said mac 'n' cheese or Top Ramen are bland and boring? They can become the backbone of a memorable and nutritious meal, if you simply add a few choice ingredients. Dried or canned fish or shrimp, pre-cooked meat (such as sausage or pepperoni), dried mushrooms or peas, chopped onions and peppers, etc. can make pedestrian fare scrumptious and satisfying.

This principle works in lots of ways by combining your favorite starch—mashed potatoes, instant rice, couscous, pasta, or other grains—with your favorite dried and chopped meats or veggies, then adding your favorite packaged sauce. The potential for delicious combinations is enormous. So is the potential for *yuuuck*. Be careful. Here are a few of my favorite accessorized meals:

➤ Instant oatmeal with handfuls of dried fruit pieces and nuts.

➤ Packaged ramen with dried fish, shitake mushrooms, and peas.

➤ Mac 'n' cheese with canned tuna and dried peas.

➤ Dried black bean soup with fresh jalapenos and cilantro, dried corn, precooked and dehydrated beef, large handfuls of cheddar cheese, and hot sauce.

Bland meals on the trail are common, but you can fix this by bringing an assortment of pizzazz. Carry dry spices in baggies or film canisters, and carry liquids in screw-top or otherwise well-sealing plastic containers. Here are a few ideas of what to include:

➤ Salt and pepper to liven up the blandest foods.

➤ Spike: My favorite savory spice for rice, veggies, and egg dishes.

➤ Cayenne pepper or hot sauce. Make dinner a four-alarm, adrenaline kick, or at least a warming trend.

➤ Curries: Flavorful and sometimes hot, for rice, soups, potatoes, etc.

➤ Fresh garlic and ginger travel well and add zing to foods. Slice them thinly and carefully once you're in camp and ready to cook.

➤ Herbs: Basil, oregano, dill, tarragon, cilantro, rosemary, sage, etc., for sauces, breads, and soups.

➤ Olive oil: Bring this for packaged recipes (hummus and mac 'n' cheese, for example), and for frying.

➤ Vanilla: Add to oatmeal, desserts, chai, cocoa, etc.

➤ Miso or bullion: You'll savor the salty goodness these provide.

Spicy note: Flavor intensifies as it cooks. Start with less; you can always add more, but you can't take it back. Make sure everyone agrees; when in doubt, have people spice their own portions to taste.

Pesto Leather

This recipe satisfies the craving for greens on the trail, and it provides vitamins, minerals, and fiber, not to mention yummy salt and cheese. It's basically pesto without the oil and with extra cheese. Substitute spinach, kale, arugula, broccoli, or other greens, if you want. Munch it as a snack on the trail, or rehydrate for pesto sauce to go on pasta, pita, or other grains.

Puree the following ingredients in a food processor:

- 1 pound basil, well-rinsed
- ½ cup walnuts or pine nuts (or more for extra fat and protein on the trail)
- 2 garlic cloves (or more if you're a garlic fiend or plan to hike with mosquitoes), baked, sautéed, or microwaved to smooth out the taste
- ½ to 1 cup grated parmesan, Romano, or other dry cheese. (The cheese helps make this scrumptious on the trail, and the fat will stoke your internal furnace. So what the heck, throw in another cup!)
- Salt to taste

- 1 cup water (or more, if needed) to help it blend

Once pureed, spread the pesto on drying trays or wax paper in dehydrator, dry (start checking after eight hours), then slice into individual sheets.

Gorp

Good ol' raisins and peanuts have earned themselves a distinguished place in the lexicon of hikers, mainly because gorp is just another name for trail mix, and it's as variable as the people eating it. The evolution of bulk food sections at many grocery stores has resulted in a delicious variety of trail mixes. Or you can build your own, starting with classic gorp, then adding whatever else is available that strikes your fancy—shredded coconut, walnuts, sunflower seeds, dried fruit chunks, etc. You'll create a delicious and nutritious snack mix to fuel your hike.

Note: Chocolate chips melt in hot weather, turning trail mix into a gooey, sinfully delicious mess. Rather than cursing your ruined snack, grab a spoon and dig in. Anticipate this by packing your gorp in a resealable plastic tub instead of a plastic bag; it will reduce the mess, give you easier access to the yum, and

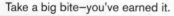
Take a big bite—you've earned it.

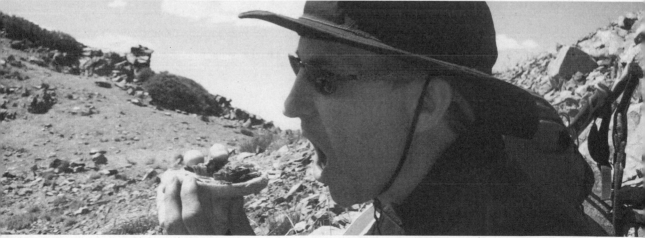

waste less chocolate (it tends to get all over the bag instead of in your mouth). When the chocolate cools and hardens, your trail mix has transformed into chunky snack nuggets—a win-win situation at any temperature!

Energy Bars

In the 1990s, PowerBar started the convenient nutrition revolution, and today, there are literally hundreds of lightweight and nonperishable energy and nutrition bars to choose from. Some are delicious; others taste like saw dust. Some are good for you, designed by sports nutritionists to provide quality carbs and sugars during your hike, or micro- and macronutrients to speed recovery after the hike. Others are little more than glorified candy bars (which can be great as a treat after miles of difficult hiking but don't provide essential nutrition). Some travel well; others melt into a gooey mess on warm days.

MY SYSTEM

Salad in the Backcountry

After my first series of weeklong wilderness trips, I discovered that not only was I craving the crunch of a salad, but my taste buds missed the fresh zing of a homemade dressing layered with the flavors of summer. Lettuce was weighty and was out of the question after the first day, so I set out to create some alternatives. The Citrus Lentil Salad has become such a family favorite that now I double the recipe when making it. That way we can enjoy it for lunch at home and then dry the rest for a lunch on one of our trips without having the effort of making it twice.

Citrus Lentil Salad

Preparation Time: 10 minutes; Dehydration Time: 5 to 7 hours; Serves 2

Salad Mixture

- 1 cup of canned green lentils, rinsed and well-drained
- 1 small carrot, coarsely grated
- 2 cloves garlic, minced
- 3 tablespoons celery leaves, chopped (see note)
- 1/3 cup roasted red pepper, chopped in 1/4-inch pieces (see note)
- 1/8 cup fresh chives or scallions, chopped
- 1/8 cup fresh parsley, chopped
- 1/4 teaspoon dried thyme
- 1 tablespoon lemon zest
- Salt and pepper to taste
- 3 tablespoons crumbled feta cheese

Dressing

- 1/3 cup extra virgin olive oil
- 1 1/2 tablespoons lemon juice
- 1/8 teaspoon cayenne pepper
- 1/4 teaspoon cumin
- 1/2 teaspoon dried sweet basil

It's up to you to choose what's right for you—everybody likes something different in their bars. I recommend variety because the same flavors can get monotonous after a few days. Speaking of which, I hope someone perfects pizza, lasagna, and curry bars soon, because I get tired of sweet bars all the time.

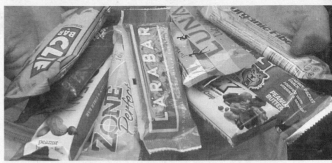

Bars provide scrumptious, quick energy for the trail.

At Home: Combine all of the salad ingredients except for the dressing in a medium bowl. Spread out the salad mixture on lined dehydrator trays and dry for five to seven hours. Time will depend on the type of dehydrator that you have. If your unit has a temperature control, set it for 135°F. Place the lemon juice and olive oil in a leak-proof container such as a small Nalgene bottle. Pack the cayenne, cumin, and sweet basil in plastic wrap or a small zipper bag. Place the salad, bottle, and spice packet inside a medium zipper bag and seal, making sure to remove as much air as possible.

At Camp: Rehydrate the salad using a formula of 1.5 parts dried mix to 1 part water. Wait five or 10 minutes and then add a little more water if needed. If you accidentally use too much water, be sure to drain the salad well before adding the dressing. Combine the contents of the spice packet to the bottle containing the olive oil and lemon juice mixture. Shake vigorously and then pour the dressing on the hydrated salad. Stir gently to combine.

Serving Suggestions: Serve the salad on its own, with lightly toasted Greek pitas, or use as a filling for a pita pocket.

Storage: If you plan to make this well ahead of a trip, do not make the oil and lemon mixture until closer to when you will leave. You can store the dried ingredients in the freezer for six months. Place the name and date on the outside of the freezer bag, using an indelible marker, and do not forget to put a comment about adding the dressing on the bag.

Roasted Red Peppers: To roast peppers, place them on a baking sheet in a 350°F oven for 45 minutes to one hour. Allow to cool before peeling off the skin. You can also grill them until the skin starts to blacken and peel. You can also buy roasted red peppers, packed in oil, at the supermarket. Just give them a little rinse first.

Celery Leaves: Many people do not realize that the leaves found on the celery stalks are good for use in salads and other dishes. Celery leaves impart a mild celery flavor. Most often, the leaves are at the top of the celery; however, if you look closely, you will sometimes find them hidden in the center of the stalks.

—**Laurie Ann March**, author, *A Fork in the Trail*, Wilderness Press

Dinner

Insta-Meal

This simple recipe provides a warm, filling meal as soon as the water's done boiling. It's a good idea to carry this (or your own variation) to warm the bodies and hearts of cold, tired hikers quickly.

In your mug or bowl, add 16 ounces of hot water to the following:

- 2 packets of your favorite instant soup
- 3 tablespoons instant mash potatoes
- Small handful of shredded or cubed cheese

MY SYSTEM

Romantic Dinner for Two

When I go backpacking with my partner, I look forward to dinner all day long. It's my big reward for the effort I've put in. As soon as we've set up camp, I start us off with mugs of hot soup. It's surprising how quickly we get chilled after we stop hiking. With something warm in our bellies, I can then take my time and make a nice dinner.

One of my favorites is fusilli with mushroom sauce and smoked chicken breast. I use dehydrated mushrooms and bring along some basil and tarragon to add to the powdered sauce mix. I usually make this on our first night because I don't trust the smoked chicken to last too much longer than that, even if it's vacuum-sealed. Then I make sure there's something sweet for dessert, like cookies, brownies, or squares of some kind. I'll make herbal tea with dessert to ensure that we're well-hydrated for a long night of indoor activities in the tent!

—**Michelle Waitzman**, author, *Sex in a Tent*, Wilderness Press

- Another small handful of cured meat, like sausage or pepperoni
- Hot sauce or other favorite and fitting spice to taste

Quinoa Pilaf

Considered the mother grain by the Inca, quinoa (pronounced keen-wa) has more protein than any other grain, as well as essential amino acids, fiber, vitamins, minerals, starches, and fats. And it's fast-cooking, to boot—done after 15 minutes of boiling (compared with 45 minutes for whole-grain rice). Like rice and other grains, there are many ways to cook it. Learn more about quinoa at www.quinoa.net

Here's what I enjoy:

- 2:1 water-to-quinoa ratio (1 cup quinoa and 2 cups water makes about 3 cups ready-to-eat quinoa)

Add quinoa to water and bring to a boil. Add stock or butter for flavor if desired. Once boiling, set stove to simmer.

Add any one or all of the following dried ingredients, according to your desires and tastes: a half cup each of meats (fish, shrimp, beef, chicken) or veggies, and a pinch of spices—onions, garlic, mushrooms, carrots, peppers, celery, oregano, almonds, or walnuts (have these ready to go before you start cooking).

Simmer for 15 minutes (longer at altitude) until done. Add salt and pepper to taste.

Pad Thai

This recipe (submitted by Christina Woo to the REI recipes web page below) hooked me immediately and quickly became a favorite. It's surprisingly simple for such a delicious dish. To avoid spoiled shrimp or sauce, plan to cook this the first night out on the trail.

Pack the following:

- ¼ cup dried bean vermicelli
- 2 cups dry rice noodles

- 1 cup bean sprouts
- 3 cups frozen, precooked shrimp (use it as an ice pack)
- 2 tablespoons sesame oil for cooking
- 1 fresh lime
- ½ cup raw peanuts, chopped and placed in a small plastic bag
- 2 cloves garlic
- 2 stalks spring onion

At home, make the cooking sauce by mixing the following ingredients and placing them in a small, well-sealing plastic bottle (you can also save big steps by ignoring the following ingredients and buying instead a jar of Pad Thai sauce at your local grocery store—pack a half cup in a well-sealing plastic container for the trail):

- 2 tablespoons fish sauce
- 2 tablespoons oyster sauce
- 2 tablespoons brown sugar or molasses
- 2 teaspoons soy sauce
- ½ teaspoon finely chopped red chili (more to taste)

At camp, soak noodles and vermicelli in 2 cups water, dice garlic and chop spring onions, then set up your stove. Heat oil in your cook pot (1.5- or 2-quart pot works fine) over medium heat for two minutes. Add shrimp, garlic, and noodles, and stir until soft, one to two minutes. Turn to low heat and add cooking sauce. Add bean sprouts, then turn up to medium high for another minute or two. Turn off stove, and top meal with chopped peanuts, spring onions, and a squeeze of lime. Yum.

More on Backcountry Chow

There's much more to learn about eating well while backpacking. Check out the following resources:

➤ *NOLS Cookery*, edited by Claudia Pearson, Stackpole Books

➤ *A Fork in the Trail*, by Laurie Ann March, Wilderness Press

➤ *Trail Food: Drying and Cooking Food for Backpackers and Paddlers*, by Alan Kesselheim, Ragged Mountain Press

➤ *Beyond Gorp: Favorite Foods from Outdoor Experts*, by Yvonne Prater and Ruth Dyer Mendenhall, The Mountaineers Books

➤ www.rei.com/cooking: This site contains great-tasting, award-winning recipes for the trail.

An exposed boulder makes a great kitchen surface.

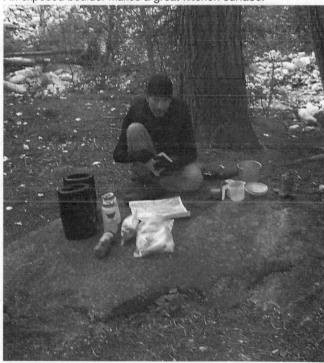

Drinks

Chai

In India, the word chai (like the word curry) describes a family of spices that go well with each other, rather than a specific recipe. You can buy mixes or make your own. A variety of the following ingredients add delicious zest to hot milk, chocolate, coffee, or tea, and big smiles to your campmates' faces: dry milk, cardamom, nutmeg, cinnamon, cloves, black pepper, cocoa, or anise.

Foods that Travel Well

Nearly every grocery store has a wide variety of dried foods that will work great on the trail. Here's a list of foods that travel well

Repackage Your Food

Before you pack your food, remove all extra packaging—foil, plastic, cardboard, etc. Not only are you cutting down on unnecessary weight, you're also reducing litter on the trail. Repackage everything into bags or other containers (I like empty plastic peanut butter jars).

For cereals, pasta, and powdery stuff, simple plastic bags work great. Tie a knot in the top to seal (not too tight!). Ziploc bags can clog. When in doubt, double-bag. Avoid twisty-ties, because they'll inevitably become litter in the backcountry.

For spices, oils, and other liquids, use small screw-top bottles (well-rinsed hotel shampoo bottles are my favorite). Avoid flip tops at all costs; they *will* open and spill over everything.

Label bottles and bags with a permanent marker.

Pack each day's meals—or all breakfasts, lunches, and dinners—together, in larger plastic grocery bags or stuff sacks. Include instructions in the bags.

to give you some ideas. The following list is by no means comprehensive; your own culture, tastes, favorite recipes, and ingenuity can easily expand this list in a variety of delicious ways.

Breakfast

➤ Cereals, hot or cold: High-volume cereals take up a lot of room, and they turn to powder when crushed. Granola, muesli, oatmeal, Cream of Wheat, Zoom, grits, and other denser cereals travel better.

➤ Powdered milk: I prefer Milkman.

➤ Bagels, rolls, muffins, tortillas, dense breads: Fluffy sandwich bread is bulky, turns stale quickly, and is fragile. Crumbs aren't good for sandwiches, but they make good additions to soup at night.

➤ Cream cheese or peanut butter.

➤ Powdered eggs with cheese, diced, dehydrated vegetables (dice onions and peppers at home and dehydrate them for the trip), and sausage or other cured meat.

➤ Hash browns.

➤ Fruit: Fresh or dried.

➤ Breakfast bars, Pop-Tarts, or other nutrition bars.

➤ Pancakes: Carry syrup in a well-sealing bottle with screw-top lid.

➤ Leftovers from last night's dinner.

Drinks

➤ Hot: Coffee, cocoa, tea, chai, lemonade and flavored Jell-O (really!).

➤ Cold: Powdered lemonade, Crystal Light, Tang, apple cider, Gatorade (or other electrolyte-replacement powders), Kool-Aid or other flavored drinks, Emergen-C.

Lunch and Snacks

➤ Energy or nutrition bars.

➤ Gorp, trail mix, nuts, or seeds.

➤ Dried fruit or fruit leather: Apple, raisins, prune, mango, papaya, pineapple, dates, coconut, etc.

➤ Rolls, tortillas, pita, or crackers.

➤ Peanut butter or other nut butters: Almond, sesame, walnut, etc.

➤ Jerky or other dried or canned fish or meat: Because of their unnecessary water weight and heavy trash from their packages, canned foods are not good for backpacking, unless you don't mind carrying a 100-pound pack. On shorter trips, canned meats and fish add savory and easy nutrition to any meal; but they're still heavy, they can leave behind serious smell, and you must pack out heavier garbage. Aim for jerkies and other cured meats instead. Textured vegetable protein (TVP) is a bland but lightweight alternative protein source for soups and sauces (bring bullion or other spices to help flavor it).

➤ Cheese: It's tasty, it helps make less-than-perfect foods more palatable (when in doubt, add cheese), and it provides welcome protein and fat—good for every meal. Low-fat cheeses like Parmesan and mozzarella travel best because the grease doesn't separate in heat and they resist spoiling better than other cheeses. If you're careful (double-bag them, and carry them deep in your pack to insulate them from the heat), you can carry cream cheese, feta, cheddar, gorgonzola, brie, havarti, and other fine favorites into the wild.

➤ Hummus, pesto, sun-dried tomatoes, and other spreads.

➤ Cookies, chocolate, muffins, and/or other sweets. Mmmm, love sugar and salt!

Dinner

➤ Pasta: Ramen and other noodles.

➤ Rice: Whole-grain rice takes time and fuel to cook; buy instant or pre-cook and dehydrate your rice at home; quick-cooking couscous is a great substitute.

➤ Tortillas, nan, chapattis, pita, and other flat breads.

➤ Other grains such as bulgur or polenta.

➤ Instant mashed potatoes: Make a mountain o' mash, and pour your favorite soup or sauce over the top, fry up potato pancakes, or use them as a thickener for soups and sauces.

➤ Beans: Black beans, lentils, etc.

➤ Powdered soups and sauces: Powdered soups, bullion cubes or packets, miso, and tomato base powder are all great for a quick, hot drink or to augment your regular soup or sauce. Pour into water as base for rice, couscous, or potatoes.

➤ Canned or cured meats or textured vegetable protein (TVP).

➤ Dried veggies: Onions, peppers, mushrooms, peas, carrots, and squash.

➤ Fresh garlic: Adds zing to food, and it keeps bugs away—other campers, too, unless you're all eating it together.

Dessert

➤ Chocolate: High in fat and antioxidants.

➤ Instant Jell-O or pudding.

➤ Cake: If you have an oven, it's easy to make many store-bought cakes mixes that require only water. From gingerbread and devil's food to cheesecake and carrot cake, numerous cake recipes are surprisingly easy and tasty.

WILDERNESS WISDOM

Not only do chocolate, coffee, and tea give you extra spring in the morning along the trail, caffeine also boosts your body's endurance. What's more, these items contain antioxidants to help your body recover from a hard day's hike.

Efficient Cooking

How quickly water boils and meals cook in the backcountry depend on many factors, including the ambient air temperature, the elevation, the amount of water and its starting temperature, and the efficiency of heat transfer from your stove to your pot, which in itself depends on several factors, including your stove's efficiency, wind (and what protection you provide against it), and the shape and color of your cooking pots. Here are a few tips to make your cooking efficient:

➤ Cover your pot and use heat reflectors, wind screens, and heat exchangers. Use caution with canister stoves because reflecting too much heat to the fuel bottle could result in unwanted fireworks.

➤ Use pots with curved bottoms, which facilitate heat transfer.

➤ Blacken your pots with soot or black stove paint (available at hardware stores), because dark surfaces absorb heat better than shiny metal.

➤ Keep liquid-propane gas (LPG) canisters warm in your jacket or sleeping bag until you're ready to cook.

➤ Clean your liquid-fuel stove. Carbon residue can clog fuel assemblies and seriously reduce efficiency.

➤ Use clean fuel. White gas and other fuels degrade when exposed to air. Store in air-tight bottles.

➤ Maintain pressure in your fuel bottle. As you burn liquid fuel, air space in the bottle increases, reducing the pressure. Keep pumping as you cook (don't spill the pot while you're pumping).

➤ Plan your meals ahead of time. Have ingredients ready, and know what to do with them once the stove is lit.

➤ For small groups and one-pot meals, boil all the water you'll need for your meal at once. Pour off water for drinks, then use the rest of the water for your main meal.

How Much Fuel to Bring

Carry too much fuel, and you're stuck with unnecessary weight. Come up short, and you face inconvenience at best, and a life-threatening situation in cold weather.

Camp stove manufacturers provide "burn time," which tells how long a stove will run at full blast with a full fuel bottle. They will also advertise "boil time," which tells how long it will take a particular stove to boil a liter of water in warm air at sea level. Although these figures will help you compare stoves, don't use them to plan how much fuel to bring backpacking; these numbers, derived in a laboratory under ideal conditions by people trying hard to get you to buy their product, are close to useless in the real world, where there are a lot of factors at play to change those numbers. The following discussion should help.

In general, it takes 3 ounces of liquid fuel (white gas or its equivalent) to boil 2 liters of water each day (a liter for breakfast and one for dinner) for quick-cooking meals and hot drinks for two people in warm to cool weather below 4000 feet. This means you can get by with one medium liquid-propane gas canister (220 to 250 grams) for two people for three days in warm to moderate conditions. Make sure you have the recommended fuel canister for your stove.

Adjust these rules after considering the following factors. When in doubt, bring more fuel until you're familiar with your typical fuel consumption.

Cold temperatures, high elevations, and wind require more fuel. Water boils about 2°F cooler for every 1000 feet you climb in elevation, which means food will take longer to cook because it's cooking at a lower temperature. High elevations also make stoves work less efficiently. Initial water temperature, air temperature, and altitude also affect how long it will take to boil water. During a recent snow camping trip at 9000 feet, with temperatures dropping into the teens, it took nearly 15 minutes to boil water—more than triple the advertised boil time of my MSR XGK stove.

If you're melting snow, plan 15 minutes to melt enough for 2 quarts of water. Plan another 10 to 15 minutes to boil that water. If you're melting snow for water for two people to drink, cook, and eat twice a day, bring 8 ounces of fuel per person per day (pppd). When traveling at high elevations in cold temperatures, bring at least 10 ounces pppd.

Also consider how many meals you will cook. In warm weather, you can cut back on fuel (and cooking time and hassle) by cooking only one meal each day—or none at all.

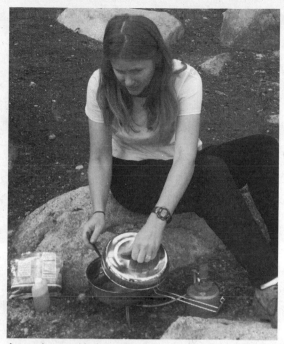

A good camp kitchen will allow you to cook almost anywhere.

How complicated are meals? Is dinner simply a matter of boiling water and pouring it into dehydrated food, or will you be simmering, baking, sautéing, etc.?

Will you need to boil water to disinfect it for drinking?

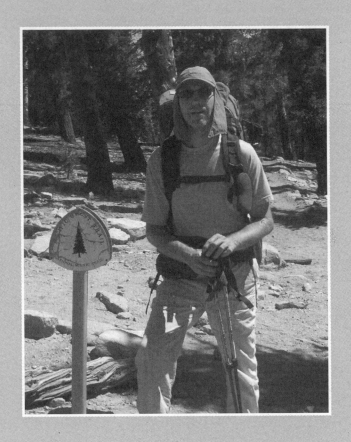

PART IV
PREPARING FOR THE TRAIL

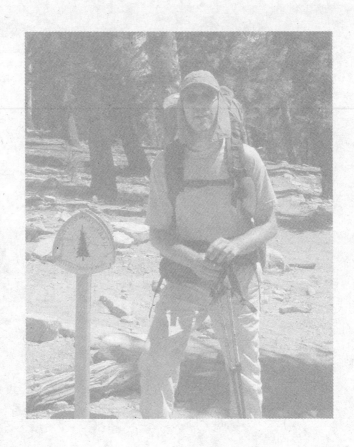

Navigating your way through the backcountry is easy on a beautiful day when you're following a clear trail. But how will you find your way after you accidentally take a wrong turn? When the sun sets long before you reach your destination? When thick fog or a storm sets in? When there's no trail and you're hiking cross-country? Or when someone else in your party gets lost, and you want to know where to start looking?

Wilderness navigation skills are essential, not for perfect days when everything's going well, but for when unplanned situations prevent you from finding the easy way. Just as you (should) have a spare tire, jack, and lug wrench ready for those unplanned flat tires, you should also have a map and compass (and know how to use them) and otherwise know how to move safely and deliberately through the wilderness. To venture into the unforgiving wilderness without these skills is simply asking for trouble.

Choosing the Right Map

When traveling into wild country, it's important to have a map that will help you figure out where you are in the wilderness, and help you follow your chosen route to your destination and back again safely. Some maps are better than others. Here's a breakdown of the most common types of maps available:

Specialized maps. Custom publishers like Trails Illustrated and National Geographic have maps of the most popular national parks and other destinations. If you're hiking in one of these areas, one of these maps will probably suit your needs. Call rangers at your chosen destination to ask their recommendations, as there might be multiple maps from which to choose.

1:100,000-scale maps. These are good for planning longer trips because they cover larger areas (most 1:100,000-scale maps cover 30 by 60 minutes, which is between 1500 and 2200 square miles—see note below), but they may not be detailed enough to help you navigate convoluted terrain.

Note: Because longitudinal lines meet at the poles and are farther apart at the equator, there is no standard distance for one degree longitude—it can range anywhere between 0 and 69 miles. This makes mapping an inconsistent science and confusing to explain here. For example, at 30 degrees latitude, 1:100,000-scale maps cover 2240 square miles; at 49 degrees latitude, they cover 1568 square miles.

USGS 7.5-minute maps. Also called 1:24,000-scale maps, these provide useful detail for smaller areas (at 30 degrees latitude, 7.5-minute maps cover 64 square miles; at 49 degrees latitude, they cover 49 square miles), but several maps may be necessary to cover your chosen trip. If you don't find a specialized map of the area you're planning to backpack, it's likely you'll be using these maps for navigation.

Maps on CD. Publishers like National Geographic, which produces Topo!, and Mapquest, have maps on CD for entire states, as well as for specific national parks, wilderness areas, and regions. These maps on CD are helpful for many reasons: They allow you to explore entire regions seamlessly (no taping maps together on the floor), zoom back and forth between different map scales, draw in routes and add landmarks, get distance and elevation profiles for your route, and create digital or paper maps to share with your hiking partners and take on your trip.

Many outdoor equipment stores now have kiosks that let you print out exactly the map you need. Call your favorite local store to find out if there's one in your area.

Remember, maps can be wrong or poorly labeled. Trails on the map may have disappeared through nonuse, or more trails may have been created since the map was published. Also, flashy-looking maps don't necessarily provide the information you'll need on your trip. If you're choosing between different maps of your chosen destination, ask rangers or other experts which map they prefer.

It's also important to know how to use your map, otherwise it's just a piece of paper taking up space in your backpack. Before you head into the wild, make a point to learn map and compass skills, so you'll know how to read a map correctly. A basic primer follows.

How to Use a Map and Compass

Maps and compasses are valuable tools for wilderness navigation, but they're only as good as your ability to use them. Of the two, maps are far more important. Compasses can tell you which direction you're looking, but maps can tell you where you are and where to go—if you know how to read them. And if you know where you are on a map (and which way is north), you don't need a compass.

About Your Map

The basics of reading maps are straightforward: A map is a two-dimensional picture of a three-dimensional landscape. Maps have several important features you will need to understand to use them effectively:

Scale. Accurate maps are drawn to scale. For example, on a 1:24,000-scale map, 1 inch represents 24,000 inches on the ground. Larger-scale maps (1:100,000, for example)

Map key showing declination

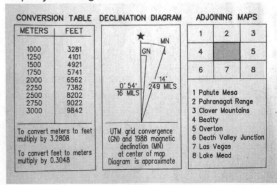

show more area but less detail; smaller-scale maps show more detail of a smaller area. Each map's scale is printed somewhere on the map's margin.

Bar scales. Usually in threes, these indicate map distance in miles, feet, and kilometers.

Adjacent map finder. Somewhere on your map, you'll find either a tic-tac-toe-style grid (usually on the margin) showing your map's name in the center and adjacent maps' names in the adjoining squares, or adjoining maps' names at the center and corners of your map's margins.

Contour lines. Topographic maps depict three-dimensional landscapes with contour lines. Each line follows a single elevation. The on-the-ground change in elevation between any two lines (called contour intervals) is consistent, usually 40 or 100 feet, or 50 meters for metric maps (the contour interval is listed somewhere on the margin of every map). Somewhere along darker contour lines, you can often find the elevation, which is marked in either meters or feet (to convert meters to feet, multiply by 3.2).

When contour lines are close together, the land is steep; when they're farther apart, the land is flatter. Peaks and summits are often easiest to identify, because they show as concentric circles. They also often have the peak's elevation and name if the landmark is prominent.

It can be challenging to differentiate ridge lines from drainages because each of these features can create similar V or U shapes in the contour lines. The key is to look for rivers and streams, which are depicted by blue solid (perennial) or dashed (seasonal) lines running perpendicular to V- or U-shaped contour lines. Because water never runs down the nose of a ridge, you know you've found a drainage.

When your trail runs parallel to contour lines, your hike will be level. When it cuts perpendicularly across contour lines, you'd

better have strong legs and lungs, because the trail is steep!

If you're still confused about contour lines, the following exercise might help: Choose a rock that is the size of your fist or larger. Dip it halfway into water, then use a crayon or pencil to trace the waterline. Dip it one inch deeper, then trace the water line again, and so on until you've submerged the rock entirely. Now take it out, let it dry, and look at the rock from above. Each line represents a different elevation and follows the contours of the rock. If the Great Flood returns, fills the world, then retreats in 50-foot increments, the remaining water lines would look like a topographic map in 3D.

Real Terrain vs. Map Terrain

Both the 1:24,000-scale map and photo below show the same terrain on the northern slope of Mt. Whitney in Sequoia National Park. By comparing them, you can see how the map depicts the landscape.

This photo was taken roughly where the diamond is on the map, looking in the direction of the arrows. Notice how the contour lines depict the features on the land—the small lakes with the steep ridge and peak beyond them. Notice how the contour lines are farther apart at the bottom of the valley and closer together when the land gets steep.

Notice also that maps don't tell you everything you need to know—whether the walking will be smooth and easy or rocky and treacherous to ankles and knees, as it was here.

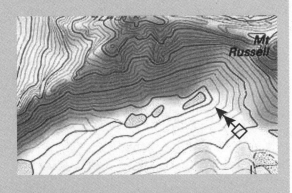

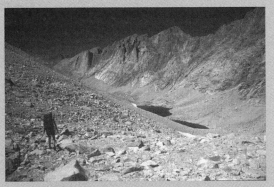

Latitude, longitude, and UTM coordinates. Cartographers long ago covered the globe with a grid that allows any spot on the planet to be described with precise coordinates. All quality maps will have lots of little numbers along their margins to indicate these gridlines. There are two standard grids: Latitude/Longitude (lat/long) and Universal Transverse Mercator (UTM).

Latitude, denoted along the left and right margins of the map, mark the distance north or south of the equator. Latitude measurements are somewhere between 0 and 90 degrees. Longitude, marked along the top and bottom sides of the map, is the distance east or west from an arbitrary (but standard) line running between the poles through London. Longitude measurements are somewhere between 0 and 180 degrees west (North and South America and other places west of London) or east (Europe, Asia, Australia, and other places east of London). For mapping navigation, each degree of latitude and longitude is divided into 60 minutes, and each minute is divided into

UTM grid

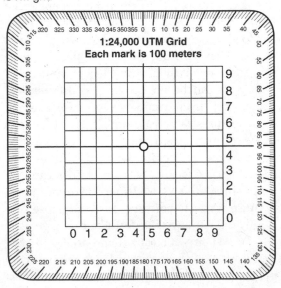

10 decimal-minutes, to help make coordinates more precise.

For instance, the lat/long coordinates for the summit of California's Mt. Whitney (the Lower 48's highest peak, and a great hike!) would look like this:

Latitude 27° 59' 17" N; Longitude 86° 55' 31" W

At each corner of quality topographic maps are the lat/long coordinates at that point. Lat/long coordinates are measured along the edges in 1- or 5-minute increments, depending on the scale of the map.

The UTM system is a metric grid that divides the world into 60 north-south zones. Within each zone, a coordinate is measured in meters north from the equator (called a northing) and in meters east from a central meridian (called an easting). UTMs are preferred by some because they experience less distortion than lat/long measurements. Maps show UTM gridlines spaced 1000 meters (1 kilometer, or 0.62 mile) apart. Use vertical UTM lines to measure your position east and west; use horizontal UTM lines to measure your position north and south. Knowing your UTM zone is most important when using your Global Positioning System (GPS) unit. (It's also important to know which map datum your map is based on, especially if you're communicating your coordinates to other people. Learn about this in the section on setting your map datum on page 135.)

The UTM coordinates of Mt. Whitney's summit (using NAD 83, a term that will make sense once you read about map datum) would look like this: 38.664 E; 40.486 N.

For more about using your GPS, see page 134.

About Your Compass

A compass consists of a base plate, needle (the moving red needle always points to magnetic north, or a nearby piece of metal), the rotating compass housing (marked with degrees and the four cardinal directions—North/0°, East/90°, South/180°, and West/270°), and an arrow-shaped box in which you can frame the compass needle. These are the only parts you need for basic navigation. Any other features on your compass are bells and whistles that are not necessary for most backpacking needs and require explanations beyond the scope of this book.

One of the most important things to know about your compass is that the red needle does not point to the North Pole; it points to magnetic north, which is in the Canadian Arctic about 1000 miles south of the North Pole. Magnetic north is not a giant magnetic rock or other geological feature. Rather, it's a focal point of energy—a complicated interaction between the Earth's mass, rotation, gravity, and the larger electromagnetic forces of the universe—a topic that's *waaaay* beyond the scope of this book.

This map is aligned to true north.

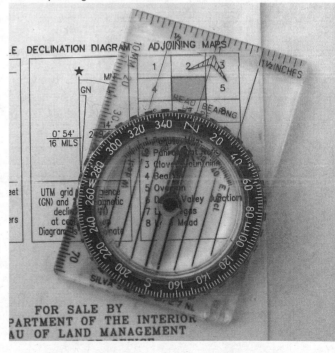

Luckily, these grander details don't matter when it comes to using your map and compass, as long as you can determine the difference between "true" north at the North Pole and magnetic north, which is pretty simple.

In some places, there's little difference between where the vertical lines on your map are pointing (i.e. "true north"/the North Pole) and where your compass needle is pointing (magnetic north). In other places, the difference can be significant enough to get you lost. Consider this extreme example: You're wandering on the sea ice somewhere between magnetic north and the North Pole. Your compass needle will be pointing south and away from true north, despite the fact that you are hundreds of miles south of the North Pole. Most of us will never have this problem to solve.

Maps help you compensate for this difference between true and magnetic north by providing a declination diagram, which is located somewhere in your map's margin. It can help you orient your map to true north, the North Pole.

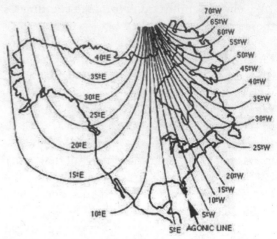

This diagram shows how inaccurate your compass needle will be in different locations in North America.

Putting Map and Compass Together

Orienting your map. Adjusting for true north is easy: Lay your map flat (make sure it's not near any metal objects that might fool your compass needle and you, such as car hoods, metal posts, or bolts on a picnic table). Then place the straight-edge side of your compass base plate directly along the "MN" (magnetic north) line of your declination diagram, located somewhere in the margin of your map. Turn the rotating compass housing until the arrow-shaped box points forward (at this point, the arrow on your housing, the arrow on your base plate, the edge of your compass base plate, and the "MN" line on the map should all point in the same direction). Now rotate your map and compass together until the red compass arrow is framed neatly by the arrow-shaped box on the housing (and pointing the same direction

as the arrows on the compass, the edge of the base plate, and the MN line). Your map is oriented to "true" north (i.e. the North Pole).

If you're a stickler for precision, prepare to be frustrated. If your map is more than a few years old, its magnetic declination isn't accurate because magnetic north travels about 25 miles each year. If you have an older map, your declination symbol could be off by a few degrees. Luckily, for most places on the planet, close is good enough. (The illustration above shows the general declination for different parts of North America. It's helpful to note that everywhere east of the agonic line shown on the diagram (on this line, true north and magnetic north are the same), compass needles point too far west; everywhere west of the agonic line, needles point too far east.)

Taking a bearing. This is an easy way to take a bearing of an object (a mountain, other landmark, or your destination) in the distance. This works whether the landmark is visible or not, as long as you know where you are on the map.

First, orient your map and compass to true north as described earlier. With a pencil, draw a line from the center of the desired landmark to your current location (fold down the edge of your map to use as a straightedge). While keeping both map and compass oriented, place the center of your compass dial on your exact location on the map. The number on your compass dial where it meets the line you just drew is your bearing. It might be 47 degrees (roughly northeast), 225 degrees (roughly southwest), or another number on the dial.

Bearings are most useful for cross-country travel (where there is no trail) or for figuring out your position on a map through triangulation (more on this next). If you are navigating using a bearing, sight a landmark on this bearing, hike to it, then repeat to the next landmark until you arrive at your destination. If you cannot see your landmark, hike while following the bearing number on your compass.

Triangulating your position. If you're not sure where you are on a map, but you have a clear view of prominent landmarks in the distance, you can triangulate your position to determine where you are on a map. Here's how:

First, using your compass, orient yourself to true north. Next, find a prominent landscape feature (major mountains and other formations make this part easiest) in the distance and determine the direction of the landmark relative to north by reading the number on your compass. Let's say that you have determined that your landmark is at 35 degrees. Now, with your map oriented to north, find that landmark on your map. Next, take a pencil and draw a line from the landmark across your map at the angle of your bearing (which would be 35 degrees, in the example above). Next, find another major landmark somewhere else on the horizon (it's helpful if the new landmark is at least 45 degrees away from the bearing line you just drew). Take its bearing, then draw a

second line from the second landmark across your map along the new bearing you've established. Where the two lines intersect is your position. If you're unsure about your position, add bearing lines from additional landmarks, all of which will converge at your position.

Finding your map coordinates. Assuming you know exactly where you are on your map, and that latitude/longitude and/or UTM coordinates are marked along the map's margins, this method will help you establish the precise coordinates of your position. You can then communicate these coordinates to rescuers to help them find you, or to partners when planning a rendezvous. You can also use this method to determine the coordinates of a desired destination in the wilderness, then enter the coordinates of your destination into your GPS unit, and have it lead you reliably to your location—an advantage when hiking cross-country.

First, use a pencil to mark your position. Second, fold the map down so the top edge of the paper lies horizontally across your exact position. Square the fold—no diagonal lines allowed! Third, mark the point where the top edge of the paper meets either the right or left margin of the map, where the coordinates are printed, then unfold the map. Now, fold the map vertically from the left or right so the edge lies vertically across your position. Square the fold, and mark where the edge crosses the top (or bottom) margin of the map.

Next, read the lat/long or UTM markings along the edge of the map, and write down the coordinates of each mark, doing your best to estimate where the marks are between the nearest UTM or lat/long coordinates along the edge. All coordinates along the top and bottom margins of your map run east-west; all coordinates along the left and right margins run north-south.

This method will help you determine coordinates that are precise enough for most needs. If accuracy is important, get yourself a UTM grid overlay and map ruler—available for $3 to $5 from www.maptools.com. Make sure these tools match the scale of your map.

The best way to improve your map and compass skills is to practice. The next time you're in dramatic country with a large, unobstructed view, pull out your map, orient it, and see how everything matches up. Make this a regular habit during your backpacking trips (good excuse for a rest stop!). This practice will help you get better at seeing the landscape through the lines. Compare the peaks, ridges, rivers, canyons, and other major landmarks with the map to see how they are depicted. Study the trail on the map. Figure out where your route will take you in relation to the real-world landmarks you can see. Note rivers, creeks, peaks, trail intersections, and other landmarks you can use as "handrails" to help you gauge your progress and stay on route. While you're hiking, frequently ask yourself and others, "Which way is north?" Regular practice of this develops a stronger sense of direction.

Finally, keep in mind that no map precisely represents terrain. What looks like a gentle slope on the map might be covered with impenetrable shrubs. Or what looks like a gently sloping canyon might in fact be a series of impassible 20-foot cliffs and ledges that don't register on a map with 40-foot contour lines. And yes, the trail that's clear on the map might long ago have disappeared through nonuse—or new trails might have been created that don't appear on your map.

About Global Positioning Systems

First, a warning: These modern tools can make navigation easier, but they also pose definite risks because they are subject to failure in several different ways. Satellite readings are often inaccurate. Reception can be difficult in thick forests or narrow canyons. And what will you do when the batteries run out, if you drop the unit, or if it otherwise malfunctions? Although GPS units have many valuable uses, I don't like them for backpacking; they draw my attention to the LED readout and not to the landscape. Many people rely too much on GPS, only to find themselves frighteningly lost when the device fails. I never carry one when backpacking recreationally, which saves me weight and money.

A GPS unit is no substitute for a good map and map-reading skills. When it works correctly, it will give you coordinates for where you are, but you need a map and the skill to plot those coordinates and determine your position. For backpacking at least, every GPS unit should carry the following warning: For entertainment purposes only.

Warnings and grumblings aside, here are instructions on how to use your GPS unit.

Using Your GPS Unit

This section explains the general steps necessary to navigate with a GPS unit. For details on operating your particular device, refer to the manufacturer's instructions.

The Global Positioning System originally was developed by the US military to track the positions of ground troops. GPS units communicate with satellites to triangulate the unit's position on the ground. By plotting the coordinates your GPS unit receives from satellites on an accurate topographic map, you can determine your position relatively accurately.

Initialize your GPS. After turning on your unit, initialize it by entering your approximate latitude and longitude, date, and time. (If you don't know your latitude and longitude, go to www.maporama.com, enter your address in the maps section, click go, and presto! It will appear on the map that pops up.)

Choose either latitude/longitude (lat/long) or UTM coordinates. You can set your

GPS to read and display one type of coordinates over the other. Check your map to see if it uses one or the other. Most modern maps have both. Also, check with other people who might be using a GPS in the same area to make sure you're both using the same type of coordinates.

Look at the lower right-hand corner of your map, where you'll find the lat/long coordinates at that point. Changes in lat/long or UTM are measured along the edges of your map—top and bottom for east-west changes, and left and right edges for north-south changes.

Set your map datum. All maps are produced to meet lat/long and UTM standards, but standards change depending on the map you're using and where you are. Most maps in North America use either North American Datum (NAD) 27, NAD 83, or World Geodetic System (WGS) 84. Quality topo maps will tell you which datum they use. Follow your GPS's setup instructions (your manual might be helpful here) to make sure it reads the same datum as your map.

As an example of how confusing things can be if your map and GPS are each set to different datum, let's look again the UTM coordinates of Mt. Whitney, which I mentioned earlier. Using NAD 83, the UTM coordinates of Whitney's summit look like this: 38.664 E; 40.486 N. But using WGS 84 datum, the UTM coordinates of Whitney are 36.578; -118.292—not at all the same. If you need precise coordinates—and why bother with coordinates if you don't need to be precise?—it's important to make sure your map and GPS unit are both using the same datum. Wherever you travel in the world, you will need to reset your GPS map datum to agree with the map you're using.

Set your GPS unit to read true north. Using the navigation setup screen on your GPS unit, you can program your unit to read according to true north. Now your unit agrees with your map and compass.

Set the waypoints. Waypoints are simply the recorded coordinates of a particular place. You can record a waypoint in your GPS unit's computer in two ways: by entering the coordinates of a desired destination, or by recording the coordinates of your current location.

The GPS "go to" function. This function points the way to any waypoint programmed into your GPS, telling you which direction to go and how far away it is. This is useful for finding your way to a chosen destination, or for finding your way back to camp (if you marked it as a waypoint) after a dayhike.

To save batteries, use your GPS to establish distance and bearing to a waypoint, then use your compass to keep you on that bearing until you get there.

If accuracy is important, take a few extra minutes to confirm that your GPS, compass, and map agree by orienting your map to true north, using your GPS to measure your current coordinates, finding those coordinates on your map, then using your compass to double-check your bearing to your waypoint.

It's important to remember that all compass and GPS bearings are "as the crow flies." Actually getting to your destination can be difficult if mountains, cliffs, thick brush, or steep ravines are in the way.

Your brain is the most important thing you carry into the wilderness. Your body simply follows orders, and the rest of your equipment is limited by how well you use it. Your safety and happiness on the trail come down to how well you prepare for contingencies, and the decisions you make while you're out there. This section will discuss different skills you can practice to ensure your safety and enjoyment while backpacking.

Developing a Wilderness Mindset

The best cure for backcountry disasters is prevention—anticipating and being prepared for contingencies and making safe choices. Most wilderness injuries and fatalities occur because people make unsafe decisions, which are easy to make when hunger, fatigue, frustration, confusion, or panic are preventing you from thinking clearly. Sometimes accidents come out of the blue, but often awareness and caution allow you to avert danger before it happens.

To assess and evaluate risk in the backcountry, think about your backpacking trip as a mathematical equation. Whitewater rafters and kayakers, rock climbers, and some backcountry skiers assess the difficulty and risk of their activities on a scale of 1 (low difficulty and low potential for serious consequences if something goes wrong) to 5 (high difficulty and high potential for serious consequences if something goes wrong).

Using this same 1-to-5 scale, assign a number to every variable on your next backpacking trip—your fitness level, experience, equipment, level of preparedness, knowledge of the area, hiking partners (and their fitness levels, experience, and preparedness), the terrain, weather, season, elevation, types of plants and animals in the area, etc. The more 1s and 2s you have, the lower the risk; the more 4s and 5s you have, the higher the risk. Compensate for higher risk values by preparing better and being more cautious while you're out there.

WILDERNESS WISDOM

Rock climbers use the term "exposure" to describe the level of risk they face when climbing. High exposure means there's nothing but a whole lot of empty space between you and the ground far below—meaning dangerous, possibly fatal, consequences if you fall. When you're backpacking, think about your exposure to danger based on poor fitness, poor planning, bad decisions, weather, terrain, wildlife, etc. How can you minimize your exposure to these dangers?

Next, think about specific risk factors:

Watch the weather and react accordingly to minimize the risks it presents. Is it sunny and clear? Put on sunscreen. Cold and windy? Put on extra layers. Are thunderheads building, or is there a winter storm blowing in from the north? Get off exposed ridges. Make camp low before the storm hits. How soon is the sunset, and can you make it to camp before then? Either pick up the pace or plan to camp sooner if you can't.

Assess and react to other environmental risks. Are you on a wide, well-marked trail, or traveling cross-country over rough terrain? Are you only a few miles from the trailhead in a popular national park, or days from anywhere in the middle of nowhere?

Assess your equipment. Does your stove work reliably, or is it sometimes uncooperative? Would your tent offer superior protection against a surprise blizzard, or is it old, tired, and flimsy? Are you limping along with broken boots or a ripped backpack? Did you forget your rain shell?

Assess human factors. Are you and others in your party in good shape? Are you all experienced backpackers? Do you know the area well, or is this unfamiliar terrain? How is everyone getting along? Is your leader capable and responsible? Are their rivalries, tensions, or fears that might contribute to poor decisions? Is everyone cold and tired? Is anyone sick?

With each of the risk factors described above, what can you do to minimize risk by planning better or reacting differently to changing conditions? Keep in mind that accidents happen suddenly. You're walking along on a beautiful day, everything's fine, then all of a sudden, everything changes—you twist your ankle, slip on a wet rock, trip over an exposed root, or round a bend in the trail and come face-to-face with a bear. Attention and awareness can keep safe and stable situations from turning dangerous.

The Value of Preparing Well

Only three types of events happen in the wilderness: things you can predict—cold weather in winter, heat and mosquitoes in summer, dirty hands, etc.; things you can't predict but which shouldn't catch you by surprise if they happen—twisted ankles, surprise storms, having the sunset catch you far from camp, rockfall, animals getting into your food; and out-of-the-blue situations that no one can predict.

Although it's impossible to plan and prepare for everything this complex universe might throw at you, proper planning and preparation will arm you to manage most, if not all, situations that occur in the backcountry. That's a pretty good start.

Planning well for the unique demands of backcountry travel also lessens the impact you leave on the land. For example, neglecting to bring warm clothes into the mountains might force you to build a large fire to keep yourself warm, creating a visual scar on the landscape, depleting wood, and risking the possibility of wildfire.

Each landscape has its own unique character. Wherever you plan to travel—whether to a lush rainforest, labyrinthine desert canyon, high-mountain meadow, a forested river, or coastal wetland—each landscape will respond differently to your presence. Become knowledgeable and aware of how each environment is sensitive so you can travel lightly, make sound judgments, and avoid unnecessary impacts. Regardless of where you're planning your next backpacking trip, contact Leave No Trace (www.lnt.org; 800-332-4100), which publishes pamphlets about the character and demands of particular environments—rivers, deserts, forests, and high mountains.

In dynamic situations, and situations that have high potential to shift suddenly in a dangerous direction, use particular caution.

Is your situation relatively predictable, or is it capable of changing quickly? Are you hiking across a meadow, or fording a deep river? Enjoying a sunny afternoon, or is a storm rolling in?

Quickly changing situations carry more risk than stable ones. And when multiple high-risk factors conspire (if you have lots of 4s and 5s in your risk equation), your level of risk increases dramatically. For example, inexperienced hikers in cold weather, with no map, poor equipment, and no water left is a recipe for disaster. Your old boots might hold well on dry granite, but mossy rocks in the rain?

After evaluating your risks, work to minimize them. Trust your instincts. Make certain you can walk away from your mistakes.

Leave No Trace

In 1800, the US population was about 5.3 million people; in 1900, it was roughly 76 million. In 2006, it passed the 300-million mark. The Earth's population is now 6.5 billion.

As our population grows, we convert our natural landscapes into houses, farms, asphalt, and strip malls. To escape these modern

Avoid trampling fragile plants and soils.

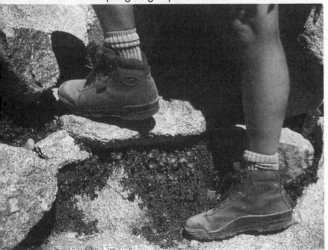

conveniences, increasing numbers of people venture into our last wild places to enjoy the beauty and challenge of nature. In the good old days, it was possible to find solitude, beauty, clean water, and little trace of other people in the backcountry. Today, those luxuries are getting harder and harder to find.

Annual visitation to Yosemite National Park exceeded a million in 1954. In the mid-1990s, visitation topped 4 million per year. Annual visitation in Yellowstone National Park grew from 5438 in 1905 to more than 3 million annual visitors in 1992. More than 4 million people visit the Grand Canyon each year. Great Smoky National Park, the nation's most-visited national park, experiences nearly 9 million visitors each year.

These parks experience more visitors than other places, but the trends are similar in wild places everywhere. Wherever visitation increases, so do the scars people leave in the backcountry—litter, trampled plants and trails, distressed wildlife populations, trashy-looking campsites, and polluted water. Although pristine landscapes still exist, they're disappearing like snow in the hot August sun, trampled by millions of pairs of adoring, well-intentioned people in hiking boots. We can preserve the quality of our last wild places only by minimizing our impacts when we visit.

Since 1965, the National Outdoor Leadership School (NOLS) has worked to develop practices and methods backcountry travelers can use to leave no trace when traveling in wilderness. This backcountry wisdom has been distilled into seven principles of wilderness ethics to minimize our impacts on the backcountry.

Principles of Leave No Trace

The following Leave No Trace principles were developed by NOLS and are currently maintained and improved by the Leave No Trace Center for Outdoor Ethics. Details on how these apply in the backcountry are incorporated into the relevant chapters in this book. By taking these principles to heart, you are arming yourself with the power to leave a beautiful world to your grandchildren and theirs.

Plan ahead and prepare. Know the regulations and special concerns for the area you'll visit. Prepare for extreme weather, hazards, and emergencies. This will help you prevent unnecessary impact by cutting down a tree for a signal fire, for example. Schedule your trip to avoid times of high use and visit in small groups. Split larger parties into groups of four to six. Repackage food to minimize waste. Use a map and compass, or GPS, to eliminate the use of marking paint, rock cairns, or flagging.

Travel and camp on durable surfaces. Durable surfaces include established trails and campsites, as well as rock, gravel, dry grasses, or snow. Protect riparian areas by camping at least 200 feet from lakes and streams. Good campsites are found, not made; altering a site is not necessary.

In popular areas:

➤ Concentrate use on existing trails and campsites.

➤ Walk single file in the middle of the trail, even when it's wet or muddy.

➤ Keep campsites small. Focus activity in areas where vegetation is absent.

In pristine areas:

➤ Disperse use to prevent the creation of campsites and trails.

➤ Avoid places where impacts are just beginning.

Dispose of waste properly. If you pack it in, pack it out. Inspect your campsite and rest areas for trash or spilled foods, and pack out all trash, leftover food, and litter. Deposit solid human waste in cat holes dug 6 to 8 inches deep at least 200 feet from water, camp, and trails. Cover and disguise the cat hole when finished. Pack out toilet paper and hygiene products.

To wash yourself or your dishes, carry water 200 feet away from streams or lakes and use small amounts of biodegradable soap. Scatter strained dishwater.

Leave what you find. Preserve the past: Examine but do not touch cultural or historic structures and artifacts. Also leave rocks, plants, and other natural objects as you find them. Avoid introducing or transporting nonnative species. Do not build structures, furniture, or dig trenches around your tent.

Minimize campfire impacts. Use a lightweight stove for cooking and enjoy a candle lantern for light. Campfires can cause lasting impacts to the backcountry. Where fires are permitted, use established fire rings, fire pans, or mound fires. Keep fires small. Only use sticks from the ground that can be broken by hand. Burn all wood and coals to ash, put out campfires completely, then scatter the cold ashes.

Respect wildlife. Observe wildlife from a distance. Do not follow or approach them. Never feed animals. Feeding wildlife damages their health, alters natural behaviors, and exposes them to predators and other dangers. Protect wildlife and your food by storing

Learn More About Leave No Trace

➤ Leave No Trace: 800-332-4100; www.lnt.org

➤ *Soft Paths*, by Bruce Hampton and David Cole, Stackpole Books

➤ Leave No Trace Skills and Ethics booklet series, each of which addresses LNT challenges of particular regions, such as Rocky Mountains, Southeastern states, western river corridors, temperate coastal zones, desert and canyon country, rock climbing, Alaskan tundra, Northeast mountains, and the Sierra Nevada.

rations and trash securely. Control pets at all times, or leave them at home. Avoid wildlife during sensitive times: mating, nesting, raising young, or winter.

Be considerate of other visitors. Respect other visitors and protect the quality of their experience. Be courteous. Yield to other users on the trail. Step to the downhill side of the trail when encountering pack stock. Take breaks and camp away from trails and other visitors. Let nature's sounds prevail. Avoid loud voices and noises.

Knots You Need to Know

For years, I never bothered to learn any knots, figuring my "granny knots," and whatever variations I could come up with on the spot would meet any needs I might have to tie or secure things in the backcountry. That laziness cost me countless hours of frustration, not to mention the occasional collapsed tent and fallen food bag. Several years ago, I finally decided to learn basic knots to help me perform important common tasks. The following five knots have helped me in a variety of backcountry uses, and I've been thankful ever since. You will be, too.

If you're planning to rock climb, fish, boat, or rescue people in extreme situations, you will need to learn many more knots. But these are a good start for basic backpacking applications. Copy these pages and practice tying these while you're sitting around in camp until you can tie them quickly and easily. Your friends will be impressed by your outdoor skills.

Half-hitch. This quick-and-easy knot, and its simple variations, has many uses—securing light loads, tying off the line that hangs your food in camp, and adding security to existing knots (like a couple of the ones below). Here's how it works:

1. Send the free end of your line around a tree (or through a grommet) to create a bight.

2. Cross the free end over the standing end to create a loop.

3. Send "the rabbit through the hole" by wrapping the free end around the standing end and sending it through the loop you just created. Then cinch it tight by pushing the knot tight up against the tree or grommet to which you're tying.

Variation 1: Double half-hitch. Stack another half-hitch on top of the one you just made. Do this by creating a second loop: Wrap the free end around the standing end once again, this time outside of, or on top of, the knot you just created. Pull the free end through the loop and cinch tight by pushing the second half-hitch tight up against the first.

Variation 2: Quick-release double half-hitch: This is the same as the double half-hitch in variation 1, but with one key difference: Instead of pulling the free end through the second loop, make a bight on the free end, then pull only the bight (not the end) through the loop and cinch it tight, leaving the free end hanging. A quick tug on the free end, and your knot is released. This is a great way to finish off knots yet make them easy to undo when it's time to untie everything.

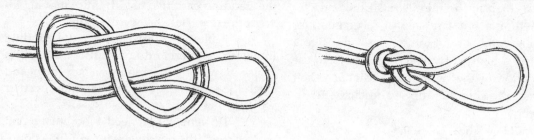

The figure eight on a bight creates a quick, reliable loop.

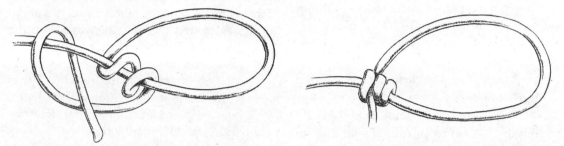

The taut-line hitch allows you to adjust tension on your rope—perfect for tying down tents and shelters.

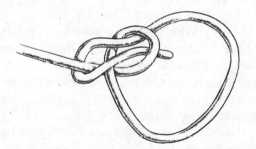

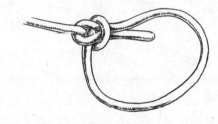

The bowline creates a loop that won't slip closed.

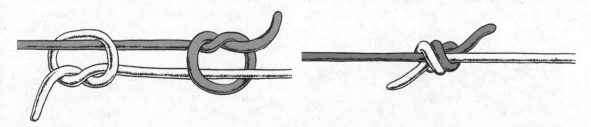

The fisherman's knot is helpful to tie two lengths of rope together.

Figure eight on a bight. If you need a quick loop in the middle or at the end of a rope—to attach a carabiner or other item, for hanging food, or for other uses—the figure eight on a bight is for you. Rock climbers use a variation of the figure eight to attach their harnesses to climbing rope—a testament to its reliability.

Here's how to do it:

1. Fold the line in half to create a bight (the folded end of the rope), with the standing lines pointing up and the bight pointing down.

2. Create a loop by crossing the bight behind the standing lines.

3. Make another loop by crossing the bite in front of the standing lines.

4. To complete the knot, send the bight through the bottom loop. You now have a figure eight knot with a bight at the end.

Taut-line hitch. The taut-line hitch is great for securing tent or shelter guy lines to a stake or a tree. You can slide the knot easily up and down the line to adjust tension, but it holds tight when the line is strained. To make a taut-line hitch:

1. Wrap the free end of your line around a tree or stake, bringing it back to the standing end, creating a bight.

Learn More About Knots

➤ *The Klutz Book of Knots*, by John Cassidy, Klutz

➤ *Knots for the Outdoors*, by Cliff Jacobson, Globe Pequot Press

➤ *Knots for Hikers and Backpackers*, by Frank Logue, Menasha Ridge Press

➤ www.animatedknots.com: This website has helpful animated diagrams to help you get the knots right.

2. Wrap the free end of your line around the standing part, two to four times moving toward the tree/stake inside the loop.

3. Next, tie the free end to the standing line with an overhand knot outside the loops. Finish it with a quick-release half-hitch and cinch the knot by squeezing the knot together with one hand.

Bowline. If you need a loop that won't cinch closed, the bowline is for you. It's popular with rock climbers and rescuers who need to fashion a rescue loop or safety harness. You've probably heard how the rabbit comes out of the hole, goes around the tree, then back into the hole. This is the knot where that happens, and here's how to do it:

1. Several feet from the free end of your rope, wrap the rope once around one hand, while holding palm and fingers flat. Remove your hand, leaving a small loop.

2. Hold the loop level in front of you with one hand (the standing hand). Make sure the rope closest to the free end is crossing over the top of the standing end.

3. With your free hand, grab the free end of the rope (the rabbit). The amount of rope between the small loop in your standing hand and the free end will determine the size of your working loop when the knot is complete. Send the rabbit up through the loop, around the backside of the standing end ("tree"), then back down into the loop.

4. Cinch the knot tight by pulling on the standing end above the knot with one hand, and on both parts of rope from step 3 (the part coming up out of the hole to the tree, and the part going from the tree down into the hole) with the other. Practice will help you make the size of loop you need.

If you don't want a free-hanging loop, but want the bowline to tie off to a branch or post, go back to step 3 and send the rabbit around your branch or post before it goes through the hole and around the "tree." For safety, leave plenty of free end dangling after tying the knot. Add security to slippery plastic or nylon ropes by finishing with a half-hitch or two with the free end/rabbit.

Fisherman's knot. This knot is good for tying two ropes together. Not only do they have a clean, symmetrical look, but the harder you pull on the two ropes, the more secure it becomes. If your ropes are slippery, add a few more loops to each knot to increase security. Note: This doesn't work well with ropes of different diameters. Here's how to make it:

1. Place both lines in front of you, parallel, running left to right, and overlapping by about 18 inches

2. With the free end of line 1, tie an overhand knot around line 2. When done correctly, the free end of line 1 will point toward the standing end of line 2.

3. With line 2, now tie a mirror-image overhand knot around line 1. In true mirror fashion, the free end of line 2 should now point toward the standing end of line 1.

4. Grab the standing end of each rope and pull them apart from each other, cinching the knots together.

Fording Streams

During spring runoff and in well-watered climates, there might not be a bridge over every swollen stream and river, and you might have to ford it to continue on your journey. Here are a few things to consider and a few ways to cross streams and rivers safely:

Make safety your primary consideration. Don't cross above waterfalls, dangerous rapids, submerged trees, or in deep, swift current. Wide and shallow spots are safer than narrow, deep ones. If it looks treacherous, can you go around? Consider hiking up- or downstream to look for safer places to cross—a several-mile detour is better than drowning. If the water is treacherous and you can find no safe crossing spots, consider canceling your plans to cross. Again, changed plans are better than dying.

If you decide to cross, before you enter the water, change into your camp shoes to keep your boots dry. If you don't have camp shoes, decide whether to keep your boots on and protect your feet (soggy boots!), or take your boots off and increase the chances of falling and possibly injuring your feet (if you remove your boots, hang them around your neck, or tie them securely to your pack—hiking barefoot back to the trailhead is no fun if you lose your boots).

Before entering the water, undo your hip belt and loosen your shoulder straps. If you fall, you'll want your pack to come off easily, lest it drag you down to a watery grave.

Trekking poles give you stability when fording streams.

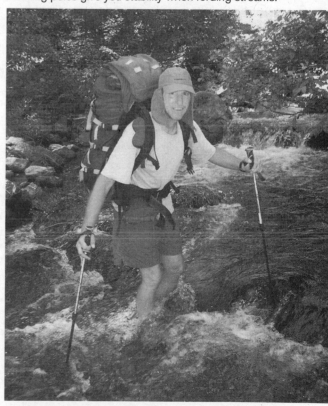

Here are a few ways to cross safely:

Send the strongest member across with a rope. Tie the rope to a tree, so everyone has a taut, secure handrail; cross on the downstream side of the rope, so you don't get tangled up if you fall. Or use a stick or your trekking poles as support. Face upstream, plant your pole(s) firmly upstream before taking each step and lean into it/them for stability.

On riskier crossings, place another member of the party downstream with a long stick or throw-line in case a rescue is needed.

During spring runoff, cross early in the morning, when water levels are lowest; later in the day, the sun will melt more water and raise the level of water and risk.

If you fall in deep, swift water, turn and float head up, facing downstream, and feet first, so your feet can cushion you from rocks or other obstacles. Keep your feet up off the bottom to avoid getting your feet trapped by a submerged rock or log. Swim to shore as you are able.

Preventing Backcountry Crime

When hiking in the backcountry, you're more likely to become a victim of dehydration, hypothermia, or a twisted ankle than the victim of another person. Most trails see less crime than most downtowns. But in rare instances, violent crimes do happen in the wilderness, especially on popular trails near urban areas. Proximity to cities can mean higher rates of alcohol, drugs, and weapons violations. The Angeles National Forest near Los Angeles has a reputation for being the most dangerous national forest in America. Because of their proximity to the Mexican border, Anza-Borrego Desert State Park in California, Organ Pipe National Monument in Arizona, and Big Bend National Monument in Texas are seeing increasing levels of illegal immigration, drug smuggling, and associated violent crime.

The most common crimes in the backcountry are crimes of opportunity, which means your highest chances of becoming a victim are at or near the trailhead (human predators are most often lazy and prefer to drive rather than hike). According to the US Forest Service, the most prevalent crimes at trailheads are car burglaries. Minimize your risk of this by leaving any unnecessary valuables at home.

Luckily, once you're a mile or so down the trail, you're quickly putting distance between you and 99 percent of society's psycho weirdoes (bad intentions are often too heavy to carry in by foot). Although assaults on the trail are extremely rare, you can minimize the risk of becoming a victim in the following ways:

➤ Don't hike alone. Hike with a friend or a large dog.

➤ Be aware. Strange people often act strangely. Trust your instincts. If a situation seems uncomfortable, take steps to avoid or leave it quickly.

➤ Be discreet. Avoid the most popular trails and campsites. Camp off the beaten path.

➤ Maintain psychological distance. Don't reveal much about yourself to strangers.

➤ Consider protection. Pepper spray is a lightweight and affordable way to ward off attackers. And everyone should know a few self-defense tactics to repel attackers.

➤ Report suspicious activity to local law enforcement.

17 GETTING FIT FOR THE TRAIL

Backpacking is rewarding partly because it requires no particular skills. But it is far more demanding than just walking. Carrying your gear on mountain trails requires physical strength, balance, and endurance.

The following exercises will help you get into shape to explore wild and beautiful country, or keep you in shape over those long months until you hike again. They will also help you live longer, look and feel better, fight sickness off with a robust immune system, reduce stress, and enjoy more peace of mind. The exercises in this chapter have been chosen for people of all fitness levels and do not require expensive exercise equipment. So what are you waiting for?

Cardiovascular Exercise

Backpacking requires your muscles, heart, and lungs to work at higher levels for extended times. To do so, your body must be aerobically fit (i.e. it must efficiently convert oxygen from the air into energy for all of your cells). Cardiovascular (cardio = heart; vascular = vessels) fitness requires many things to happen at once: strong lungs and breathing muscles must pull oxygen from the air; blood that's rich in hemoglobin must carry the oxygen; a strong and efficient heart must pump the blood to every cell in the body, delivering nutrition and collecting wastes; and robust blood vessels must manage the heavy traffic. Cardiovascular health means you'll breathe more easily, your heart won't pound itself out of your chest, and your muscles will be less fatigued. In short, your hike will be easier and more enjoyable.

There is no way to prepare for increased cardiovascular activity except through increased cardiovascular activity. Luckily, any exercise that raises your heart rate (see sidebar on page 146 for a discussion on target heart rates) for at least 20 minutes will do the trick, such as walking, jogging, running, bicycling, or your favorite Stairmaster, treadmill, elliptical trainer, rowing machine, or other device. Pick your favorite exercise, or mix them up to keep things interesting. The only equipment you'll need for walking or running is comfortable clothes and proper shoes. Adding music to the mix can put a bounce in your step and help pass the time.

If you've led a sedentary life until now, start gently—two to three times a week, for example. Increase the speed and intensity gradually as you improve. Although any exercise is better than no exercise, three days a week is the accepted minimum for real results; five to six times a week will bring the quickest results. Never work out more than six days a week—always give yourself a day of rest, especially after a hard workout.

Follow Your Heart

It's important to listen to your body. Pick up the pace if you're feeling strong. If you're tired or sluggish, slow down or take a day off. Sometimes, however, how you feel doesn't tell you how hard your body is actually working. If you don't work hard enough, you will never challenge your body enough to get in better shape; push too hard, and you risk burnout or injury.

The best way to tell how hard your body is working is to listen to your heart. Like the tachometer on your dashboard, your pulse tells you how hard your internal engine is actually working. Abundant sports research has shown that working out at 50 to 70 percent of your maximum heart rate (MHR) will most efficiently help you lose weight and get in shape for hiking.

To estimate your MHR, subtract your age from 220. For example, I'm 40 years old. My MHR is 180, so my cardiovascular workouts should keep my heart rate between 90 and 126 for at least 20 minutes. This equation is simple but crude; it does not account for your particular fitness level and medical history. For a more accurate evaluation of your heart rate, consult a personal trainer. If you have concerns about your health, consult your doctor.

After 10 minutes of exercise, take your pulse to determine your heart rate: Stop, place your second and third fingers on your wrist, in the notch between bone and tendon at the base of your thumb (this is your radial pulse). Count your heart beats for 15 seconds, then multiply by 4 to determine your heart rate. If the number is between 50 and 70 percent of your maximum heart rate (220 minus your age), you're making progress toward hiking fitness.

Strength and Balance Exercises

Strength training is an excellent way to build strength and endurance, burn calories, and recover from injuries. As we age, strength training helps maintain bone density, preventing osteoporosis. It will also help you meet the challenges you'll face along the trail. (A note for those of us hoping to trim our waistlines: Because muscles weigh more than fat, you might not lose weight with strength training. But because muscles are trimmer than fat, you'll peel off the inches and look better.)

The muscles around your middle—abdomen, hips, buttocks and back—initiate and support every step, twist, throw, lunge, jump, lean, and reach you make in life. If these core muscle groups are strong and balanced, you will make every move with more power, precision, grace, balance, and confidence. Strong abdomen and back muscles also improve posture and protect your back from twisting and lifting injuries. They also help you look good in a bathing suit. The following exercises will help.

Sit-ups. Sit-ups strengthen your upper abdominals, which support many upper-body movements.

Lie on your back on a firm surface with your legs bent comfortably and feet flat on the floor. With your arms crossed across your chest, slowly curl your chin to your chest, then continue curling your back until your shoulder

Sit-up

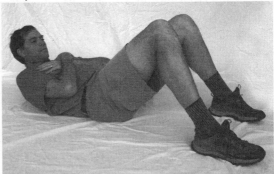

blades are off the floor. Slowly reverse the curl back to starting position. Aim for 20 repetitions.

Penguins. Penguins strengthen the abdominal muscles down your front and sides, which help with sitting, side-to-side motion, and balance.

Penguin

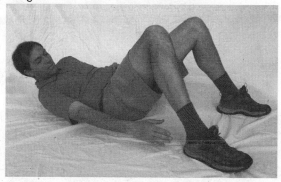

Again, lie on your back on a firm surface with your legs bent comfortably, feet near your buttocks and your arms resting on the floor by your hips. Lift your shoulder blades off the floor. With your right fingertips, reach down and touch your right ankle. Then touch your left ankle with your left fingertips. Back and forth, left, right, left, right. Aim for 20 repetitions on each side. For greater challenge, place your heels farther from your butt.

Easy bridge. This simple yoga pose will help to strengthen your lower back, butt,

Easy bridge

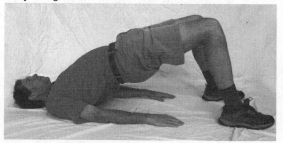

and hips, providing balance to the six-pack you're developing in the front with the exercises already described.

Lie on your back with your legs bent, feet near your butt, and arms straight and flat by your sides. Now lift your pelvis up, squeeze your buttocks and push your pelvis toward the sky. Breathe deeply, and count to 10. Then lower, rest, and repeat three times.

Leg lifts. Leg lifts train the muscles you'll need to lift your boot-heavy legs up a steep trail.

Lie on your back on a firm surface with your legs bent comfortably, feet near your buttocks, and arms straight down by your sides, with palms pressing downward (you'll need your arms for stability). Slowly lift one leg at a time toward your chest, then lower it. Then lift both legs at once. Aim to do each of these

Easy leg lift

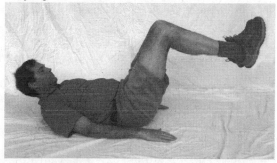

Advanced leg lift

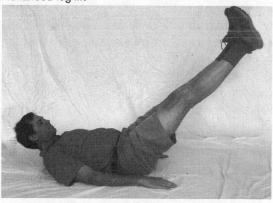

20 times. Pull your belly button toward your spine, and keep your lower back flat on the floor during these lifts to ensure proper form and avoid injury.

For an advanced version of this, straighten your legs. Slowly lift them 3 feet off the floor, then ease them down. Do not attempt if you have lower-back problems.

Bicycles. After a few weeks of sit-ups, leg lifts, and penguins, you should be ready for this advanced ab-burner. Lie on your back with legs straight and hands lightly touching (not grasping) your ears. Curl your head and shoulders up off the floor, then raise your left knee toward your chest until you can touch it with your right elbow. Extend your left leg (don't let it touch the ground) while bringing your right knee up until you can touch it with your left elbow. Then extend the right leg and bring the left leg back to meet your right elbow. Back and forth, over and over—left elbow to right knee, then right elbow to left knee—extending each leg between reps, and all the while keeping head, shoulders, and feet off the floor, and hands lightly touching your ears. Aim for 10 repetitions on each side, then increase the reps to 25, then to 50. Don't be surprised if this burns like the dickens. Lie flat and take deep breaths until the burn fades.

Squats. Squats strengthen many muscle groups and teach them to work as a team— your quads, buttocks, hips, and back. They also build support strength around your knees, which are prime candidates for hiking injuries.

Stand on a firm surface, legs shoulder width apart and weight evenly distributed. While maintaining proper posture (look up toward the ceiling to help with this), bend your legs and lower your buttocks a few inches, then stand back up. Keep your knees in line with your toes.

Beginners should start with shallow squats. Advanced squatters can squat deeper, and/or add weight (start with 3- to 5-pound

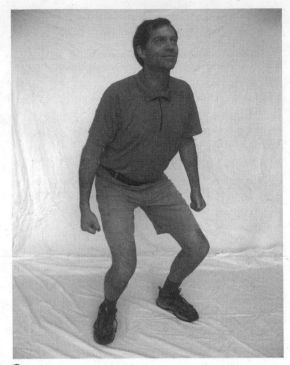

Squat

dumbbells, then increase as you gain strength and confidence. To protect your knees, do not bend them past a 90-degree angle. If your knees hurt, do shallower squats. You can also reduce the weight by supporting yourself with ski or hiking poles. Do this five to 10 times. Stop if you feel pain in your knees or back.

Lunges. Like squats, lunges help your body work as a unit for acceleration and deceleration on the trail. They also improve balance and coordination.

Stand upright with your feet 8 to 12 inches apart. Step forward, placing one foot 12 to 18 inches in front of you, then sink into that position and hold it for a count of three, keeping your knees in line with your toes. Then reverse the motion until you're in the starting position. Do the same for the other side. Aim for 10 repetitions with each leg.

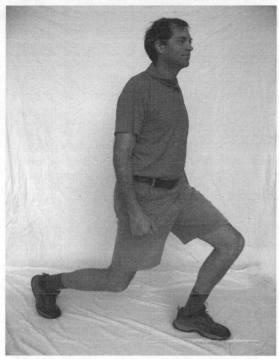

Lunge

For advanced versions, step farther forward, deepen the bend, hold weights, or wear a backpack. To improve your balance, pretend you're standing in the center of a clock face, lunge out to the 1, 2, and 3 o'clock positions.

As with squats, protect your knees—don't bend your knees past 90 degrees. If your knees hurt, don't step as far out, don't bend your knees as far, and add support with ski or hiking poles. Do this five to 10 times. Stop if you feel pain in your knees or back.

Calf raises. There are two great reasons for doing calf raises: They strengthen your lower legs for uphill hiking, and they build support for your ankles, which are prime candidates for hiking injuries.

Stand either on the floor or with your toes on a stair, heels hanging over (for full range of motion and greater stretch). Gently hold onto a rail or the wall for balance, if need-

ed. Push up with your toes, raising your heels high, then lower your heels slowly. Do this in three positions: toes straight ahead, toes pointed in, and toes pointed out. Try for five reps in each position, for 15 reps total. For more challenge, increase reps, hold weights, or put on a backpack.

To balance strength in this region, complement ankle raises with toe raises, which will strengthen the much smaller and weaker muscles along the front of your shin. While sitting on a chair with one leg extended comfortably in front of you, point your toes, then pull them up toward your knee, bending only at the ankle. Add resistance by pressing down on your toes with your other foot, or by placing something heavy on your toes (such as a sand bag or the edge of an ottoman).

Training Tips

A healthy training regimen balances cardiovascular and weight training. A good example might be three days of cardiovascular training, at least 20 minutes each day, then two to three days of strength training, alternating between the two to rest the muscles from the day before.

The repetitions here are only recommendations. Do fewer if you need to in the beginning; add more as you improve. For faster results, do multiple sets of the repetitions—with a minute of rest in between, because your muscles respond quickly when they're fatigued.

Also follow these general training tips:

Warm up. Cold muscles are prone to injury. Do the first 10 minutes of your cardiovascular workout at a gentler pace until your muscles are warm and ready for more challenge. Do 10 minutes of cardiovascular activity before strength training, too. Full-body warm-ups are best; use an exercise machine with moving arms, or simply do bicep curls and arm lifts

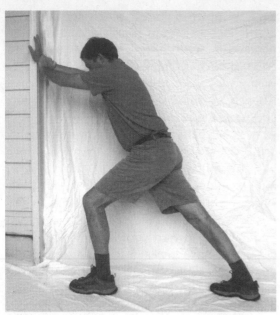
Calf stretch

Take baby steps. Rome wasn't built in a day, and your favorite athlete didn't become superhuman in a week, so don't be in a hurry. Focus on the journey, not the destination. Start with a pace that gets you used to this new activity and helps you avoid injury from pushing too hard. The first weeks can be difficult; many people get frustrated by the initial discomfort, fatigue, and sore muscles. Push through, and your enjoyment level will rise with your fitness. Before long, you'll be admiring yourself in the mirror and relishing your wonderful new levels of energy, balance, and fitness.

Balance muscle groups. Your body is a single unit, and balance is important to health and fitness. When training, exercise the opposing muscle groups in each part of your body—front/back, flexors/extensors, biceps/triceps, quadriceps/hamstrings, abdomen/back, etc. Muscles never work alone but in groups. Working front and back will strengthen muscles that support as well as those that do most of the work. This provides balance and overall stability to your body and movements.

with 1- to 3-pound weights on a walk around the neighborhood. This advice applies to your first steps on the trail each day, as well.

Hamstrings stretch

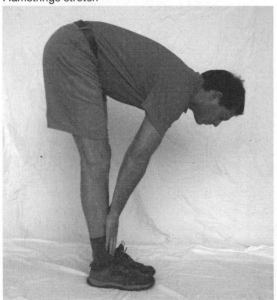

Stretching the hamstrings a little more

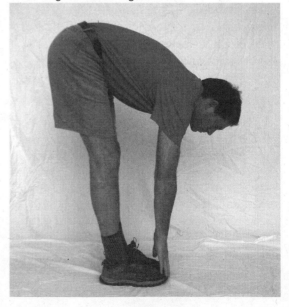

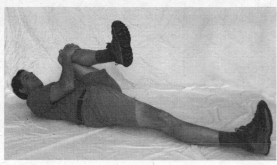
Knee hug

Create a routine. Create a checklist of all the exercises described here (and more!), then check them off each time you do them. If you're a busy person, schedule your workouts into your calendar and create a regular routine to keep other distractions from pre-empting these important activities.

Breathe! Breathe deeply during all exercises—oxygen is life.

Listen to pain. Don't worry about the good pain:

➤ The burn of working muscles (caused by a buildup of lactic acid and other toxins in the muscle—this should dissipate quickly after you stop exerting).

➤ Stiff and sore muscles in the days after a hard workout. The pain will fade after a couple days, leaving you with stronger muscles.

➤ Painful cramps that form in your muscles during a workout; massage, stretching, and drinking something can relieve the pain.

Pay attention to bad pain. If sharp pain comes suddenly, it could indicate sprain, strain, or bruise to muscle, tendon, or ligament. If you experience breathing difficulty or chest pain, stop immediately, find a comfortable position, and relax. If pain doesn't go away or gets worse, seek medical attention immediately. Learn more about pain in the chapter on first aid.

Be a good mechanic. Proper body mechanics will help you achieve results and avoid injury. When lifting weights, always use good posture and good spine position. If exercise is forcing you into a bad or struggling body position, you're doing too much. Back off by doing fewer repetitions or using lighter resistance to ensure good form. A professional trainer can help you develop good form from the outset.

Stretch. Stretching tired muscles will help flush out toxins, improve healing, and ensure greater flexibility and range of motion. It's a great thing to do after each day's hike while backpacking. See the additional resources below for more information.

Buff or lithe? The amount of weight and number of repetitions you do will determine your ultimate strength and looks. Low weight with high repetitions will give your muscles endurance and tone with less bulk. Fewer repetitions with more weight brings brute strength and impressive bulk. Until you have a personal trainer, however, don't attempt any strength exercise that you can't repeat 15 times comfortably and in good form. If you don't know what good form is, you need a trainer.

Additional Resources for Fitness and Exercise

➤ *Staying Fit Over 50: Conditioning for Outdoor Activities*, by Jim Sloan, The Mountaineers Books

➤ *Conditioning for Outdoor Fitness*, by David Musnick and Mark Pierce, The Mountaineers Books

➤ *Stretching*, by Bob and Jean Anderson, Shelter Publications

➤ www.fitnessonline.com/getfit/

➤ www.justmove.org/myfitness/

Gathering all the food and equipment you'll need for your expedition into the backcountry is one thing. Packing it well so you can find everything when you need it, and so nothing get ruined (so your cooking fuel doesn't leak all over your food, or your sleeping bag doesn't get wet from rain, for example) is another thing entirely.

The same careful planning that went into gathering your food and equipment should also go into packing it into your backpack.

MY SYSTEM

Packing Sleeping Socks

Dry, warm, and comfortable feet are more than a luxury; they're a necessity. One way to guarantee happy feet is to change into warm, dry socks when you get to camp or before you climb into your sleeping bag at night. Pack a pair of clean, fluffy socks with your sleeping bag, so you know right where they are when you unroll your bag. If wet weather threatens, pack both your bag and socks in a plastic bag to keep them dry.

–Brian Beffort, author

The Art and Science of Packing

When packing your backpack, here are a few things to consider:

Make a list. It happens often: You're at the trailhead (or worse, setting up camp), and someone groans in frustration because they forgot something—toothbrush, headlamp, hat, or, worse yet, boots, sleeping bag, or poles for the tent. Avoid this frustration by making a list and checking items off as you pack. It also helps to pack a few days ahead of time. Waiting to pack until late the night before puts you in a rush—you're tempting your own forgetfulness to leave something important out. You'll find packing lists in Appendix I. Make a copy, add or delete items to suit your needs, then use it to make sure you bring all you want and need. After each trip, fine tune the list, then store it where you can find it easily (fold it into this book, for example). You'll be one step ahead for your trip.

How many clothes to bring? Pack only what you need, plus a few extra items for surprise cold or storms. Backpacking is not a fashion contest. If you're backpacking, you're automatically stylish no matter what you wear, as long as it's comfortable and functions appropriately against the elements. With this in mind, consider bringing only one pair of pants, one pair of shorts, a long-sleeve shirt, and a couple T-shirts. The weather will dictate how many other layers you need (long-sleeve shirts, vests, fleece jackets, storm shells, etc.). Socks are one item to indulge in; bring three pairs for a weekend and five pairs for a weeklong trip, not counting liners. This allows a fresh pair each day. After day three, wash three pairs, wear the fourth, and keep an extra pair in a bag for sleeping or emergencies.

What will you need when? Easy access is important for essential items, such as sunglasses, hat, sunscreen, water, snacks, map, first aid kit, headlamp, and extra layers for changeable weather. Keep them in the top or outside compartment of your pack, so you can get them quickly when you need them. Other things—food for dinner, tent, toiletries, and the rest of your clothes—can be buried deeper. Sleeping bags work well at the bottom of your pack; in too-large stuff sacks, or none at all, sleeping bags conform to any pack's shape. In rainy weather, pack your tent so it's easily accessible, so you can pull it out and set it up quickly, creating a dry refuge for everything else.

Be a creature of habit. Pack everything in the same place every time—first aid kit, headlamp, toothbrush, map, etc., so you'll always know where things are when you need them.

Balance. Your pack needs to move with you, not pull you in unwanted directions. Pack the heaviest items close to your back—higher up if you're on open trail, lower if you need agility for climbing or cross-country travel. Center the pack weight over your hips. If the weight is too low, you'll have to lean forward awkwardly to get the weight over your hips; if it's too high, you'll feel top-heavy and out of balance. Women in general have a lower center of balance than men; packing weight lower and closer to the body often works best for them. Balance your weight left to right as well, or you might end up walking in circles.

Share the load. Divvy up items with your partners to share the load. One can carry the tent, while another carries the stakes and

MY SYSTEM

The Checklist

The year I started backpacking, I forgot a critical piece of gear on several trips. I work as a data analyst at an environmental organization, so I figured I could use a little computer technology to help me keep track of my backpacking gear. I developed an Excel checklist to consult when packing for each backcountry adventure. I have all the gear I need to consider categorized in a spreadsheet. When I pack, I simply consult my list and then mark each item as either "not taking" or "packed." I add all the "packed" items to a gear pile next to my backpack. This approach not only keeps me organized, it dramatically speeds up the packing process.

My list is divided into categories of similar items: essential gear (pack, tent, sleeping pad, etc.), kitchen (pot, lighter, stove, cup, etc.), clothes (convertible pants, fleece, thermals, etc.), toiletries (toothpaste, toothbrush, etc.), food, and extras. Since the list is electronic, I can easily add new items, notes, or ideas about what to bring for future trips. I can also consult it to see what I brought but never used so I can plan to go lighter next time.

On a recent trip, I was feeling overconfident and didn't check my list. When I prepared to make dinner that night, I realized I had forgotten my stove, which is pretty critical to the dining experience. Luckily, I was car camping not backpacking, and there was a Chinese restaurant a few miles away. It was an embarrassing lesson, but at least I wasn't stuck eating crunchy, freeze-dried, veggie lasagna in the backcountry.

—**Mathew Grimm**, environmental activist and outdoor enthusiast poles; one carries the stove, while the other carries the fuel. Split your food. However you divide your load, always make sure each member of the party has food, water, and shelter, just in case you get separated.

Internal compartmentalization. Top-opening internal frame packs can seem like gaping black holes that make it hard to find gear. Put different types of items in color-coded stuff sacks—a red bag for first aid, a small blue one for toiletries, a bright-yellow sack for clothes; green for food, etc. The colors will help you find what you need quickly, and the bags will keep everything relatively tidy as you pull everything out while looking for what you want. Light colors will be easier to see in a big, dark pack.

Streamline your pack. Pack as much as you can inside your pack; items attached to the outside can fall off, catch on passing branches, look silly, and annoy fellow hikers with clanking and clanging.

Items attached to the outside (sleeping pad, etc.) should be secured well with a trim profile, so they don't get ripped up by branches or rocks. In this instance at least, appearances are everything—you are only as sleek and streamlined as you look.

Carry a quarter. When fully packed for the trail, your pack should weigh no more than 25 percent of your body weight. But even that can be too much. For example, on a really good day, I weigh 200 pounds (I'm tall and thin, not obese). But a 50-pound pack is far more than I want to carry, so I strive to keep my pack weight below 40 pounds in winter, and less than 30 pounds in summer.

These are challenging goals for me, as I am a notorious over-packer. On long trips in cold weather, a heavy pack might be necessary. If this is the case, make sure you're in shape to handle it.

Going by Plane

Flying with backpacking equipment presents unique challenges. Do not pack fuel canisters in your luggage. They are forbidden and can be confiscated before you get on the plane, even if they're empty. Camp stoves may be restricted as well. Call your airline ahead of time to check on these and other security restrictions, as rules change often in this post-9/11 world. Call outdoor stores near your trailhead to make sure you can obtain fuel and other prohibited items after you land.

Backpacks, with their many loose straps, can get torn apart by airport conveyor belts. Secure all loose straps before you check your backpack. Even then, the airline might require you to put the pack in a large plastic bag or tub, and then sign a form absolving them of responsibility if the pack gets damaged.

Shoes and boots with thick soles and/or steel shanks in the soles will cause delays if you wear them through airport security metal detectors. If you can, pack these shoes and wear lightweight shoes on your flight.

Goodies for the Road

When packing for your trip, bring extra supplies in your car—not to pack with you on the trail, but to enjoy once you get back to your car days later. These items might include extra food and drink (include some favorite treats that you'll relish when you get back to the car), a clean, comfy, nice-smelling change of clothes, and some comfortable shoes.

Having supplies waiting in the car also provides extra protection against emergencies—if you run out of food or water on the trail, if you encounter an emergency on the trail, or if your car gets stranded between civilization and the trailhead, the extra supplies will provide needed relief and security.

It's also a good idea to camp at the trail-head the night before you begin hiking (giving you an early start in the morning), or the night after you get back to the car (to avoid driving back home at night when you're exhausted).

Keep an extra sleeping pad waiting in the car, a stash of good food, a camp chair, an extra-thick sleeping pad, or other comforts that are too heavy for the trail.

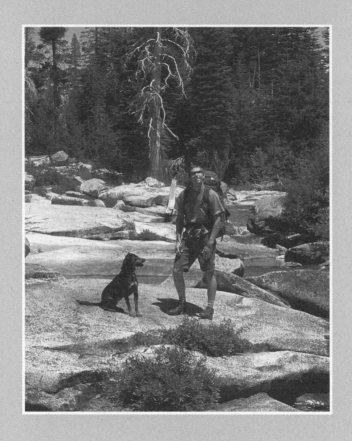

PART V
JOY ON THE TRAIL

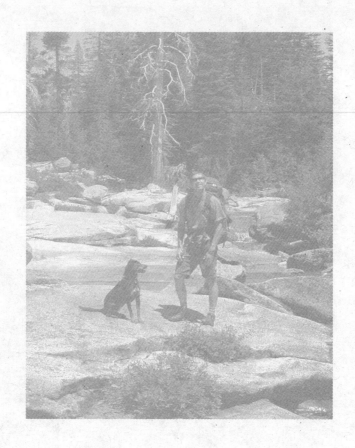

19 THE HIKE IN

This is it, the moment you've been waiting for—your first steps into the wilderness. It's a last chance to evaluate how well you've planned and prepared for the trip ahead of you. Once you've done this, it's time to trust your planning and instincts and start hiking. This section will cover everything you need to know while in the wilderness.

At the Trailhead

Before you start hiking, you have one last chance to make sure you have everything you'll need in the wilderness. Take a few moments now to give your gear and yourself the once-over to make sure you're prepared for your trip.

Start with your person: Dress for the warmest part of the day, even if you're starting your hike in the early-morning chill; before too long, you'll be working hard and generating a lot of heat once you start hiking with that pack on. Wear warmer layers that you can peel away as the day heats up. Keep extra layers handy in your pack for windy ridges and sudden rain.

Care for your feet. They'll be carrying you (and your heavy pack) over miles of trail, and if you take a moment now, you can spare yourself pain later. Start by cutting your toenails. You'll save your socks and neighboring toes, and you won't lose your toenails after miles of pounding down hills in boots that

aren't quite right. Make sure there are no wrinkles in your socks or creases in your boots, and check that your boots are laced snug, but not too tight.

Next, apply sunscreen. Sunscreen takes 20 to 30 minutes before it begins working. Don't wait until your skin starts to turn pink, and don't neglect sunscreen if it's cloudy.

Well-prepared and ready for the trail

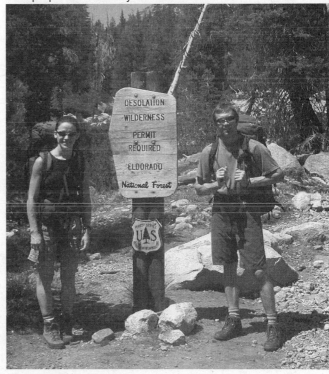

Saying No to the Sun

In my earlier camping days, I lost many nights of good sleep due to the residual effects of the sun. I hated to invest in expensive sunglasses because I always broke them within weeks of their purchase. As a result, I'd often head out to bright, high-altitude destinations wearing cheap, $8 gas-station sunglasses. Nine hours of power squinting through cheesy plastic lenses often left me with a "mysterious" headache. After finally investing in a good (and slightly expensive) pair of glasses with effective lenses, the headaches went away! Light eye colors are especially susceptible to bright-sun-induced headaches (I have green eyes), so they can make a difference to lighter-eyed folks.

My other sun-induced ailment was mild sunburn, not quite sufficient to make the skin bright pink but strong enough to give me an achy and sore feeling after the sun had gone down. Your body, probably already low on water, needs to hydrate your skin to keep it healthy. Subtle sunburn can make it hard to sleep and bring about annoying headaches. Try to put on sunblock at all your major snack breaks, summits, or restroom breaks. It only takes a few seconds and can make the difference later on when you're trying to get a good night's sleep.

–James Dziezynski, author, *Best Summit Hikes in Colorado*, Wilderness Press

Ultraviolet rays can still penetrate through clouds, and sunscreen helps protect your skin from drying and chapping from wind.

Now turn to your gear. Begin by inspecting your pack. Double-check your list (better now than when you get to camp and realize you forgot your X, Y, or worse, your Z). If you don't have a list, flip to the back of this book and check the gear lists in Appendix I. Make sure you have everything you'll need for your trip—tent, sleeping bag, boots, stove, and food, as well as essentials like your map, compass, fire starter, first aid kid, etc. Then fasten all pockets and cinch down all compression straps to secure and stabilize your pack before you put it on.

When your pack is all set to go, double-check your car; make sure everything is stowed, stashed, and locked. Leave an itinerary on your dashboard, so law enforcement folks know whether to worry about you, and when and where to start their search if you don't return.

Before you set off, make sure you're on the right path. Orient yourself with your map and compass: Lay out your map on the ground or picnic table (but not on the hood of your car, because your compass arrow will be disoriented by the metal in your car). Orient the map to true north (see page 132 to learn how). Make mental note of east, west, and south while you're at it.

If you can see the landscape around you, compare the peaks, ridges, rivers, or other major landmarks with the map to see how they are depicted. Place the center of your compass dial on your exact location on the map, if you know it. Look across the compass toward a peak or other landscape feature in the distance. You will find it on the map directly on the imaginary line between your compass and the landscape feature itself.

Study the trail on the map. Figure out where your route will take you in relation to the real-world landmarks you can see. Note rivers, creeks, peaks, trail intersections, and other landmarks you can use as "handrails" to help you gauge your progress and stay on route. Maybe even locate a nice spot for your first rest stop or for lunch. If you're following a trip from a guidebook, review the route description to help get a mental imprint of the route.

Now you're ready to put on your backpack. Lifting a heavy pack up over your shoulders can be difficult and awkward. Here are a few ways to make it easier:

➤ Lift the pack onto a picnic table or rock, then put it on and adjust straps before you take on the pack's full weight.

➤ Start with the pack on the ground, holding the shoulder straps; lift it onto one knee; wiggle one shoulder in, swing the pack onto your back, then put on the other shoulder strap. Easy.

➤ Have a friend help you. (Don't forget to return the favor.)

Once your pack is on, adjust straps in the following order:

1. Shrug the pack high up on your back, or have your partner hold it so the hip belt is well above your hips. Clasp and tighten your hip belt, then let the pack settle down into position on top of your hip bones. The great majority of your pack's weight should rest on the top of your pelvic bone or your hips. This allows your legs to support the weight instead of your shoulders, because your legs are much stronger. It also keeps your center of gravity low.

2. Tighten the shoulder straps, but not too much; they are designed to keep the pack weight upright and close to your body, not to support weight. When fully weighted, you should be able to slip a finger or two easily under the top of the shoulder strap. If your shoulders get tired after time on the trail, they're carrying too much weight. Ease their burden by lifting the pack higher, then tightening your hip belt to transfer weight to your hips.

3. Snap the sternum strap. One of the subtle yet wonderful innovations of pack design, the sternum strap helps pull your pack's weight forward, closer to your body, saving your shoulders from unnecessary burden. The

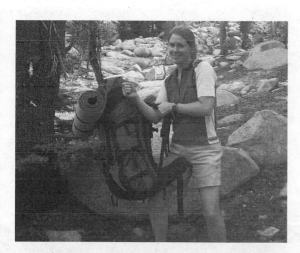

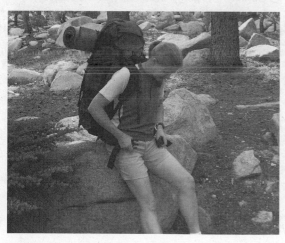

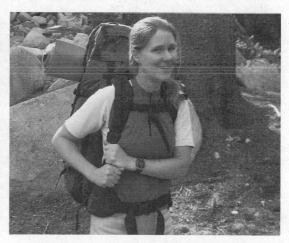

sternum strap should be about the level of your armpits. Too high, and it will feel uncomfortably close to your windpipe; too low, and it will interfere with your breathing.

4. Above the top of your shoulders, reach up and tighten the load-lifter straps, which connect the pack to your upper shoulder straps. This helps pull the pack closer to your body and lift the shoulder straps up off your shoulders. When adjusted properly, load-lifter straps should run from your shoulders up to your pack at a 45-degree angle.

5. Where the hip belt meets the backpack, tighten the straps that run between your hip belt and the pack, which should snug the backpack closer to your body. You can always nudge, fiddle, and otherwise adjust your pack along the trail.

Finally, just before you go, don't forget to stash your car keys in a safe place!

First Steps

Before you start hiking, stop, turn around, and inspect the area for anything you might be leaving behind. This is a good habit before you start hiking at every point on your trip—after rest stops and when leaving camp to hike back out. Your goals should be to remember everything, and to leave the spot cleaner than you found it (pick up other people's trash—but if you're just starting your trip, don't carry this garbage with you the entire time; put it in the trash, or leave it by the car to pick up on your return).

Finding Your Pace

Everyone has a pace at which walking is most efficient and comfortable. Each person's pace will change with elevation, terrain, weather, fitness, nutrition, and pack weight. Pace isn't speed, it's how much energy you're using. Start hiking slowly. Not only will this give your muscles an opportunity to warm up so you don't get injured, it will give your cardiovascular system (lungs, heart, circulation, and muscles) time to find a comfortable, efficient pace; it might take a few miles.

Rhythm is important to a good pace, and that rhythm will change depending on your load and the difficulty of the trail. A cheerful song or a little drummer in your head can

You know you have a good pace when your lungs, legs, and heart are working together.

keep you bouncing along. Avoid using your iPod while you're hiking, however, as it takes you away from your surroundings; not only does it distract you from the sights and sounds around you, it might make you miss the important sounds—rockfall on the slope above you, the elk bugling in the meadow, the rattlesnake buzzing under the bush ahead, the distant cry of someone lost, or that cougar padding quietly up behind you.

You know you've found a good pace when you're able to carry on a conversation, you're not sweating buckets or breathing too hard, and you have some energy left to set up camp and enjoy your destination. It's enjoyable when your pace syncs up with someone else's, but it doesn't always happen that way. If different hiking speeds among the group are a source of tension, you can adjust loads; transfer some of the turtle's load to the rabbit, which should help equalize your hiking speeds. If this doesn't work, don't feel obliged to hike with others if their pace doesn't match yours. Make arrangements to meet them at a prearranged spot ahead on the trail, so you can each hike in comfort. For gosh sakes, however, don't lose your hiking partners.

Heed the tortoise. On the trail, slow and steady often wins the race over those fast out of the gate. Rabbits sprint ahead for a few minutes, then need to rest to let the burn in their legs subside and their lungs catch up. They also tend to sweat more, which can be dangerous on cold days. And they're inefficiently using their energy. It's more efficient and more comfortable to find a steady pace you can keep for long distances without tuckering out. Take your time. Be comfortable. You'll get there. If you're not first, who cares? It's not a race, is it?

Difficult Steps

Long, steep trails at high elevation require the right pace. When even a few steps are making you suck wind on steep terrain, use

MY SYSTEM

Pacing Myself

I'm about 10 inches shorter than my partner, and every time we backpack, I'm reminded of what a difference it makes. Climbing or descending steep slopes, fording streams, and scrambling over boulders are way more difficult for those of us with little legs! I figure I take at least 50 percent more steps than he does over the course of a day. To make sure I don't burn myself out trying to keep up with him, I take the lead during long climbs and descents.

If the day's hiking is going to last for more than four hours, I like to take a break every hour (or 90 minutes at the outside) with my pack *off*. It may seem like more of a pain than it's worth, but I've discovered it's way easier to keep my back and shoulders in working order if they get a break every time my legs get one. By taking regular breaks and going at my pace rather than his, I can tackle long trails and multi-day trips with the same vigor as my much-taller man!

—**Michelle Waitzman**, author, *Sex in a Tent*, Wilderness Press

the mountaineer's rest step: After each step, straighten your rear leg and rest on it for a breath, then lean forward into your next step. Slowly. It takes practice and patience, and it can seem aggravatingly slow. But slow and steady reaches the summit.

When hiking up steep terrain, large steps place a lot of strain on your knees. Smaller steps are better. If you must take a big step up, place both hands on your knee and push down to add strength and support.

It's easier to climb up than down. Remember this when you're tempted to climb up that cool rock, tree, cliff, or glacier. Many

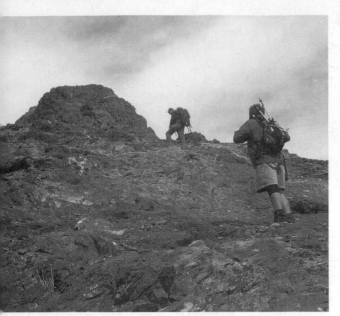

Take your time; you'll get there.

Rest

Everyone needs time for a little "ahh"… but for how long? Sometime in the first hour after leaving the trailhead, stop and scrutinize how everything is going so far. Are your shoulders beginning to hurt? Does the pack need adjusting? Are your feet happy? Are there any hot spots (annoying rubbing or pinching) on your feet that could become crippling blisters hours from now? This is the best time to readjust your boots or socks, and apply duct tape or moleskin to hot spots. Prevention is the best cure.

Shorter, frequent rest stops are best. Stop for a few minutes two or three times each hour to catch your breath, enjoy the view, check the map, or eat a quick snack. Take longer midmorning and midafternoon breaks and a healthy break for lunch. Never stop so long that your body cools off and you lose momentum. Only you know what works for you.

For quick stops, keep your pack on (sit while resting it on a rock or log, if available). Take a few minutes to sip some water, eat a quick snack, and let your lungs catch up. For longer breaks, find a cozy spot off the trail where you can take your pack off, sit down, and enjoy the view. These rest stops can be highlights of your entire trip.

search-and-rescue operations are formed to get people off cliffs and out of other tight situations caused by their poor judgment on the way up.

The same is true for simple hiking: Downhill can be more difficult than up. It's harder on your feet and knees; there's greater risk of twisted ankles, banged up toes, different blisters than you got on the climb, and a lot farther to fall if you slip or trip. I'd rather hike up than down any day. On mountain climbing trips, many accidents happen on the way back down. After you bag your peak, don't let your guard down. Take your time. Watch your step. Trekking poles help a lot.

It's easier to step over a log in one big step than to step up onto it and then down, which can be hard on the knees. Either way, make sure there isn't a rattlesnake napping peacefully on the other side.

When walking on rocks or boulders, assume they're unsteady. Step on the uphill side of a boulder rather than the downhill side; if it slides or rolls, you'll be on top rather than underneath.

Packs make good back rests.

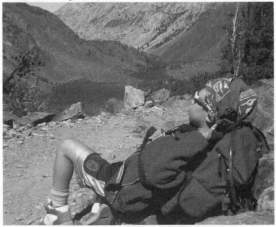

On thru-hikes in warm weather, I'm a big fan of the siesta. Get an early start, and get good miles under your belt in the morning. When the heat of the day comes, find a comfortable, shady spot, and stop for an hour or longer. Eat lunch, take off your boots, maybe even snooze a little. Then pick up and get a few more hours of hiking in before the day ends. That's my idea of fun!

Blisters

These small, red, fluid-filled, and painful sores are the most common backpacking injury, and a leading cause of misery on the trail. Although small, blisters can be extremely painful and debilitating, preventing any further movement up or down the trail. As with most injuries, prevention is the best cure.

Blisters are caused by friction against your skin by your boot or sock. Prevent blisters by avoiding the friction. Here's how:

➤ Make sure your socks and boots are comfortable and snug, and that there are no wrinkles in your socks, or annoying protrusions on the inside of your boots. Sock liners might help.

➤ Keep your toenails trimmed.

➤ Wear dry, comfy socks. Change into clean, dry socks at least once a day.

➤ Be alert for hot spots (sore spots that lead to blisters). Pay attention to how your boots are fitting and moving with your feet during the first 30 minutes of your hike. If you feel rubbing or tight spots, stop, sit down, and take off your boots.

➤ If you cannot relieve the rubbing or tight spot by adjusting your socks or retying your laces, then place a large piece of duct tape on your skin where the rubbing occurs (moleskin works, too, but it's more expensive and thicker, which means it can interfere with the fit of snug boots). This will allow the rubbing to take place against the smooth surface of the duct tape and not against your skin.

➤ Let your feet dry every day, if possible. Wetness creates friction, and it breaks down the skin, predisposing you to blisters. Keep your feet dry by changing socks and using foot powder regularly.

➤ Put your feet up during rest stops or at camp to reduce swelling and improve circulation.

➤ Wear lightweight shoes in camp if your hiking boots are big, heavy clompers.

➤ Avoid cracked feet at balls and heels (which can be painful and lead to infection) by keeping your feet well-moisturized. Cure it by applying a thick layer of petroleum jelly or other lotion to the bottoms your feet, then cover with socks, before you go to bed at night. The cracks should heal within a couple days.

➤ Get to know your boots and hiking style. My current boots are comfortable, with one exception: When I hike uphill, my heels slip against my boots, and I'm guaranteed blisters there if I don't take precautions. Luckily, the cure is easy—I prevent them by putting a big piece of duct tape on each heel when I know I'll be hiking uphill.

Perhaps you and your boots will have a similar relationship. Blisters are common on the back of heels when hiking uphill, on toes when hiking downhill, and on the sides of the ball of the foot almost anytime. Get to know your boots and where they don't fit exactly right, then actively protect those areas from blisters by placing duct tape or moleskin over those spots before you start hiking.

➤ If your boots are too tight around your toes, but too loose around the ankles, create a dual lacing system. Use two shoe laces on each boot: one through the bottom two or three sets of eyelets; one through the top set. You can tie each set as tight or as loose as you need for just the right fit.

Beating (and Treating) Blisters

I hate blisters. They are a nuisance—and, yes, a minor injury. My favorite prevention techniques are a small dab of BodyGlide or Hydropel between my toes and a liberal coating of Zeasorb powder in my moisture-wicking socks.

In the rare case of a blister, I clean the skin with an alcohol wipe and drain the blister with several small needle holes where ongoing foot pressure will expel fluid. I stretch the needle holes sideways to expand the hole since punctures often reseal). Then I apply a light coating of sticky tincture of benzoin and allow it to dry. I am careful to avoid getting any in the blister because it will burn like crazy for 30 seconds. The blister patch goes over the top, covering the blister. My favorite blister patches are Spenco's QuikStik or Sport Blister Pads.

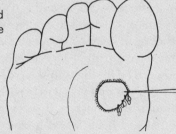

Use a sterilized needle to make several small holes on the outside edges of the blister.

My blister-patching kit includes a few alcohol wipes, a tincture of benzoin swab, several sizes of the patches, a small vial of Hydropel, and 2 feet of waterproof Kinesio-Tex tape. I use the tape over hot spots and to protect toes. The whole kit in a Ziploc bag weighs less than 2 ounces.

—**John Vonhof** fastpacked the John Muir Trail in 1987 in 8.5 days, is the author of *Fixing Your Feet: Prevention and Treatment for Athletes* (Wilderness Press), and publishes several newsletter on foot care at www.fixing-yourfeet.com.

The sooner you catch a blister, the easier it will be to treat it and continue walking. If the blister is small and intact, do not puncture it. Cut a piece of moleskin or Molefoam (the same as moleskin, but thicker) at least twice the size of the blister. Round the corners off with scissors to prevent them from rolling up once you start hiking. Cut a doughnut-hole slightly larger than the blister in the middle of the moleskin. Make sure skin around blister is clean and dry, then apply the moleskin or Molefoam. A small amount of tincture of benzoin applied to the skin will make the moleskin stick better.

Cover the entire area with a large piece of duct tape to reduce friction over blister. Place a smaller piece of duct tape on the larger one, sticky sides together, so the area of tape over the blister won't stick to the blister.

For large blisters, if the bubble is intact, use a sterilized safety pin or needle (hold over a flame or wipe with an alcohol swab to sterilize) to puncture the blister at the base. Massage out the fluid, which can delay healing if left in place. Clean the area with an antiseptic wipe or soap and water, and dry well. Apply antiseptic ointment, aloe vera, vitamin E oil, or Spenco 2nd Skin to blister area. Cut a hole in the moleskin or Molefoam, apply it over blister, and cover everything with tape or bandage as described earlier.

It doesn't take much of a blister to cripple you. If walking is necessary, consider cutting a large hole in your boot to minimize aggravation and allow you to walk (this is an extreme solution to an extreme problem; prevent such a situation by treating your blister before it occurs, or at least when it's small). Inspect the wound daily for redness, swelling, pus, increased pain, or other signs of infection. If infected, clean and disinfect again, then reapply ointments, moleskin, and tape or bandage. If infection does not go away, seek medical attention quickly.

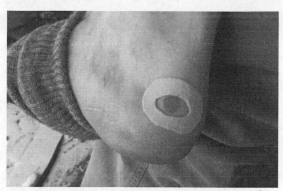

Place a pad around the blister.

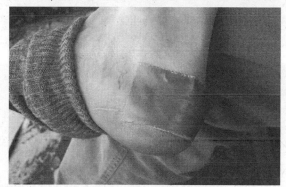

Cover the entire area to reduce friction.

Time

We live in a world with two times: natural time and human time. Natural time is measured by the rising and setting of the sun, the phases of the moon, the passing of seasons, the migration of birds and animals, the blooming of flowers, the turning of leaves, and our own breathing, heartbeats, and bodily cycles.

Humans have chopped these natural rhythms and cycles into arbitrary pieces. Days clearly match the natural cycles of daylight, and our yearly and monthly calendars are based loosely on the solar and lunar cycles. But hours, minutes, and seconds, not to mention dates and the names of days and months, are arbitrary; they have no bearing on, or relation to, the natural world. Why 24 hours in a day, and not 17 or 12? Why divide hours into

60 minutes, with 60 seconds marking each minute? Why not metric time, with 10-hour days, each divided into 10 deci-minutes, each of those divided into 10 centi-minutes, each of those into milli-minutes?

There is a value to knowing how long it took you to hike a particular trail, so you can better estimate your trail travel time in the future. But wilderness doesn't care whether it's 2:45 or 4:15. When you're backpacking, all that matters is how long you have until sunset, and whether everyone is together, safe, sheltered, and nourished when night comes. How many minutes are there in a sunset? In a clearing storm? In a blooming flower?

If you want to tune into nature while backpacking, leave your watch at home; it's a handcuff to civilization, meetings, schedules, and deadlines. The whole point of backpacking is to leave these things at home—hard to do if you keep looking at your watch.

It's not easy to let go. If you've worn a watch for years, you might feel deeply connected to it and find yourself looking at it frequently. If you're like many people, you'll have to look again moments later if someone asks you what time it is. Challenge yourself, take a risk, and try not to worry what time it is, even if just for a few days.

It might take a while, but in forgetting about human time, you'll become more aware of deep time—the cycles of days and seasons, the slow creep of millennia. You'll be able to think more like a mountain, a tree, or a marmot.

You can still coordinate schedules with people without a watch; just be less precise. Plan to be at the lake by midday, or to meet your party back at camp by sunset, with ample wiggle room in the schedule.

If it's important you be back somewhere at a certain time on a certain day (back at the trailhead to catch the shuttle, for example), keep your watch lonely and neglected in your pack until that morning. Before you look, have everyone guess what the time is; it's fun to see how accurate people's guesses are after not knowing for days.

Hiking Time

It can be difficult to judge your hiking speed, because it depends on many factors. In general, you'll be doing well to average 2 miles an hour. Your speed will drop closer to 1 mile an hour when any of the following factors come into play: poor fitness, hot weather, high elevation, heavy pack, steep trail, beautiful views or flowers that keep distracting you, or a large group (because you're only as fast as your slowest hiker). As a rule of thumb, add an hour for every 1000 vertical feet you must climb.

WILDERNESS WISDOM

You don't need a watch to know when the sun will set; the answer is in your hand. To estimate how long until sunset, hold one hand at arm's length toward the horizon under the sun, with palm flat and facing you. The width of your hand equals about an hour of daylight; each finger, about 15 minutes. For example, if there are three hand widths between the horizon and the sun, you have about three hours of daylight left. In summer, you'll get another hour of light after the sun sets—more in high latitudes, less in winter.

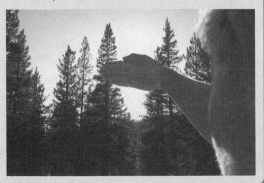

For example, assuming you're in decent shape, give yourself six hours to hike 8 miles to your destination 2000 feet higher than the trailhead. If you make it faster, great!

The first day is always the hardest and slowest, especially if you drive from a lower city to your higher-elevation trailhead. After a couple days of hiking, you should be moving faster than you did on the first.

Snacking and Hydration

When you're inactive—sitting at home watching bad daytime TV—your body can lose a quart of water a day through urine, perspiration, and exhalation. On mildly active days, you can lose more than 2.5 quarts of water per day. While backpacking, you'll lose even more. How much water should you drink while backpacking? The easy answer–lots! In hot weather, drink at least a quart an hour.

If you're not sure whether you're drinking enough water, check the color of your pee. You should piss clear. Dark-colored urine is a sign of dehydration (although some vitamins and medications can turn urine dark).

Backpacking can take a lot of energy. Snack and drink frequently to stay hydrated and keep your energy high. When you're bonking—you have no energy at all—low blood sugar is probably the culprit. Eat something. Salt, potassium, and other electrolytes are also important, because you lose them when you sweat—Cheez-Its produce big smiles when you pass them around on the trail.

Find a spot to stop, take off your pack for a few minutes, and eat something (energy bars, candy, trail mix, and other quick-and-easy foods are perfect for quick boosts of energy). You'll be surprised how quickly that spring returns to your step and you can keep hiking.

Trail Etiquette

One of the primary reasons people go backpacking is to get away from other people—which means you. It's nothing personal; it's just difficult to enjoy the solitude of nature when you're surrounded by others. Regardless of whether you feel the same, it's important to recognize that people feel this way, and have respect for other people's desire for solitude.

Solitude is a wonderful part of the backcountry experience. Help others enjoy the same solitude you're seeking by hiking in a group of no more than six people and remaining unobtrusive. Choose a campsite off the main trail that is screened by trees or rocks. Plan your trips to popular areas during off-peak days and seasons. Consider entirely avoiding areas that are particularly fragile or over-visited.

Here are some other rules of the trail to make you and those around you happy campers:

➤ As with driving, let uphill climbers have the right of way, unless circumstances dictate a different policy, or the uphill hiker needs an excuse to rest while you pass.

➤ Always give horses the right of way. If horses approach, step off to the downhill side of the trail (predators attack from above, so horses get skittish if you're looming above them, even if you're polite about it). Remain visible (horses need to be able to recognize you as a person, not a threat). Hold your dog or child safely out of the way, and say a few reassuring words, so the horse knows you're a nice person.

➤ Mountain bikes are supposed to give you and horses the right of way. Sometimes, however, they zoom right past before there's time to think about it, so stay alert.

➤ Camp and travel on durable surfaces. Many soils and plants are sensitive to a bunch of people tromping across them with big boots and heavy packs. In many places, the landscape is so sensitive, or there are so many people, the backcountry cannot recover from the damage caused by visitors before the next group arrives. Avoid undue impacts by traveling and camping on durable surfaces such as rock, sand, and established trails and campsites.

Use existing trails. Staying on designated paths helps minimize the chance of wide or multiple trails forming. Walk through muddy sections and trails instead of skirting around them. Stay on switchbacks; cutting corners causes erosion and doesn't save time. When traveling off-trail, seek durable surfaces and avoid sensitive vegetation and unstable slopes.

Staying Found

Prevention is the best way to manage emergencies. Avoid the fear, cold, danger, and search-and-rescue costs. (Some search-and-rescue authorities charge to look for you. How much do you think a rescue helicopter costs per hour?). Follow these tips to avoid getting lost in the first place:

Use your map and compass. Make sure you have the knowledge of how to use them. Study your map and plan your route at the trailhead, before you hit the trail. Try to use the most up-to-date map available. Find north with your compass and try to remember where that is in relation to where you are. Look around at the major landmarks, and see how the map represents them. Which directions do the rivers flow? Finally, see where the trail goes on the map and see where in the terrain it will take you. This will help orient you to the landscape, minimizing chances you'll get lost.

Use handrails. These are features such as rivers, streams, roads, canyons, and ridges, which you can use to keep yourself going the right direction. For example, if you know the trail follows a river into the mountains, then you know you're off course if you're no longer near a river. You know you'll find the trail if you can find that river again. Similarly, if your trip will take you up onto the west slope of a mountain range, you'll know you're off course if you find yourself on the eastern slope.

Popular trails are often marked by blazes (marks cut into the bark of trees along the way) or by cairns (also called ducks), which are piles of rock set up to mark your way.

Survival Rule of Threes

➤ Without oxygen, your brain can die in three minutes.

➤ Without shelter in harsh conditions, you can die in three hours.

➤ Without water, you can die in three days.

➤ Without food, you can die in three weeks.

Remembering these threes will help you focus on what's most important during emergencies.

With care, you can keep from getting lost in this very big world.

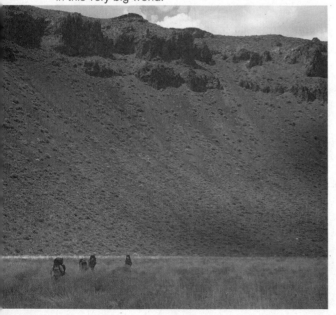

Cairns are particularly useful when there's not much of a trail to follow.

Watch your back. Do you remember Flower, the skunk from Bambi, who always traveled backward so he could see where he had been? From time to time while hiking, turn around and look back at what you just hiked through. Terrain looks different from the other side. This will help it look familiar to you on your way back to the trailhead.

Watch the time. If you're traveling in unfamiliar terrain, mark the time and check the map at prominent landmarks or when you rest. If you suddenly discover that you're lost, you'll have a decent idea of how long you have traveled since you were last "found."

If You Get Lost

Best-laid plans and years of experience aside, everybody eventually gets lost (or shall we say "temporarily disoriented"). Being lost is most dangerous to those who are unable to find themselves again. Here are a few tips to make sure that being lost remains a temporary problem and to keep it from getting dangerous.

As soon as you think you might be lost, S.T.O.P. Here's how:

Sit. Find a comfortable spot, and give yourself a few minutes to catch your breath and collect your thoughts.

Think. How might you have gotten lost? When was the last time you knew you were on the right track?

Observe. Look at the landscape around you. Are there any familiar landmarks? Are there landmarks that look unique enough that you can find them on your map? Before you make a plan based on what you see, make sure you're certain that mountain over there is indeed the mountain you think it is on the map.

Plan. If there's plenty of daylight and you're confident you can make it back to being found, then give it a go. But if little light remains, and/or you're pretty darn disoriented or injured, then make camp and settle in for the night.

The following rules are important to follow if you're lost:

➤ Stay put. Wandering around when you're lost only saps your strength and morale, and it increases your chances of injury. It also creates a moving target for rescuers, which makes you harder to find than if you were in one place.

➤ Find shelter or set up your tent somewhere that will be visible to rescuers or close to a visible area where you can run out to signal passing planes or searchers. Alternatively, you can make a large X with sticks or rocks near your shelter.

➤ Stay warm. Huddle together for warmth, wear everything you have, eat well, and drink a lot to provide fuel for your warmth. Your brain and body are your best tools for survival. Keep them warm.

➤ Stay dry. This is crucial to staying warm. Water steals body heat very quickly, making you prone to life-threatening hypothermia at cool temperatures. Stay out of wet and cold weather, change into dry clothes, and build a fire to dry out, if necessary.

➤ Signal. Signal with your whistle or yells when you first decide you're lost, in case others are nearby. But don't continue yelling and exhaust yourself. Find a clearing and build a large X with rocks, sticks, or logs. Hang a brightly colored jacket or other flag near your location. Build a fire.

At night, fires can be seen for miles; use dry wood that burns hot. During the day, the best signal is a smoky fire made with green wood. Keep a low fire burning with a pile of appropriate wood ready nearby. If you hear or see a search plane, pile on the wood and hope they see it.

Wilderness, almost by definition, is inhospitable to human comfort and safety. Here and there, however, nestled among the rocks, trees, snow, ice, beasts, and wild winds, are pockets where living is easier, softer, safer, and more comfortable. These are the places to camp. And if your pocket of safety and comfort happens to be beautiful, you've just found your little corner of paradise.

But don't be fooled by beauty. That perfect-looking campsite on the edge of the lake, or snug among the trees, might not be the right place to camp for numerous reasons. This chapter will help you make your camp in the backcountry as safe and enjoyable as possible—all paradise and no purgatory.

Choosing the Right Campsite

Congratulations, you've arrived at your destination! Or perhaps you're just running out of daylight. Either way, it's time to set up camp and settle in for the night. There are a number of things to consider when choosing the best campsite.

First, look for a place that is remote—away from the trail and other people. Avoid campsites directly on, or too near, the trail. You and other hikers will enjoy it more if people aren't tromping through your camp. Choose instead a discreet site well off the main trail.

While you're at it, see if you can find a spot with a nice view. Can you situate your tent or shelter to face the sunrise or to look over a misty lake? Here's your chance to get the best real estate for your "home" without having to pay for it.

It's also nice to have convenient water (that misty lake might serve a dual purpose), but don't trample or pollute riparian areas and water sources to get it, and don't prevent wildlife or other people from getting to the water. Wildlife are attracted to water, so if you camp near it, you'll probably have more visits from locals—mice, mosquitoes, snakes, bears, and other animals—than you would by camping farther away.

If you do camp near water, follow Leave No Trace principles and many state laws, which require that people camp at least 200 feet (70 steps) from water sources. This helps protect the water quality from the contamination threats we pose from our cooking, washing, peeing, and pooping. Many well-established campsites at popular destinations ignore this rule, leaving you to use your best judgment. If you do choose to use such a site, make every effort to avoid contaminating the water with your food, soap, or bodily wastes.

Also make sure your site is safe. Look up to make sure no widow maker (a dead tree or branch) is above you, waiting for that special moment in the middle of the night to earn its name. Falling rocks, big pinecones, an avalanche path, and other hazards can be equally dangerous. If your campsite is in the path of potential disaster, choose another site.

By the same token, you also want to keep the area safe from you. Avoid trampling sensitive ecology. In well-traveled areas, choose existing campsites that are already impacted, rather than spreading impacts to new, undisturbed sites. In remote, more pristine areas, choose open sand, rock, or thick grass for your campsite.

Unless you're trying to increase your chances for an epic adventure, seek a place that is sheltered from weather. Which direction do prevailing winds blow? A look around at the trees can answer that for you. If the trees are lopsided, with most of the foliage on one side, then strong, consistent, prevailing winds have blown them that way. Winds also tend to change direction during the day, blowing up the canyon during the day, and down-canyon at night. Once you sort this out, back your tent into the wind.

Also consider nighttime temperatures. Valley bottoms, lakeshores, and other low places tend to be colder at night because cold air settles to the lowest point. Ridge tops can be too windy. A spot in between might help you avoid the most severe chill.

If you enjoy (or maybe require) a little sunshine in order to get out of bed, situate your shelter so you have exposure to morning sun. Face your tent east, toward the rising sun, which will quickly melt away the night's chill. In the heat of summer, however, you might choose a spot protected from the morning sun for more time in cool shade in the morning.

No one wants to share their bed with insects and other critters. Look around to make sure no ant hills or rodent nests are under your proposed sleeping spot. Mosquitoes tend to be thickest near water and in woods. They're less bothersome in open areas, where there's a breeze to keep them away. Face your tent door into the breeze, as mosquitoes tend to congregate on the lee (downwind) side of objects (yes, this contradicts the "back your tent into the

Sometimes it takes work to find the right campsite; sometimes they find themselves.

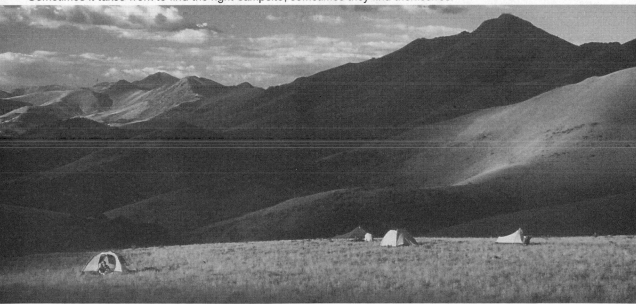

wind" advice earlier; it's up to you to decide which is worse, the weather or the bugs).

Once you're certain your spot is free of bug nests, check out the condition of the bed sites. Soft pine needles or grass make great beds. Look for the smoothest, flattest spot. Move aside any sticks or loose rocks that might pop your sleeping pad or poke you. Avoid low spots or drainages, which can collect water or turn into rivers during a storm. If you don't have a free-standing tent, look for convenient trees, to which you can tie your shelter, tarp, or hammock.

Once you've got your campsite picked out, look for a nice kitchen/campfire site. Find rocks or logs that can serve as tables, seats, or

wind blocks for your stove. A killer view provides the ambiance during dinner. But keep in mind that bears, raccoons, mice, and other rodents are attracted to food (as well as other scented items, such as toothpaste, lip balm, gum, perfume, scented toilet paper, and salt stains on your clothing or pack). So don't keep your food in your kitchen overnight. You must find a place to hang or store your food. Read more on page 178 about storing food properly.

Remember, campsites are found, not made. Resist the urge to cut trees, remove rocks, dig trenches around your tent, or otherwise alter a campsite to make it better. Your goal should be to enjoy the beauty of a particular area, not shape it to fit your needs.

A room with a view

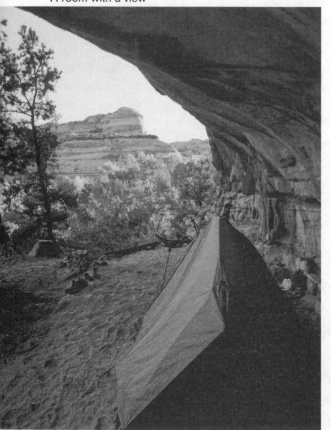

Setting Up Camp

It's a lot easier to set up camp while you still have light. Before you get into relaxation mode, set everything up, so you know where everything is and you're prepared for night. Then you can focus on the fun stuff.

Set up your tent, including your rain-fly and guy lines to hold it down if you anticipate heavy weather. Close the tent after you're done to prevent bugs, other critters, and weather from getting in. If you chose not to set up your tent, or add your rain-fly, at least have them ready to deploy when you feel those first, surprise raindrops on your face in the middle of the night.

If you do own a tent, make sure to stake it down well. In a strong wind, it can be nothing more than a big kite, even with your

WILDERNESS WISDOM

If the grommet rips from your tarp, or you want to improvise a tarp shelter, place a small rock in the corner of the tarp fabric, then tie your cord around it.

stuff or small children in it. Place stakes leaning at a 30-degree angle away from the center of your tent for best strength. If the ground is too rocky to stake your tent down, use cord to tie it to large rocks at the corners, or tie each tent corner to a stick, which you can bury under snow, sand, or large rocks.

Next, roll out your sleeping pads and bags; give them time to fluff up before you go to bed. Don't blow up your self-inflating pad; instead, open the valve and let it inflate on its own. Top it off with a gentle puff or two. Blowing in more than necessary sends unneeded water vapor from your breath into the pad, which can freeze on cold nights, making you colder; the moisture also weighs down your pad the next time you carry it. Plus, mold can form inside the pad, and how do you clean that out? During the day on hot days, open the valve of your sleeping pad. An inflated, closed pad on a hot day can delaminate or burst.

Once your tent is up, set up your kitchen and food storage (if you need to, hang your food from bears and/or rodents; read how on page 179). The kitchen area should be free of clothes or other items that don't belong in the kitchen.

If you haven't done so already, find your headlamp. Put it in your pocket or hang it around your neck so you know where it is when dark comes. Also arrange bedtime clothes,

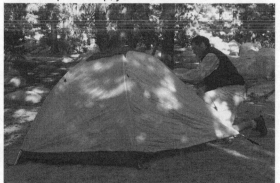

Once camp is set up, you can relax.

Tentiquette

Your tent is your home away from home, and in order to keep it comfy, follow these rules:

➤ Take your shoes off before you get in the tent. This will keep the tent's interior more comfortable and enjoyable, and it will keep your tent in good shape for longer—dirt and other materials can grind in and ruin tent fabrics. Put your footwear in the vestibule or just inside, so it's handy when you need to get out. Do not walk around barefoot in camp, especially at night.

➤ Be careful with food and drinks in tent. Tasty crumbs and morsels attract animals; spills ruin technical fabrics.

➤ Ventilation: The average person exhales up to two pints of water each night. Open your tent's doors, windows, or other vents a tad (keep the mosquito netting closed) to reduce condensation on your sleeping bag and other gear, not to mention the stuffy smell from multiple dirty bodies in a small space.

➤ Dry stuff each day. When you're blessed by sun in the morning, hang your sleeping bag and clothes outside to dry them before putting them back in the tent or into your pack for hiking.

socks, toothbrush, and other toiletries so they are easy to find when you need them. Always change into dry clothes and fresh socks before bedding down at night (in cold weather, I enjoy extra-thick sleep socks or down booties).

If it's already dark when you get to camp (don't feel bad; everyone has done it), just be glad you know your equipment well because you've done this all before (practiced at home at the very least), and that you've packed well, so you can find everything ("Now, where is that darn headlamp?").

Cooking and Dining Alfresco

Eating a delicious meal overlooking a gorgeous view, or by a darling lake, can be a memory that lasts a lifetime. Cooking in the backcountry isn't difficult, but it does call for planning, ingenuity, some experience using camp stoves, pots, utensils, and wilderness-friendly recipes, not to mention a high tolerance for dirt. Here are some tricks to make it go smoothly:

Before each meal, evaluate your party's situation and needs. Is everyone cold, hungry, and tired? Do they need not only the warmth,

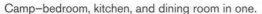
Camp—bedroom, kitchen, and dining room in one.

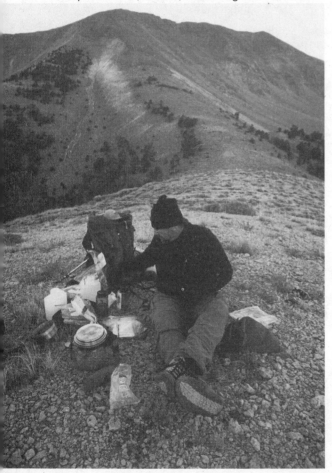

but the morale boost of a quick, hot, filling meal? Or are they content to snack on trail mix while you prepare a more elaborate meal? If planning an elaborate, time-consuming meal, will the weather cooperate? How about the daylight (will dinner be ready soon after sunset, or will it be 11 p.m. before the food's ready)? Is there anything you can do to get the process going earlier, such as rehydrating vegetables while you hike, or at least while you're setting up camp before you start cooking?

Here are a few other ideas to make food preparation enjoyable and safe:

➤ Organize everything: Have all food, pots, utensils, and dishes prepped and ready to cook before you light your stove.

➤ In bear country, put your kitchen area at least 100 yards downwind of camp. Hang your food. Make every effort to leave everything that smells good in that bag away from camp.

➤ In your pack and in camp, always separate food from cooking fuel.

➤ Wash your hands. Before handling and/or sharing food, make sure your hands are clean. Carry a small tube of alcohol-based hand sanitizer to kill germs that might make people sick.

➤ Share cooking duties. Make each person responsible for a different meal. Pitch in to make sure no one person is stuck doing all the work.

➤ Watch your meal closely as it cooks; food burns quickly with high-output camp stoves and thin cooking pots. No amount of spice will save a burned meal. Turn or stir your food often, or use a double-boiler to avoid burning foods by placing a smaller pot on top of 1 to 2 inches of boiling water in a larger pot.

➤Don't spill fuel. Soils made of broken-down plant matter (often called duff) can burn. Avoid burning down the forest while you're out there; it'll be a tough thing to explain to your parents (and authorities) when you get home.

➤ Never step over food. This prevents spills and keeps dirt and twigs from getting in your food.

➤ Cover pots and open food. Food cooks more quickly when covered, and covers keep dirt and bugs out.

➤ Tidy up. Never leave a mess—food or dirty dishes left out, or socks, shirts, or other clothes strewn about. Smelly stuff attracts animals, loose items can get lost, and it's easier to find things and more enjoyable when you develop good habits. Pack stuff away, straighten up, and batten down camp before you leave for a dayhike.

➤ Do not feed wildlife! Animals that get used to eating human food become more aggressive and dangerous; they often have to be killed by rangers to keep future campers safe. Small rodents may carry bubonic plague. Coyotes, skunks, and raccoons can carry rabies. Bears are big and dangerous when they insist you share the food in your pack. Avoid trouble by keeping your food to yourself. (More on wildlife in the "Where the Wild Things Are" chapters later in this book.)

Campfires

Campfires are going out of fashion these days, for lots of reasons: Fires leave unnecessary impacts on campsites and on the land (Leave No Trace recommends using a stove instead); in some popular backpacking destinations, the wood has been picked over; in others, especially at high elevations, there simply isn't any to begin with; during fire season, fires are often prohibited.

But nothing beats the crackle of a fire and the chance to stare into glowing embers under the stars. So if you have the opportunity (or need) to build a fire, here's how:

Use already-established fire rings, if available. If one's not available, build your fire on a mound of mineral soil that won't burn (sand, rock, etc.). Dirt, especially in forests, has a lot of plant material (a.k.a. duff) that can catch fire easily. Do not build a fire ring unless necessary. When you're ready to break camp, make sure the fire is dead out, scatter the ashes, and otherwise remove all evidence you built a fire there. This Leave No Trace technique will help avoid attracting further impacts to the site.

Build small. Unless you're building a signal fire for rescue, build a compact fire. If you have to stand back because it's too hot, then it's too big. Leave some wood for the rest of us.

For heat, build a fire so you are between it and a large rock, tree, or log that can reflect some heat back at you. For cooking, build small, so you can approach the fire without burning yourself. Coals are more reliable for cooking than open flames. Be aware that once your pots are black, the soot is nearly impossible to clean, and it will spread that soot to everything in your pack, unless you have a stuff sack for your pots. Luckily, black pots absorb heat better and will heat food more efficiently in the future.

Never leave a campfire unattended, even for a few minutes.

I was horrible at building fires for decades, until I figured out the following two reliable methods. Each works for large and small fires. Now I am more confident in my manliness:

Lean-to fire. Start with one main log set against the back of the fire ring (call it a turd, backbone, or anchor, whichever pleases you most). Place paper along the base, then small kindling on the paper. If you have fire starter, place it on top of the paper. Build a lean-to of kindling, leaning sticks from the ground over the paper against the turd. This creates a chimney effect, encouraging airflow to feed the fire with oxygen. As the fire builds, lean larger pieces of wood as the small pieces burn.

Tepee fire. Place a crumpled ball of paper in the center of the fire ring, then put your fire starter on that. Lean two small twigs together, making a triangle over the paper. Lean two more twigs perpendicular to the first two. Keep adding sticks, filling in the circle until you have a tepee-shaped structure. This creates a chimney effect to encourage airflow and reliable fire. Keep adding sticks as the fire continues. With both methods, the chimney effect is of utmost importance; you need a structure that will pull new oxygen in to feed the fire as the heat escapes up and out the top. Don't pack kindling too tightly. Air needs to move freely to supply the fire with needed oxygen.

Fire Starters

There are several things you can use to give your fledgling fire a boost:

➤ Woodchip-based fire starters can be found next to firewood in any store that carries firewood or artificial fire logs. Although easy to find, these are the heaviest options.

➤ Candle shavings or drippings can give a needed boost to stubborn fires.

➤ Gauze soaked in wax. Do this at home, then keep a small roll handy in your pack.

➤ Boy Scout's helper. When I need a fire now, a *small* splash of white gas from my fuel container does the trick. Stand back when you light it! Some people call it cheating. I call it being prepared. Name aside, this method is not approved by Boy Scouts of America or any other rational, competent organization.

Storing Food

Bears, raccoons, mice, coyotes, squirrels, ants, and other animals are opportunists; they will take food that's available. If you leave food sitting out or in your pack, you might as well put it on a silver platter. Your pack itself might be a target if there are salt stains from your sweat on pads and straps. To avoid swearing up a storm at local residents for raiding your pantry, you'll need to store it properly.

Everything that smells good (including gum, toothpaste, lip balm, sunscreen, unwashed pans, and utensils from meals) will attract bears, raccoons, skunks, squirrels, ringtailed cats, mice, and/or other locals. In the parlance of public-lands agencies, fed bears are dead bears. Feeding bears and other animals makes them more aggressive toward people in the future, and it disrupts their natural diet and feeding habits. Aggressive animals are often destroyed by authorities. If you care about local wildlife, do not feed them.

Three Reasons Why It's a Bad Idea to Cook in Your Tent

➤ Cooking fuels create carbon monoxide and other toxic fumes. Being in your tent with them will kill many brain cells you'll wish you had later on. The fumes also soak into fabrics, creating a toxic atmosphere every time you get into your tent in the future, even after you air it out.

➤ Cooking can be messy. At least I'm a messy cook, and I don't enjoy sleeping in oatmeal and spaghetti sauce. Many backpacking stoves are also precarious and top heavy; spill risk is high.

➤ Stoves have been known to burn tents. It's only a matter of time before yours flares up unexpectedly. I never realized how quickly tent walls and mosquito netting can melt into big holes (sorry about your tent, Beau!).

So what do you do in foul weather? Cook under the shelter of a tree or rock (don't burn the forest down!) or cook under a well-ventilated tarp or shelter.

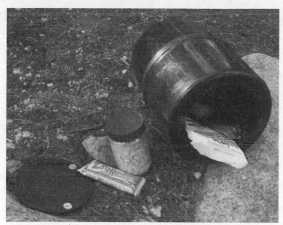
Bear canisters are fool-proof and bear-proof.

Often, bear-proof lockers are provided in campgrounds by trailheads where bears are active. In some areas, your car doesn't count. Bears in Yosemite National Park, for example, are good at opening cars: Claws make handy tools for tearing off doors and windshields, and a big bear's determined jump on the roof of a small car will pop the doors right open. Try explaining that to your insurance agent.

Proper food storage depends on where you backpack. Bear canisters are required in many bear hot spots, where bears know how to get your hanging food, or where there's nowhere to hang food. Canisters can hold three to five days' worth of food for one person, and they cost $60 to $80. They're also available for rent near trailheads in many locations. Call officials where you plan to hike about requirements and availability. Canister manufacturers include BearVault, Counter Assault, and Backpacker's Cache.

Hanging food is the most common way to protect it from wildlife. Some national parks and other destinations provide cables at designated campsites to make this easier. If cables aren't available, find a good, strong branch that sticks out. Make sure food is at least 10 feet out from the nearest tree trunk and 12 feet off the ground.

Tying off one end of your cord to a nearby tree trunk often doesn't work. Bears are smart, and they'll figure the puzzle out quickly. Instead, counterbalance your food to ensure its safety. Here's how:

➤ Tie a rock to one end of your cord and throw it over a branch or cable.

➤ Put half your food in a stuff sack, then attach it to one end of the cord (small carabiners are useful here), and hoist it all the way up to the branch or cable.

➤ Make a loop on the other end of the rope, as high as you can reach. Attach the other half of your food here, then push it up with a stick or trekking pole, so both bags are hanging side by side and well out of reach from any wildlife. You'll need that stick or trekking pole to get it back down (a foot-long loop of extra cord hanging from one of the bags will give you something to grab with the stick or pole).

Rodents will be after your food if bears aren't. Hanging food helps, and it doesn't need to be as high. Squirrels and mice can climb down the cord to enjoy a hanging picnic. Prevent this by tying a knot in the cord a few feet above the food, and stringing the cord through a tin can or Tupperware lid, so the lid rests on the knot above the food. Rodents won't be able to get past this on their way down the cord from above.

Before You Go to Bed

Just as your pack needs to be streamlined and items secured before you start hiking, everything in your camp needs to be cleaned and tucked away securely. This way, animals won't be attracted to food, wind won't blow away loose items, and rain or snow won't soak boots, clothes, or other items you left out. Good planning will also make your morning much more enjoyable.

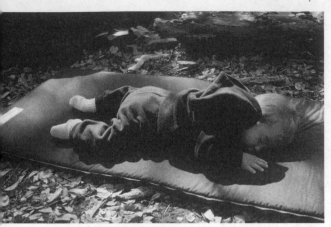
Some folks fall asleep before camp chores are done.

➤ Clean up camp, wash dishes, and secure food and other items that might blow away overnight.

➤ Set up stove and a pot of water, so it's ready to fire up first thing in the morning.

➤ Have your water bottle, headlamp, and other emergency items waiting in your tent.

➤ Set shoes ready to deploy near the door, in case you need to get out in the dark.

➤ Light sleepers might enjoy ear plugs, which minimize the impact of snoring tent mates or other unfamiliar noises at night.

➤ Pee bottle: It's a drag crawling out of the tent at night in cold or buggy weather to pee. Consider the following alternatives: Men, use a wide-mouth bottle that has a totally different shape and feel than your water bottle—mix-ups are no fun. Gatorade bottles work well. Empty them in the morning, when you're dressed and ready to face the elements. Women can use a wider-mouth Tupperware-style container with a tight-fitting lid, or a TravelMate, which is designed to help you aim into a normal bottle, or pee standing up when you're on the trail.

Germs surround us every day, in improperly cooked or stored food, on dirty counters and sponges, on infected handshakes, and on money that's been who-knows-where. At home we combat these germs with soap, hot showers, municipal water-treatment plants, flushing toilets, and other modern conveniences.

In the backcountry, such conveniences are nearly nonexistent. When backpacking, it's possible to go days without bathing; water sources are untreated, and human waste is often improperly disposed. In such conditions, it's easy to get sick and pass it to others. No wonder colds, flues, and digestive troubles commonly spoil the fun in the backcountry.

People are the leading source of diseases in the backcountry; we carry them in and infect water sources, which in turn infect wildlife and future people visiting the area. There is a direct connection between the number of visitors to an area and your risk of getting sick.

That beautiful babbling brook you're about to drink from might have *Giardia lamblia* or cryptosporidium donated by an infected person or animal who pooped or peed too close to the water. Your hiking partner might infect you with the flu the next time he sneezes, or pass you botulism or E. coli in the sandwich he made for lunch.

Before you barricade yourself in your tent from all those malicious threats, take a look at your hands. Where have they been lately? Did you thoroughly wash them after pooping and before you made lunch? What about all the doorknobs, payphones, money, and other people you've been touching? Our hands are our most important tools. They're also the most likely carriers of disease into your body. Pass food to your mouth, rub your eyes, or touch an open sore, and you're inviting germs to infect you.

Luckily, we can significantly reduce our chances of getting sick by cleaning up our act on the trail and in camp.

Know Your Enemies: Bacteria, Viruses, and Protozoa

There are several types of organisms that can make you sick:

Viruses. These super-tiny packets of genetic material invade cells, then hijack them to manufacture new virus particles. Viruses are responsible for the common cold, most flues, mumps, measles, meningitis, encephalitis, herpes, chicken pox, shingles, hepatitis, and HIV.

Luckily, most viruses cannot survive for long outside of living tissue (lessening your chance of getting any of the above from the trailhead toilet seat), although hepatitis and other viruses can be swallowed with fecal-contaminated foods, water, and utensils, or by exchanging bodily fluids (you'll begin to feel sick days to weeks later). High heat (boiling), extended exposure to ultraviolet radiation, and sufficient chemical treatment will destroy viruses. No water filter can remove viruses—they're simply too small.

Bacteria. Thousands of species of these one-celled organisms live around us, in us, and on us. Many species perform essential functions, such as the decomposition and recycling of dead tissues into nutrition for other life. Unlike viruses, they do not need a host cell to reproduce, although some are dependent on living tissue to complete their life cycles.

Bacteria are responsible for infected wounds, staph, and strep infections. Tetanus, anthrax, bacterial meningitis, E. coli, botulism, and salmonella are among the nasty bacteria you should avoid. Because they breed and mutate so quickly, bacteria are becoming resistant to antibiotics.

Bacteria infect wounds and slip past weakened immune systems; we ingest them with contaminated food, water, or utensils, or when we exchange bodily fluids with someone who's infected. Bacteria cannot survive high heat, chemical treatment, extended exposure to ultraviolet light, and dry conditions.

Protozoa. These tiny, mostly one-celled parasites are responsible for an array of sicknesses you'd prefer to avoid. Giardia and cryptosporidium infect many backcountry water sources. Ingesting them can cause severe stomach cramps, epic flatulence, and explosive diarrhea.

Amoebas living in warm water sources are responsible for amoebic dysentery. Luckily, boiling and filtration will kill or remove protozoa. Giardia and cryptosporidium cysts have thick shells; chemical treatment can eat through that shell to destroy the cyst, but only with enough time and the right chemicals.

Defending Your Castle

To best protect yourself, friends, and family from getting sick, you need to stop germs at the source, whether it be an infected water supply, a rancid sandwich, or a sneezing friend. Because you never know who's carrying what illness into the backcountry (people can carry pathogens without ever showing symptoms), follow these tips to avoid passing sickness among fellow campers, to wildlife, or into nearby water sources:

Wash your hands. Use hot water, lather, and scrub well, especially under your fingernails. Dry your hands with a bandanna or towel packed especially for that purpose. Always use biodegradable soaps (such as Campsuds or Dr. Bronner's), and wash at least 200 feet from fresh water sources to avoid contaminating them. Wash your hands before dinner each day (and always after you poop).

Sanitize your hands. If hot water isn't available, if you're the camp cook, or if someone in camp is already sick, cleansing gels with alcohol will kill most of the germs you didn't get with your hand wash.

Cover your mouth. Sneeze into your elbow or a handkerchief, not at your campmates.

Avoid sharing food. That big bag of trail mix that everyone's reaching into is nothing but a germ fest. Avoid sharing hydration nozzles, cups, utensils, or drinking bottles. Instead, pour individual portions into people's cups or other containers.

Avoid passing germs. If someone in camp gets sick, have them wear a bandanna, bandit-style, and relieve them of any kitchen duties.

Don't infect the water. Pee, poop, and wash hands and dishes at least 200 feet from water sources.

Break it up. Divide larger groups into smaller units of three to five, each with its own sleeping, cooking, and cleaning arrangements. If one person gets sick, only a few others will get sick and not everyone.

Don't share. That is, when it comes to bodily fluids.

Avoid leftovers. They can spoil easily. Instead, plan better and cook less.

Keep clean. While we're on the subject, how long has it been since you washed your pocket knife or multitool? Open it up and give it a good washing. Lube the hinges with lightweight oil after to keep the knife working smoothly.

Luckily, you are your best defense. With skin that keeps out most unwanted visitors and white blood cells that attack intruders, your immune system is designed to keep you healthy. But you must do your part to keep it strong.

➤ Sleep well. Fatigue weakens your immune system.

➤ Eat well. Quality foods, vitamins, and minerals fuel a healthy body.

➤ Relax. Stress weakens your immune system.

➤ Stay fit. A strong, active body keeps your immune system strong.

➤ Practice good hygiene to prevent germs from spreading.

➤ Drink water. Proper hydration boosts immune resistance.

➤ Keep vaccinations up to date.

Backcountry Water

Nothing beats plunking your head into a cold stream on a hot day and drinking deeply. But is it safe? Backcountry water sources can make you sick. Popular backpacking destinations have higher rates of water-borne diseases lurking in water sources than do less-visited locales. Yes, it's true; we bring our diseases with us, and then pass them to other people, wild-life, and water sources through our own poor hygiene.

How can you determine whether backcountry water sources are safe? Many streams, springs, and lakes look clear, cool, and refreshing. But unfortunately, without a scientific testing laboratory, it's hard to tell if they really are. You may need to resort to educated guesses based on the information that follows.

The closer you are to people, cattle, and wildlife, the more suspicious you must be about how safe the water is. Water sources in well-visited areas, and in areas with lots of cattle and/or wildlife, are statistically the most polluted and the most likely to make you sick.

Likewise, remote water has a higher chance of being safe. If you're at high elevation, off the beaten track, and most important, at the source of a water supply (such as the source of a spring, or near water trickling from the bottom of a snow field), there's a decent chance that the

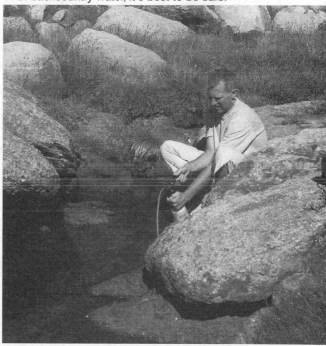

With backcountry water, it's best to be safe.

Poop Pack

Make wilderness pooping easier by carrying a "poop pack." Put everything you need for this activity–trowel, toilet paper (in a Ziploc), hand wipes or sanitizer, and plastic bags (if you're packing out your TP)–in a stuff sack. Carry it in an easy-to-grab spot in your backpack.

–**Brian Beffort**, author

water is safe. Remember, however, that a single poop from a passing bird, deer, or other animal might have contaminated what you're about to drink. It takes only a little to make you sick. The crystal-clear stream in front of you might be mostly pure, but it only takes a few microscopic organisms to make you sick.

Snow is not necessarily safe. It, too, might be contaminated by bird or animal poop. And at least 60 species of snow algae have been identified in the western US, the most colorful of which is *Chlamydomonas nivalis*, often called "watermelon snow" because it turns the snow bright pink. Anecdotal evidence suggests that consuming some types of snow algae can cause diarrhea.

Unfortunately, there's no way to know for sure when you're standing by the water. The better-safe-than-sorry bet is to disinfect the water anyway. There are three ways to disinfect suspicious water sources: boiling, mechanical filters, and chemical treatment. Each has its own advantages and disadvantages. For a detailed discussion of these, see page 90.

Here's how *not* to infect backcountry water:

➤ Camp at least 200 feet (70 steps) from water.

➤ Never use soap at a water source (it can kill fish and other organisms). To wash dishes or yourself, fill a container with water, then carry it 200 feet from water (and camp, to avoid attracting wildlife to camp). Use only biodegradable soap, such as Dr. Bronner's or Campsuds. Once done washing yourself, scatter the water; after washing dishes, scatter or bury the food waste and water.

➤ Never poop or pee within 200 feet of camp or water. In most soils, make it even farther; pathogens can travel with water underground.

Shitting in the Woods

Everyone does it, but we often avoid this stinky subject and face unpleasant consequences as a result—in the form of ugly and smelly toilet paper "lilies" sprouting up behind bushes and increased levels of disease in the backcountry. Boldly face your dark side, and follow these tips to keep our trailheads, campsites, and backcountry water supplies clean, appealing, and disease-free:

➤ Use a bathroom or outhouse, if available.

➤ If there's no toilet, choose a spot at least 200 feet (70 steps) from water, camp, or other people.

➤ Bury your poop. Dig a hole 6 to 8 inches deep, by 8 inches across, using a stick, rock, or lightweight, plastic trowel. Do your business, then bury it. Pack out your toilet paper in a Ziploc bag. If you insist on leaving your TP, bury it with your poop. Please use dye- and perfume-free TP for backcountry use.

➤ Learn more by reading *How to Shit in the Woods* by Kathleen Meyer (Ten Speed Press).

➤ Don't use toilet paper. Who needs it? Toilet paper in the backcountry poses several challenges: It doesn't break down well by the natural organic processes in the soil, and perfumes and dyes in toilet paper can attract animals. Leave No Trace recommends packing out your TP in a Ziploc bag, and how fun is that? Avoid these problems by leaving the TP at home, and instead use one of the following items common to the outdoors (you might discover a newfound sense of peace knowing that you're making this process purely organic and natural):

Local plants. Big handfuls of grass or wide, thick leaves are best. Sagebrush, other shrubs, a sprig of pine needles, and soft pinecones work well, too (make sure to wipe in the right direction with some of these to avoid getting poked). By all means, avoid thorns and poison ivy.

Rocks. Choose ones that fit your personal contours.

Snow. It's not really as cold as it seems. Make a pile of small, pointy snowballs ahead of time, so they're ready when you need them.

Hint: Think about availability of good wiping materials when scouting a spot, not after you're squatting there, pants down around your ankles.

Bathing in the Woods

Refreshing face- and hand-washes are great ways to start or end each day. Every few days or so, the rest of your body will need some scrubbing, too. Soaping up in a pond, lake, stream, or river might seem like a good idea, but it contaminates the water with chemicals, your own naughty bits, and possibly disease, which are all bad for wildlife and other people. Instead, fill a pot with water (heat it if you wish), and take a sponge bath using biodegradable soap and a washcloth somewhere you won't infect the water source.

Women-Specific Hygiene

The physical exertion of backpacking, not to mention the disruption of schedules and habits, can alter women's menstrual cycles. Yours might start early, or it might not happen at all while you're backpacking. Neither should

MY SYSTEM

Periods

It never fails; every time I go on a wilderness adventure, I get my period. I often travel in a group where I am the only woman, so it can be a bit embarrassing. For years, I took a small black garbage bag and diligently packed out my feminine-hygiene products. It was a pain, to say the least, and I was always worried about odor from the bag, even though the contents were in a zippered freezer bag concealed inside the larger black bag. Then I discovered a solution to my problems—the menstrual cup.

The menstrual cup has made dealing with my period on backpacking and paddling trips much more comfortable. It collects the fluids, I empty it, cleanse it, and reinsert. It's made of surgical silicone, which means I can wear a menstrual cup for six to 12 hours, depending on how heavy my period is. The menstrual cup is very comfortable, does not leak, and moves with me. I can hike, swim, or paddle and not have to worry about my period. To add even more benefit, I am putting less into the garbage. Let's face it, all those applicators and tampons really add up to a lot of refuse.

If you decide to make the switch from tampons, just search the internet and you will find several suppliers. The menstrual cup is not for every woman, but it certainly has made my life on the trail easier.

—**Laurie Ann March**, author, *A Fork in the Trail*, Wilderness Press

be cause for alarm (if you're still concerned after you get home, consult your doctor). Bring supplies with you, so you're prepared if your period starts, even if you're not planning to hike when it's your time of the month.

Every woman has her preference—either pads or tampons. In the wilderness, tampons are often preferred because they are more comfortable when hiking. Pads can also be chillingly cold when wet in cold weather. With tampons, however, it's important to keep your hands clean, or you can minimize contact by choosing tampons with applicators. Pack out your used pads or tampons in a Ziploc bag (place a tea bag or some tea tree oil inside to control odor), then place the plastic bag in a paper bag or colored plastic bag. Do not bury or burn tampons or pads.

Wash yourself daily to avoid infections. Sweat and poor hygiene make conditions prime for yeast infections. Sponge baths are convenient for this. Hand wipes are quick and convenient for this purpose; they're also nice for a quick face and hand wash each morning or night.

Your backpacking trip has been either a wonderful joy or pure misery. But now it's time to pack up and go home. This part is often easy because there's less food now, and everything fits into your pack more easily.

There are two main goals in breaking down camp and packing up to go: Don't forget anything, and leave camp un-impacted and cleaner than you found it.

Before you start packing stuff up, dry everything out, if you can–sleeping bags, tent, pack, clothes, etc. Your pack will be lighter, you'll be warmer when you use them again, and damaging mildew will have less chance to form. In humid and/or rainy climates, this might be impossible.

Final check. Before you leave, take a good look around to make sure you aren't leaving anything behind, especially small stuff, such as wrappers, tent stakes, or your sunglasses. Earn extra karma points by picking up after others. Leave your campsite as clean as you would like to find it.

Debrief and Reorganize

Once you get home, and while your trip is still on your mind, think about what went well and what didn't. What would you

Once you break down camp and leave, there should be no trace of your stay.

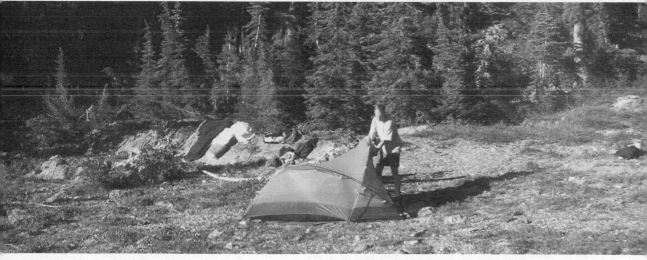

do differently next time? Add things to your packing list you wish you had brought. Cross off things you brought but didn't need (always bring your 10 essentials and appropriate clothing for the weather, even if you didn't need them last time). Clean your equipment and repack it before you put it into storage, so it's ready to travel the next time: Pack your tent complete with ground cloth, poles, stakes, and rain-fly; store your stove complete with windscreens, pot supports, matches, or lighter; keep your 10 essentials together in one bag that you can grab next time without having to assemble every single piece.

Large plastic storage tubs are great for keeping all your backpacking gear in one place. Simply write "Backpacking" across the side, then throw everything you'll need to backpack into the tub(s), so it's ready to go the next time you are. By planning and preparing well, you'll save a great deal of time pulling things together the next time you want to hit the trail.

Giving Back

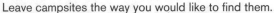

Now that you have wonderful memories from your special place, do something to keep it beautiful for you and others to visit again and again in the future:

➤ Pick up trash when you're backpacking, so you can leave it better than you found it (how beautiful would this world be if everyone did this?).

➤ Donate to a conservation organization working to protect an area you love. There are numerous regional and national nonprofit organizations working to do good for the land. Find one that's working on an area you care about, then write them a generous check. They'll become stronger with your support.

Leave campsites the way you would like to find them.

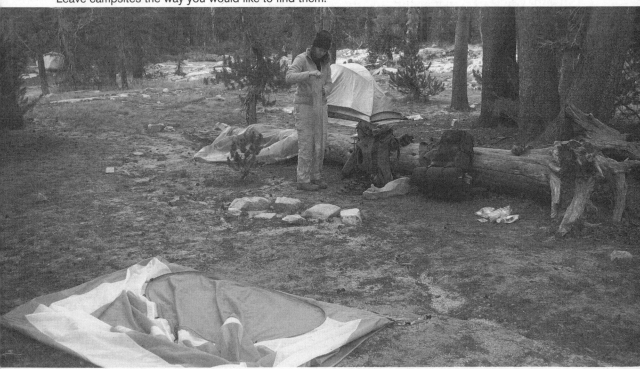

➤ Volunteer your time to restore or protect your favorite places. Ask land-management officials in an area you love about volunteer activities. Or perhaps one of the nonprofit organizations is planning a work trip or needs help stuffing envelopes at the office.

➤ Write or call decision-makers, be they land-management agencies who are drafting management plans for the area, or elected officials. Tell them how much you love a particular place, and encourage them to make decisions that will protect that area, not destroy it.

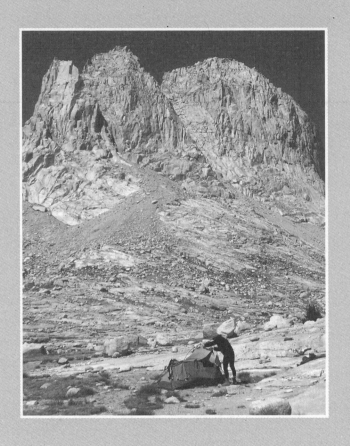

PART VI
SAFETY AND COMFORT
IN THE BACKCOUNTRY

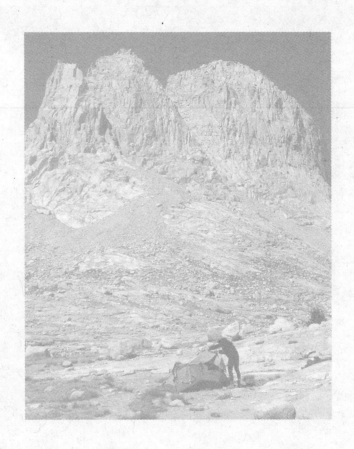

There is no such thing as bad weather—it simply is. Weather is bad only relative to our hopes and expectations. The same woman who whines about a rainy day also curses when her lawn turns brown in summer. A raging blizzard will get a different reaction from the guy who has to commute on snowy roads than it will from the skier who's itching for fresh powder.

Wild, harsh, and violent weather in the wilderness can be horrible—a true emergency—if we fail to prepare for it. It can also be exciting and breathtakingly beautiful if we're prepared—few things are more beautiful than clearing storms.

Don't let "bad" weather happen to you. Prepare to endure every kind of weather, because you're going to have to live with whatever the sky throws at you. All veteran backpackers have a story about getting caught by that surprise snowstorm in July, or that torrential downpour they simply didn't expect. This is especially true in high mountains, which create their own weather—rain, snow, high winds, lightning, and bright sun can happen on any day of the year at high elevations.

It helps to be able to anticipate the weather, which isn't always easy—ask any TV meteorologist. But there are general weather characteristics, trends, and patterns that can help you get a better idea of what's going to happen in the next day or two. These patterns and trends vary by region and season. It's helpful if you know the general weather patterns of an area well, so you'll know when weather strays from the norm. If you're planning to hike somewhere unfamiliar, ask local rangers or other experts about what to expect. What follows is a quick lesson on some general concepts.

Basic Weather Rules

The sun powers weather around the world. Air warmed by the sun rises and expands, creating low-pressure zones. Cold air settles and condenses, creating high-pressure zones. These differences in pressure mean air is always on the move—from areas of high pressure to areas of low pressure, seeking to balance the differences between night and day, and between the relative high pressure at the poles and the relative low pressure at the equator. Cold air at the poles sinks and spreads toward the equator to fill the low-pressure zone created by sun-warmed air, which rises and spreads toward the poles.

This air movement—what we call wind—is affected by three major forces: the Coriolis effect, the friction of land dragging against the air, and temperature, all of which add incredible complexity to weather around the world.

The Coriolis effect, caused by the spinning of the Earth and the friction of land dragging against the atmosphere, forces high-pressure masses to spin—generally clockwise in the northern hemisphere and counterclockwise in the southern hemisphere (low-pressure systems spin the opposite way). Differences in air pressure between high- and low-pressure systems send winds whooshing across the land. When the pressure differences are great (they're greatest in winter) winds can pack a real punch.

Another factor affecting air movement is temperature. Warm air rises, and cold air falls. Warm air holds more moisture than cold air. It is also less dense and lighter than cold air. Warm summer days will blow winds up mountain slopes; in contrast, cold air will flow

Weather Lore

The following observations have stood the test of time. Does it mean they speak true, or are they proof that we're all suckers looking for easy explanations? Read them with a grain of salt and find out for yourself.

➤ **Campfire smoke:** If the smoke from your campfire rises straight and high into the sky, you can expect fair weather; if the smoke stays low, lingering close to the ground or in the trees, barometric pressure is low, and you should expect wet weather.

➤ **Coffee:** If your hiking partner is staring into her coffee, she might just be waking up. Or maybe she's forecasting the weather. Strong coffee in a cup with vertical sides (slanted sides don't shape the surface well) can act as a barometer.

Give the coffee a vigorous stir and watch the bubbles, which will rise to the highest point of the coffee's surface. If they gather in the middle, high pressure has rounded the surface of the coffee, meaning fair weather will dominate. If they scatter to the sides, low pressure has made the surface concave, and you might be in for rain.

➤ **Birds:** Our feathered friends fly high in high pressure and low in low pressure. Mariners often watch birds to learn what weather is waiting out at sea. If birds fly out to sea in the morning, weather will be fair; if they stay on the beaches, foul weather is on its way.

➤ **Mist:** If it rises in the morning and clears to a sunny day, fair weather will prevail.

➤ **Sunrises and sunsets:** Remember the saying, "Red sky at night, sailors' delight; red sky in morning, sailors take warning." Prevailing storms in the northern hemisphere come from the west. Red sunrises can illuminate the leading clouds of an approaching storms, and if you can see a sunset at all, then there is no storm approaching.

➤ **Hair:** Like rope and other fibers, hair tends to contract when humidity is high, and it expands when humidity is low. If your hair is suddenly getting wavier or curlier, humidity is rising, and a storm may be approaching. If your hair is straighter, drier weather will dominate.

➤ **Pinecones:** If pinecones are soft and pliable, they're absorbing moisture from the air. Have your rain equipment handy.

➤ **Smell:** If the forest seems suddenly more fragrant, prepare for rain, because humid air transmits smell better than dry air. Plants also release more oils when the humidity climbs. Winds preceding a rainstorm often carry the fresh smell of wet ground where it is already raining. Lightning produces ozone, which carries a distinct, almost metallic odor.

downhill like water, then gather in canyon and valley bottoms. Remember this when pitching camp in the bottom of a lake basin before a cold night; you might be warmer camping upslope.

The dew point is the temperature at which moisture in the air condenses into visible droplets. This is when clouds form, and when you can see your breath when you exhale on a cold day; dew on the grass and your sleeping bag in the morning is a sign that temperatures overnight dropped below the dew point. The dew point changes with the weather, but knowing about it will keep you from being surprised when you wake up wet after falling asleep on a clear, dry night.

Meteorologists often refer to air pressure as barometric pressure, because they track changes in air pressure by measuring the height of a column of mercury in a barometer. Barometric pressure is expressed using two scales:

1. **Inches of mercury (Hg).** Aviators and television weather forecasters measure air pressure in inches of mercury. "Normal" atmospheric pressure at sea level is 30 inches. High pressure might be 30.7 inches; extreme low pressure, like in a hurricane, might dip to 28 inches.

2. **Millibars (mb).** Meteorologists express air pressure using this metric scale. "Normal" pressure at sea level is 1013.25 mb; high pressure might measure 1039.00 mb; low pressure might dip to 950.00 mb

In general, when barometric pressure drops, weather becomes less stable, and you might be in for a storm. The greater and faster the drop, the more intense that weather will be. Knowing this, you can use a barometer to help forecast impending storms. Note the current barometric pressure, then check back again in a few hours. How quickly the pressure drops can tell you how fast that storm is moving—a drop of 0.02 to 0.03 inch per hour indicates a slow-moving storm; 0.05 to 0.06 inch per hour indicates a fast-moving storm. Remember that barometric pressure drops as you gain elevation. Speaking of elevation, you can also use your altimeter to measure the air pressure; altimeters measure air pressure to track changes in elevation. If overnight your altimeter shows that camp has gained elevation, you know the air pressure has dropped, and a storm might be on its way.

Higher elevations mean cooler temperatures. Temperatures tend to drop between 3°F and 5°F with every 1000-foot climb in elevation, something meteorologists call the adiabatic lapse rate.

Mountains create storms. Because high-elevation air is cooler, and cooler air can't hold as much moisture, mountains often receive more precipitation than low country. When wind meets mountains, the air is pushed upslope and it cools to its dew point (called orographic lift), creating clouds and a greater chance of precipitation than in low lands. Often, the windward side of mountain ranges receives more moisture than leeward slopes.

Many deserts sit in the rain shadows of mountain ranges. For example, the Sierra Nevada squeeze most of the moisture out of prevailing winds, which explains why Donner Summit in the Sierra Nevada can get more than 450 inches of snow in a winter, while Reno, Nevada, just 30 miles to the east—on the leeward side of the Sierra—receives, on average, only 7 inches of precipitation each year.

In summer, the exposed soil and rock of high mountain peaks heats quickly in the sun, producing thermals that carry moisture upward, fueling thunderstorms while the valleys below are dry. Wherever you are in summer, know that the three Hs—heat, humidity, and hazy weather—can breed thunderstorms. In the mountains, a fourth H—high altitude—can further boost thunderstorm activity.

Fronts are large, moving masses of air. When warm and cold fronts meet, the warm air rises over the cold air. Depending on the size and intensity of the fronts, precipitation can result. The extreme thunderstorms, hail, and tornadoes across America's Midwest are often a clash between warm fronts from the Gulf of Mexico and cold fronts swooping down from Canada.

Any meteorologist will tell you that weather forecasts become far less reliable the further out the prediction is made; 48 hours is the upper limit of reliable forecasting. Beyond that, being prepared for anything is the best way to face the weather.

Seasonal Patterns

Despite our atmosphere's complexity, weather follows basic regional patterns, which explains why Hawaii, Florida, northern Arizona, the southern tip of Africa, and coastal California each has its own unique weather patterns.

Weather patterns tend to be seasonal. Each season has its rules, and rules can flip-flop between summer and winter. For example, in the Pacific Northwest, summer winds from the southwest or west indicate stable, dry air and continued fair weather. In winter, winds from the west and southwest often precede wet

Watch the sky to avoid being surprised by storms.

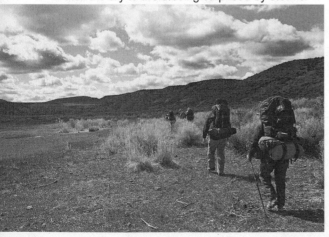

"Pineapple Express" storms out of the central Pacific. Northerly winds indicate colder storms moving in from the northern Pacific.

In New England, the Southeast, and the Midwest, summers tend to be hot and humid, punctuated by thunderstorms. In winter, however, storms can come from the Arctic or the Gulf of Mexico. Northerly winds in winter mean cold storms, while southerly winds bring warm, wet, soaking storms.

If patterns in summer and winter can be called predictable, all bets are off in spring and fall, when seasonal patterns are flip-flopping between summer and winter rules; almost anything can happen, and weather is a lot harder to predict.

The key to understanding regional weather patterns is to spend years watching the weather in one place—difficult if you're just passing through for a weekend backpacking trip. Seek out locals who know the patterns and ask them what they expect in the coming days. They might not be right, but they'll be a lot closer than your wild-card guesstimate.

Clouds: Weather's Writing in the Sky

One of the easiest ways to tell what the weather is going to do is to watch the clouds; no matter where you go in the world, all clouds speak the same language. They tell you how much moisture is in the air, how windy it is at different elevations, and what weather might be approaching from beyond the horizon.

There are many different kinds of clouds; knowing four main types can help you predict what the weather might bring:

Cirrus. Formed above 16,500 feet, cirrus clouds are the thin, wispy clouds that look like brush strokes. Often appearing on the leading edge of warm fronts, and sometimes resembling "mares' tails," they commonly precede precipitation by 24 to 48 hours. They can

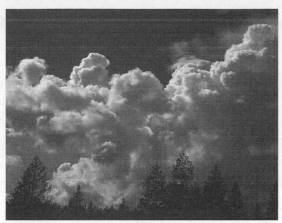
Towering clouds warn of thunderstorms.

also tell you that a storm front is passing to the north or south, blessing you with their beauty without precipitation.

Cumulus. These fluffy, cotton-ball clouds form when moist air rises until the moisture condenses into a cloud. Powered by summer thermals or colliding warm and cold fronts, these clouds can build into thunderstorms, which generate lightning, hail, and tornadoes. When you see these clouds growing and heaping, higher and higher into thunderheads, get ready for trouble—get down off ridges and peaks, and move away from tall, solitary trees; avoid being the tallest thing on the landscape. If winds are strong and blustery as thunderheads form, the storm will move through quickly; if the air is still, prepare for a lingering, angry storm. Read more about lightning later in this chapter.

Stratus. Stratus is Latin for "spreading out." These great sheets of clouds can be high (altostratus) or low (stratocumulus), and both can indicate approaching wet weather.

Lenticular. Often looking like great alien motherships capping mountains or floating stationary just downwind of a mountain range, these clouds indicate high winds at upper altitudes and can suggest approaching precipitation.

Halos. These hazy, sometimes rainbow-like rings form around the sun and moon when light refracts through ice crystals in the sky. Halos often precede approaching warm fronts by 24 to 48 hours.

Several of these cloud types can appear in concert to announce an approaching storm—high halos or cirrus might thicken and lower into altostratus, then to stratus, then to rain or snow. While this is happening, it's wise to seek a lower route or to camp, then batten down the hatches and be glad you brought a book or deck of cards to help you wait out the storm.

Although this discussion barely scratches the surface of our complicated atmosphere, it's a good starting point. Nonetheless, no matter how well you understand weather and how closely you watch the skies, you're sure to find yourself on the receiving end of surprise rain or snow if you spend enough time in the backcountry. The Earth's atmosphere is a complex system, and all of these "rules" are made to be broken. Because of this, it's always important to carry your 10 essentials—extra clothing layers, shelter, food, and water, etc., so you'll be able to avoid life-threatening situations when cold, wet weather catches you by surprise.

More Resources on Weather

► *Mountain Weather: Backcountry Forecasting and Weather Safety for Hikers, Campers, Climbers, Skiers, and Snowboarders*, by Jeff Renner (The Mountaineers Books)

► *The Nature Company Guides: Weather*, by William Burroughs, et al. (Time Life Books)

► *National Audubon Society Field Guide to North American Weather*, by David A Ludlum (Alfred A. Knopf)

Hiking Safely in Cold Weather

It can be a big, cold world out there. If you're backpacking in cold weather (intentionally or otherwise), your body heat is more precious than any jewel. Warmth is life. If your body temperature drops more than a few degrees below normal, you can fall victim to hypothermia, a potentially life-threatening condition in which your core body temperature drops below 95°F. Eventually, your body may get too cold for your brain and other crucial organs to function. Death is possible at body temperatures below 80°F.

Staying warm when the going gets cold is one of the most important things you can do. Luckily, it's not hard, if you're prepared and proactive in pursuing heat. Here are a few tips:

Stay warm. It's easier than trying to warm up after getting chilled. Add warm layers before you go outside or get to the top of that windy ridge. Inner layers help transport

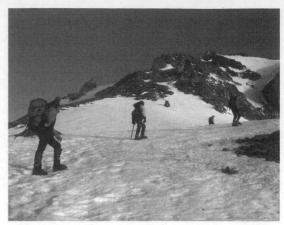

Add or shed layers carefully to avoid sweat or chills in cold weather.

sweat away from your body. Middle layers add fluffy insulation to trap warm, still air close to your body. Outer shell layers should help vent sweat while blocking wind and/or shedding rain and snow. A hat, neck warmer, and gloves will help protect those areas where heat dissipates fastest. Also, insulate yourself from the cold ground with your sleeping pad, grass, or branches in an emergency.

Stay dry. Water can steal heat from your body faster than you can say, "Jeez, Louise, it's cold." Avoid breaking a sweat on cold days. Change into dry clothes immediately after you get wet, or as soon as you get to camp. Never go to bed in wet clothes. Avoid cotton, because it absorbs water like a sponge and doesn't dry easily. Choose hydrophobic materials instead (ones that repel water, such as wool and synthetics).

Fuel up. Your internal furnace will keep you warmer if it has fuel. Sugar's quick calories burn hot and fast. If you're cold, this is the time to break into your candy stash. Fat contains more calories per gram than carbs or proteins. Throw a healthy handful of cheese into your soup, or a cube of butter into your cocoa before going to bed to keep your furnace burning all night long.

The Five Thieves of Warmth

Your body loses heat in five ways. The key to staying warm is anticipating and preventing these thieves from stealing your life-heat;

Conduction. Contact with cold surfaces, such as sitting on cold snow or rock, will transfer your precious warmth to the colder object simply through touch. What to do: Insulate yourself against the cold object with your sleeping pad, clothes, pack, even branches or grass.

Convection. Moving air carries warmth away from your body, something you'll learn quickly when you stand on a windy peak or ridge. You can also chill as warm air escapes from the top of your clothes and is replaced by cool air flowing in the bottom. What to do: Wear wind-stopping shell pants and jacket, which can deflect the wind and keep you warm (put them on before you start to chill). Snug collars and cuffs can seal the cracks where air escapes from your clothes.

Radiation. Your body radiates heats like a hot stove. This happens when your skin is not covered. What to do: Add clothing layers and find shelter to minimize heat loss. Snuggle with fellow hikers to share heat with each other in dire (or friendly) situations.

Evaporation. Water on our skin takes body heat with it when it evaporates, which is one reason we sweat on hot days—to cool off. Unfortunately, the same principle works when you're already cold: You can still sweat while hiking on a cold day. Evaporation (and hence heat loss) also happens after a plunge into water. What to do: Stay dry on cold days. Hike slower to keep yourself from sweating, and change into dry clothes as soon as you can, especially after unexpected plunges and soaks.

Respiration. With each cloudy breath on a cold day, your body loses heat. What to do: You can't stop breathing to prevent heat loss, but you can wear a bandanna, balaclava, or other face mask over your mouth and nose to minimize heat loss, and to help warm the air you're breathing in. Big, furry, Eskimo-style hoods create a tunnel of warmth in front of your face—a buffer of warm air between you and the cold.

Make muscle heat. When your muscles work, they generate heat. If you start getting cold, do some jumping jacks or push-ups for a quick burst of warmth. If you're cold in the middle of the night, you can do isometrics, sit-ups, or leg lifts without leaving your sleeping bag to generate cozy heat and help you drift back to sleep. Be careful, though—if you generate too much heat, you may begin to perspire, which will cool you off again.

Stay hydrated. Proper hydration allows blood to circulate smoothly, which keeps your extremities warmer. Hot, sweet liquids will also help you warm up if you're cold. (But stay away from the caffeine.) Drink lots of water, even if you don't think you're thirsty. Cold air is less humid, which dehydrates you quickly. Good hydration also aids circulation, which keeps you warm.

If you suspect that you or your hiking partners might be suffering from mild hypothermia—if they feel chilly, have difficulty using their hands, and have begun shivering—follow these tips for rewarming:

➤ Prevent additional heat loss. Seek shelter from that windy ridge, put on a windbreaker, or sit on a pad instead of the cold, hard ground.

➤ Swing your arms and stamp your feet to force warm blood into your extremities. If shivering is significant, wrap yourself in a sleeping bag, where the heat created by shivering will be trapped in the confined space between your body and your cozy bag.

➤ Wear thick boots and socks, but don't wear too many socks or tighten your boots too much; these restrict circulation, which leads to cold feet.

➤ Rewarm hands and feet by placing them on a campmate's warm belly. This can help prevent frostbite in dire situations, but you might need to buy them lunch or dinner when you get back to civilization.

➤ Bring a hot water bottle into your jacket or sleeping bag. Place it against areas of high heat loss, such as the sides of your chest, neck, or your groin. Your well-sealing water bottle or hydration reservoir should work fine.

➤ Bring your boots into your sleeping bag on cold nights, because it's not much fun cramming your feet into frozen boots in the morning. Gloves too, even if they're wet; they'll dry.

➤ Bring chemical heat packets for emergencies. Heat Treat disposable heat packets are convenient, quick, and environmentally friendly ways to provide necessary heat when the going gets cold. Avoid using these on a regular basis. Not only will they add weight (although lightweight, the packets work for only five to seven hours each), but your body will never develop its own ability to keep you warm if you keep adding warmth from the outside.

➤ Wear everything you have. If you're still cold, climb into your sleeping bag, hunker down, drink warm fluids, exercise, and wait for sun,

Hiking in the Rain

There's something deeply beautiful and calming about hiking on a rainy day, even if it's only the satisfaction of knowing you're comfortable despite what the sky is throwing at you. Nonetheless, it's easy to get cold in the rain. Here are some tips to help you remain comfortable when all around is wet:

➤ Always have at least one set of dry clothes, either in your pack or on your body, even if it means putting on yesterday's wet clothes before you start hiking in the morning, so you'll have something dry to change into when hiking's done at the end of the day. Keep important items dry by using waterproof stuff sacks or well-sealing plastic bags.

➤ Stay warm and dry. If you're wet and enjoying yourself in warm, rainy weather, that's one thing. But if you're getting chilled, put on extra layers. If you're dry on the inside of your shell, avoid working up a sweat, which will chill you when it cools after you stop.

➤ Make sure your tent is easily accessible. When it's time to camp, set your tent up first, so you have a dry refuge for yourself and all your equipment. Stake it taut and securely, because properly stretched fabric sheds water better than flimsy fabric.

➤ Wear gaiters over your boots to help keep your feet dry. Rain pants hanging down over the gaiters also will shed water away from your skin, whereas rain pants tucked into your gaiters will fill your boots with water.

➤ Wear a baseball cap to keep rain off your face.

➤ Avoid residual water. After the rain has stopped, don't take your shell layers off. Water can soak you as it drips off trees, or as you brush against wet plants.

➤ Take advantage of sun. Whatever your schedule, when the sun comes out, take some time to stop, dry things out, and air out your gear.

➤ Keep your furnace stoked. Lots of snacks will burn hot and keep you warm when all around is rainy.

➤ If you forget rain pants, take the emergency candle out of your pack and rub or melt wax onto the outside of the thighs of your pants. The wax will soak in and prevent your pants from soaking up water—a much more comfortable situation when you're walking into the rain.

➤ Tuck your ground cloth under your rain-fly. If it hangs out beyond the edges of your tent, you've just created a bathtub, where water can gather right under your sleeping bag.

Lightning

Few things are more impressive, more beautiful, and more terrifying than being in a thunderstorm in the wilderness. Lightning is one of the leading killers of backpackers each year. Here are a few tips to keep you off that list of statistics:

➤ Plan. Thunderstorms are relatively predictable. Although there are always exceptions, thunderstorms are common in certain seasons in certain regions, and the pattern is often predictable. Know the weather patterns where you'll be hiking (call local rangers or other experts if you're not sure). Time your hiking to avoid high peaks, ridges, and large open expanses when the storm hits. The time to head to safety is while clouds are forming and getting bigger. Once the storm starts, it's too late.

➤ If you can see it, flee it; if you can hear it, fear it. Lightning can strike as far as 10 miles from its origin in the clouds. If you can see lightning or hear thunder, the storm is close enough to strike you. It's time to seek safety. The big exception: Beware that towering thunderhead you can't see—the one that's growing on the other side of the ridge or mountain you're climbing. Estimate lightning distance by counting the time between flash and thunder. Five seconds equals 1 mile.

➤ Avoid high ground, open spaces, water, lone trees, all metal objects, and small caves when lightning is imminent. Seek instead low ground or large stands of small-sized trees.

If it's too late to flee, and you're exposed to danger, find the lowest spot you can away from metal, crouch down on your sleeping pad to insulate yourself from the ground, cover your ears to protect against point-blank-range thunder, and keep at least 20 feet from other people to avoid multiple strike victims. If one person is struck, others will be able to treat.

Treating Lightning Victims

Lightning victims do not carry a charge; it's safe to touch them. In fact, please do, because they need your help. Lightning can cause several different types of injuries. Each needs to be treated:

Respiratory system. If the patient is not breathing or not breathing adequately, administer rescue breathing.

Heart and lungs. Seventy-five percent of direct strike victims suffer cardiac arrest, but only 20 percent die; the rest can be jump-started again with prompt CPR and rescue breathing. Get to it, as time's a wasting. Continue until the victim begins to breathe on his own, someone else takes over, or you are exhausted and cannot continue.

Trauma to tissue or bones. Lighting victims often suffer cuts, bruises, and/or broken bones. The charge can cause muscle contractions that may cause a patient to fall and injure herself. Once breathing is established, perform a secondary survey (covered on page 228) to find other injuries and treat accordingly.

Burns. First- and second-degree burns are common, especially at entry and exit points (also covered in the first aid chapter)

Nervous system. Lightning can damage brain and nerve tissue, producing paralysis, tingling, numbness, amnesia, and other conditions. Seek medical attention immediately for anyone who is struck, so they can be evaluated.

Hiking Safely in Warm Weather

Sunshine is great. It helps us set our internal clocks, produces vitamin D, eases depression, and helps us forget the office for a few days. But too much sun leads to headaches, fatigue, sunburn, snow blindness, and skin cancer down the road. High in the mountains, too much sun can happen in mere minutes. Here are a few steps to preventing those maladies:

Damage from the sun comes from two flavors of ultraviolet (UV) radiation: UVA and UVB. Both contribute to skin damage, skin cancer, and damage to your eyes' sensitive corneas.

UVA rays are less harmful than UVB, but at least 1000 times more UVA rays penetrate the atmosphere. They don't burn, but they do penetrate deep into your tissues, damaging melanocytes (pigment cells), which ages your skin and in the long run can lead to the most dangerous skin cancer: malignant melanoma.

UVB rays turn you lobster red after too much sun (sometimes only a few minutes at high elevation). They can also damage the DNA in skin cells and are associated with less-

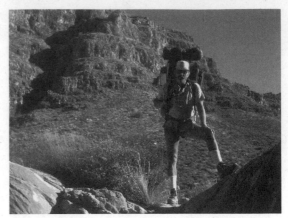

Wear sunscreen; prevention is the best cure for sunburn.

dangerous types of skin cancer: basal cell and squamous cell carcinomas.

UVA and UVB rays can also burn your cornea (the sensitive tissue over the surface of your eye). This type of sunburn is called snow blindness, because it happens commonly at ski resorts, where up to 90 percent of UV rays are reflected off the snow, nearly doubling your exposure to harmful UV rays. One Johns Hopkins University study found that even minimal exposure to the sun raises your risk of developing cataracts.

Protecting Yourself

The best way to protect yourself from the power of the sun is to avoid it—or at least to avoid exposure between 10 a.m. and 4 p.m., when the sun's rays are most intense. Yes, that's likely to be when you're going to be on the trail. Given that, use the protection strategies listed below:

➤ Use caution at high elevations and latitudes. Exposure to UV radiation increases by 3 percent with every 1000 feet you climb in elevation. At 5000 feet, for example, you're receiving about 15 percent more UV rays than at sea level; at 10,000 feet, UV rays are about 30 percent stronger. At high elevations, sunburns can happen in less than 20 minutes of exposure.

Sunburn in the Shade?

UV rays bend and bounce easily, giving you your fair share even when you're in the shade. Consider the following:

➤ Snow reflects 80 to 90 percent of UV rays.

➤ Sand and concrete can reflect 20 to 30 percent of UV rays.

➤ Water can reflect 100 percent of UV rays, depending on the angle.

Knowing these facts, take extra precautions—wear sunscreen and glasses even under your hat or while sitting in the shade, and don't forget to put sunscreen under your chin. At high elevations, be particularly cautious.

The Scoop on Sunscreen

What is SPF? The Sun Protection Factor listed on sunscreens and some clothes tells you how long you can stay in the sun without burning. If you normally burn after 30 minutes, wearing SPF 30 means you can stay out for 15 hours without burning.

Anyone who has ever spent all day in the sun will know that a single application of SPF 30 sunscreen will not protect you for 15 hours. So it's safer to treat this number with a healthy dose of skepticism. No sunscreen blocks 100 percent of UV rays. SPF 30 blocks only 96 to 97 percent of UV rays, and SPF 15 protects against 90 to 93 percent of UV rays. These numbers also don't apply in the real world, where incomplete applications combine with sweat, water, and rubbing to quickly lessen sunscreen's effectiveness.

Do not use sunscreens with SPF numbers of 15 or lower, as some don't protect you from both UVA and UVB rays. In fact, hedge your bets by using SPF of 40 or higher, because it will last longer and provide a greater spectrum of protection.

How does sunscreen work? The chemicals in transparent sunscreens enhance your pigment's resistance to sunlight by filtering the sun's energy and dispersing it as heat. Some chemicals used in sunscreens work better than others. Parsol 1789 (also called avobenzone), titanium dioxide, and zinc oxide are the heavy hitters you want batting for your team. PABA, or para-amino-benzoic acid, was one of the first effective sunscreens. It is rarely an ingredient in sunscreens anymore because it frequently caused allergic reactions.

Don't trust the marketers. Sunscreens claiming to be "waterproof" or to provide "all-day protection" simply are not and do not. Sunblocks are no more effective than sunscreens. Sunblock is just a marketing term.

Sunscreen has a shelf life. Apply sunscreen liberally this season, because when you pull that tube of sunscreen out of the drawer next year, the active ingredients may no longer be active. In extreme heat (such as in your glove compartment), the chemicals in sunscreen break down even faster.

Find out more:
www.skincancer.org
www.sunprotection.org
www.bfmelanoma.com
www.aad.org/public/Publications/pamphlets/Sunscreens.htm

Risks also increase as you near the poles, where there is less ozone in the atmosphere to filter UV rays, such as in New Zealand, northern Canada, and Alaska.

➤ Avoid exposing your skin by wearing long sleeves and pants with tightly knit fabrics (a typical white cotton shirt has an SPF of only about 8), and sunglasses rated to block at least 99 percent of UVA and UVB rays. On exposed skin, apply sunscreen with a sun-protection factor (SPF) of 30 or higher. Apply it liberally at least 30 minutes before exposure, because it takes time to start working. Then reapply it regularly (every 3 hours with SPF 30), especially if you've been sweating or swimming.

➤ Don't be fooled by clouds. Clouds filter only a small portion of UV rays, so it is possible to get sunburned on a cloudy day. If it's a full-on downpour, you might be OK.

Hyperthermia

When your body cannot keep itself cool and the temperature of your core organs rises to 101°F or above, you will begin to suffer from hyperthermia. This condition ranges from mild to sever; if your core temperature gets too high, your body's basic functions for survival will be affected. Literally, your brain bakes and is unable to control bodily functions necessary for life. Huffing a heavy load up a steep trail on a hot day is a good way to find yourself in this dangerous situation.

Muscle Cramps

When your muscles suddenly contract into a knot of searing pain during a hike, it might be a sign that you haven't been replacing electrolytes, which your muscles need to function properly. These cramps are often caused by a condition called hyponatremia. As the Latin ("low salt") implies, hyponatremia can be caused by drinking too much water, and not ingesting enough sodium, potassium, and other electrolytes. It's common during long-distance running and cycling events, and it's common on long hikes. It can happen in just a few hours after beginning a hike.

Luckily, both prevention and cure are easy. Eat or drink foods or liquids high in electrolytes. Eat salty foods (crackers, jerky, salami, etc.) or drink electrolyte-replacement drinks such as Gatorade, ERG, or other products. You can also pour a teaspoon of salt into your water bottle.

If muscle cramps happen while you're hiking, stop, stretch, and massage your muscles until the cramps subside, then rest for a while and consume electrolytes. Drink water to help flush out the toxins that caused your cramps. When you start hiking again, take it easy; try not to push your muscles too hard. They've already expressed their displeasure once.

Prevent hyperthermia by staying cool. Follow these tips:

➤ Hike early on hot days. Find cool rest during the heat of the day. Hike again if you need to in the late afternoon.

➤ Wear loose-fitting, light-colored, and lightweight clothes.

➤ Give yourself time to acclimatize to the heat. It can take days for your body to learn to cool itself efficiently.

➤ Hot and humid days are the worst. When the air reaches 95°F and the humidity is 80 percent, your body's ability to cool itself by sweating diminishes significantly. Sweat that drips from your skin without evaporating only contributes to dehydration without cooling you.

➤ Drink lots of water. Dehydration seriously limits our ability to cool ourselves by sweating. It also constricts blood vessels in the skin, preventing blood from getting near the surface to dissipate heat. Cold, tasty liquids make you want to drink more. Easy access to water makes it convenient.

➤ Replace electrolytes. Drink electrolyte-replacement drinks like Gatorade (or salted water; add a teaspoon of salt to a quart of water), or simply eat foods with sodium, calcium, potassium, and other minerals, such as cheese, jerky, salami, bananas, or trail mix.

➤ Get plenty of rest. Studies by the US military show a connection between lack of sleep, fatigue, and heat illness.

➤ Avoid certain medications. Many cold and allergy medicines decrease sweat production. Beta-blockers, ACE inhibitors, and diuretics can predispose you to heat illness. Talk to your doctor.

When we enter wilderness, we enter the home turf of other creatures. Some of them want to eat us and can give us dangerous diseases; others have annoying and dangerous defense strategies. One of the best things we can do is arm ourselves with the knowledge of how to minimize dangerous encounters. It also helps to carry insect repellant.

Insects

Mosquitoes, no-see-ums, and other insects can cause no end of annoyance to otherwise beautiful summer backpacking trips. They can also spread dangerous diseases with a single bite. Here's a brief introduction to what threats bugs can bring to us, and what we can do to minimize the danger.

Mosquitoes, Fleas, and Ticks

Mosquitoes are the most common bugs to bring bother to backpackers. And the little buggers can carry a host of blood-borne diseases, including malaria, encephalitis, and West Nile virus. Although these diseases are more prevalent the closer you get to the equator, their range has increased northward in recent years.

Ticks also carry a range of diseases, including Lyme disease, Rocky Mountain spotted fever, babeosis, ehrlichiosis, relapsing fever, and tularemia.

Fleas feeding on infected rodents living in parts of rural western America can pick up bubonic plague—the same plague that killed millions in Europe in the Middle Ages—then pass the plague on to dogs, cats, rodents, and people.

The best way to avoid getting these or other insect-borne diseases is to avoid contact with the insects that carry them. Here are a few tips:

➤ Check with rangers, local health officials, or the Centers for Disease Control and Prevention about the prevalence of insect-borne diseases where you plan to backpack.

➤ Wear long pants and shirts, with pant legs tucked into your socks or protected by gaiters. ExOfficio's Buzz Off clothing line is made with Permethrin (an artificial version of natural repellents found in chrysanthemums) incorporated into the fabric.

➤ Wear subdued colors. Studies have shown insects to be attracted to brighter colors. Wear subdued grays and browns, then sit away from your friend with the bright fuchsia jacket.

➤ Camp away from water. Water attracts insects, who will then be attracted to you if you're near. Camp farther away and they might not notice you.

➤ Keep your tent zipped up so bugs don't sneak in.

Mosquito Facts

Only female mosquitoes bite. Your blood becomes food for their egg brood.

How do mosquitoes find you? From far away, mosquitoes can detect the "carbon dioxide signature" that you leave with every breath. That signature contains unique lactic acids and other compounds that target you as a tasty meal, which triggers their feeding response. Once they get closer, they are attracted by bright colors, moisture, and movements.

Why do some people get bit more than others? Their carbon dioxide signature smells better than other people's. It doesn't help to be wearing fancy-smelling lotions.

Deet and other repellents work because they block chemical receptors in the mosquitoes, or otherwise change your carbon dioxide signature, which confuses them into looking elsewhere for food.

➤ Wear insect netting. Coghlan's makes mosquito and no-see-um netting that comes in jackets, pants, and hoods (wear a baseball hat under the hood to keep the mesh away from your face), to keep bugs away from your skin.

➤ Apply insect repellent to your clothes and exposed skin. Insect repellents containing deet are most effective. However, deet is controversial. Reported side effects include rashes, confusion, and seizures, although some studies question these reports. To be safe, avoid high concentrations of deet, direct skin contact, and prolonged use, especially on children. Start with repellents containing low concentrations of deet; save higher concentrations for when they're absolutely necessary.

You can avoid the deet controversy by first using repellents made with natural plant extracts, such as lemon grass, citronella, eucalyptus oil, and peppermint. Popular brands include Buzz Away and Natrapel.

➤ Take extra precautions at dusk and dawn, when mosquitoes are most active.

➤ Eat garlic. It's guaranteed to keep vampires, insects, and other people away. Simply triple the amount you'd regularly use in cooking. It helps if your campmates eat it too, so everyone is on equal moral footing.

➤ Avoid close calls with rodents or other wildlife that might carry infected ticks and fleas.

➤ Perform tick checks on yourself and others after hiking. If you find any ticks, then get naked and do a respectful check on everyone. Remember that ticks that pass on Lyme disease are only a millimeter or two across. It takes about 48 hours for an infected tick to pass on Lyme disease, so you might be able to wait until you get home for the naked part. Remove ticks by grabbing them with fingers or tweezers as close to the head as you can, then pull them straight out. Wash and disinfect the wound, and check it regularly for infection.

➤ Check your pets, who are also susceptible to insect-borne diseases. Check with your vet to see what prophylactic treatments are available.

Scorpions and Spiders

More than 1500 species of scorpions live on all continents but Antarctica and are most prevalent in warm, temperate to tropical climates. All are nocturnal; some are more poisonous than others (the most poisonous scorpions live in the Southwest US). Scorpion venom is a neurotoxin, which will produce burning, numbness, tingling, and muscle twitching, but usually little swelling or redness. Stings are most dangerous to pets, the very young, and the very old, but fatalities are rare. Seek medical attention quickly if you're concerned after a bite.

Although many species of spiders can bite, few species in North America are dangerous. The black widow and the brown recluse are the most notorious. Brown recluse spider venom causes extreme damage to tissues. Bites are often not noticed until a severe swollen wound forms and heals slowly. Black widow venom is a neurotoxin, which creates numbness, tingling, and more general systemic reactions, such as abdominal pain. Black widow bites are fatal in less than 1 percent of bite victims—mostly the very young and old.

A third spider, the hobo spider, lives in the Northwest region of the Lower 48. Its bite is similar to that of the brown recluse, although it's not usually as severe.

Avoid scorpion stings and spider bites with the following habits:

➤ Wear shoes, not sandals, to protect your feet, especially at night.

➤ Never put your hands where you can't see, especially when lifting rocks, gathering firewood, and clearing brush.

➤ Avoid sleeping directly on the ground (that's how the scorpion stung me at the bottom of the Grand Canyon—I won't do that again!).

➤ Shake unwanted creepy-crawlies from your footwear, bedding, and clothing. Shake out equipment and clothing that has been in storage in your closet or basement.

Treating Insect Bites

Insect bites can produce swollen, itchy welts. For most people, bites are merely painful annoyances. Some people, however, are allergic to bee stings and some spider bites. Treat insect bites/stings with the following:

➤ Remove the stinger. Bees often leave the stinger behind. Muscles surrounding the venom sack will continue injecting venom until removed or empty. With the flat edge of a credit card or knife, start at the stinger's insertion point and scrape the stinger away. Grabbing the sac with your fingers will simply squeeze all the venom into you.

➤ Apply an ice or cold pack to reduce swelling. Note: Do not apply ice to snakebites.

Ice slows circulation and keeps the venom in the area, which can result in more severe tissue damage than if you allow the venom to circulate and dilute through your body. In addition, ice reduces the circulation of needed blood, oxygen, and your body's own chemical defenses to the wound.

➤ Apply sting-relief ointment. StingEze relieves some of the symptoms of insect stings.

➤ Wash the wound with soap and water to prevent infection, especially if you're scratching it a lot.

➤ Benadryl (25 to 50 milligrams every four hours) can help relieve itching and swelling.

➤ Watch for anaphylactic shock. If the victim develops red welts (hives), redness to the skin, tightness in the chest, wheezing, difficulty breathing or swallowing, rapid, shallow breathing, and an altered mental state, he is experiencing a life-threatening allergic reaction to the sting—called anaphylactic shock. The only effective treatment is an injection of epinephrine. One-shot, spring-loaded epinephrine injectors are available by prescription, under the brand name EpiPen. If you or someone in your

Bees won't bug you if you don't bug them.

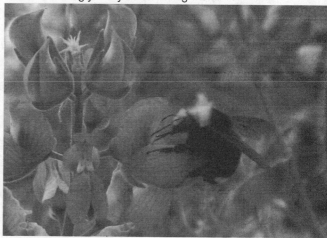

group is allergic to bee stings, having one of these on hand could save a life.

➤ Seek medical attention immediately if a sting victim shows signs of anaphylactic shock, neurological dysfunction, or if a local wound gets bigger and worse over time.

Diseases transmitted by mosquitoes and ticks mentioned above are rare and often produce similar signs and symptoms—headaches, fevers, chills, weakness, nausea, and body aches, to name just a few. They can also be fatal if not treated, so proper diagnosis is important. Unfortunately, for many reasons, proper diagnosis can be difficult: Many doctors are not experienced in diagnosing these obscure diseases; signs and symptoms can be mistaken for the flu or other maladies; multiple diseases can be passed on by an insect bite; and tests can be inaccurate.

If you experience any of the symptoms described earlier after being outdoors, or if you experience any medical condition that persists or returns after treatment, ask your doctor to consider an insect-borne disease from a mosquito, tick, or flea bite (even if you can't remember being bitten). Ask your doctor to run an infectious diseases scan on your blood. Check with the Centers for Diseases Control and Prevention or the state epidemiologist where you went camping to learn about the prevalence of insect-borne diseases in that area.

Many of these diseases respond well to antibiotics, although the debate continues over the most effective treatment for Lyme disease.

Snakes

Most snakes in the US are not venomous and pose no threat. However, there are two families of venomous snakes in the country: pit vipers (rattlesnakes, copperheads, and cottonmouths/moccasins), with heat-sensing pits in front of their eyes and fold-out fangs, and elapids (coral snakes), with fixed fangs. The risk you face from venomous snakes depends on where you hike. Here are a few interesting facts:

➤ Between 8000 and 10,000 snakebites are reported in the US each year; 12 to 15 of those victims die.

➤ A good 3000 of those bites are provoked, because of idiotic judgment, from people handling or molesting snakes. A majority of these invited bites are on the hand; many involve alcohol.

Many snakes, like this gopher snake, are harmless and beautiful parts of the natural world.

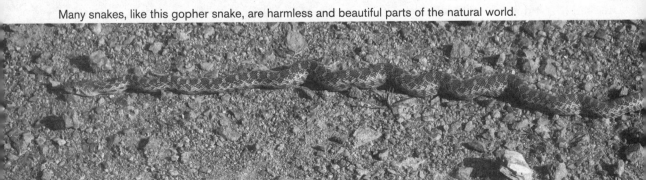

➤ Arizona, Florida, Georgia, Texas, and Alabama lead the states in snakebite fatalities; they have the most poisonous snakes, or the most foolhardy people.

➤ Eighty-five percent of legitimate bites happen below the knee.

➤ Snakes can strike about half their own length. Do not attempt to measure to confirm this.

➤ Fifty percent of bites contain no venom. Rattlesnakes can control how much venom they release. Because venom is designed to subdue prey, and humans aren't prey, snakes don't seem to think defensive warning bites to be worth wasted venom. With coral snakes, the amount of venom injected depends on the size of the snake and how long it holds on while biting.

According to renowned snake researcher Laurence M. Klauber (a.k.a. "Mr. Rattlesnake"), a rattlesnake will do almost anything it can to avoid humans. "The rattler's first wish is to get away from anything as large and as potentially dangerous as man," he has said. "If the snake strikes, it is because it is cornered or frightened for its own safety."

Avoiding Snakes

Snakes are cold-blooded; in summer, they can be found warming themselves in the sun (in the middle of the trail, usually) first thing in the morning and last part of the day. The rest of the time, they're hiding in the cool shade under a bush or rocky ledge. Because of cold nights and long winters, snakes do not live at high altitudes (the highest I've seen one was at 7800 feet). Rattlesnakes are most common during the first warm days of spring, when they emerge from hibernation. Here are other precautions:

➤ Wear tall boots and long, loose-fitting pants to protect your lower legs.

➤ Avoid walking through tall grass and along the bottom of rocky ledges.

➤ Don't put your hands where you can't see them. Don't step or jump over logs and rocks where you can't see the other side.

Snakebite Treatment

If you or someone in your group is bitten, try to identify or photograph the snake; there are many types of venom, and knowing the species will help doctors choose the right antivenin. Do not try to kill or capture the snake—don't become another victim.

➤ Remove all rings and jewelry before swelling begins.

➤ Do not cut the wound or apply a tourniquet.

➤ If you have a Sawyer Extractor snakebite kit or other suction device, apply to wound. Do not suck with your mouth (your mouth is full of germs and risks infecting the bite).

➤ Wash bite well with soap and water. Do *not* apply ice to the area.

➤ Have the patient lie supine, and keep bitten area still and below your heart to minimize tissue damage and spreading of venom through the system.

➤ Tie a snug cloth directly over the bite (if on an extremity) to reduce blood flow to the area. Splint the extremity to reduce blood flow caused by movement.

➤ Monitor vital signs (pulse, respirations, and skin).

➤ Get medical help quickly.

Learn More About Snakes

➤ *The Audubon Society Field Guide to North American Reptiles and Amphibians*, by John Behler and Wayne F. King (Alfred A. Knopf)

➤ *Rattlesnakes: Portrait of a Predator*, by Manny Rubio (Smithsonian)

Poisonous Plants

We live around poisonous plants everyday—many house and garden plants can be dangerous, even fatal, if ingested. The same is true in the wilderness, where, in addition to plants that are poisonous to eat, there are also plants that are poisonous to touch. The most famous of these are poison ivy, poison oak, and poison sumac.

The active ingredient in each of these is an oily substance called urushiol, which inspires an allergic reaction in those who touch it—an itching, oozing, burning, swelling, red rash on your skin that appears 12 to 48 hours after contact and can take two weeks to heal. Urushiol is present in the leaves, stems, and roots of these plants year-round (use extra caution in winter, when the leaves have fallen and the plant is hard to recognize). You can also get a rash by touching your pets, clothes, or backpack after they have brushed up against these plants. Contact can be particularly dangerous to people who ingest any of these plants, or who inhale smoke when these plants are burning. Your reaction to these plants can change over time; you might experience a full-blown rash one year and a minor one the next, or vice versa.

In general, poison ivy grows east of the Rockies; poison oak to the west. Each of these is easy to recognize because their leaves grow in clusters of three—hence the familiar rhyme, "leaves of three, leave them be." Poison sumac is most prevalent in the Southeast US, and its leaves grow in clusters of seven to 13. None of these plants grows in Alaska, Hawaii, or the more arid parts of deserts.

As with many accidents in nature, rashes caused by poison ivy, poison oak, and poison sumac are easier to prevent than they are to treat. If you think you may have come in contact with any of these plants or the urushiol oil they produce, wash off with soap and cold, running water. Because urushiol is an oil, any solvent—gasoline, paint thinner, or rubbing alcohol—will do in a pinch (but these are toxic to you, so soap is the preferred alternative). Without soap or a thorough washing, you might actually spread the rash rather than prevent it. Next, wash your clothes with detergent.

If you get a rash, relieve the itching with cool showers. Apply over-the-counter creams, such as hydrocortisone, calamine, or aloe vera gel. Avoid scratching the rash; contrary to popular belief, you cannot spread the rash by scratching it, but the nasty bacteria under your fingernails can infect the wounds.

For help in identifying these poisonous plants, graphic photos of what the rashes look like, and more tips on prevention and treatment, log onto www.poison-ivy.org.

One of the great thrills of backpacking is being able to see wildlife in their natural environment. Most wild animals will keep their distance or be long gone before you arrive. When you are lucky enough to encounter wild animals, please respect them from a distance. Remember that you are a visitor in their home and not part of their natural environment.

When humans and animals get too close, bad things can happen. Feeding wild animals, even unintentionally, teaches them to associate humans with food. They often become more aggressive as a result, which creates lose-lose situations for everyone involved: Animals can hurt you in their quest for your food; they often have to be destroyed because they become aggressive—a fed bear is a dead bear.

Animals can also pass dangerous diseases to you. Raccoons, skunks, bats, foxes, and rabbits can carry rabies (coyotes, interestingly, rarely carry rabies); mice in the Southwest can transfer hantavirus; chipmunks and ground squirrels in the West can carry bubonic plague. Fortunately, these diseases are extremely rare, and fatalities from them are even rarer. Nonetheless, it's best to keep your distance, because it's no fun being this kind of statistic.

Perspective also helps. It's wise to look over your shoulders for bears and cougars, but don't forget about mosquitoes carrying West Nile virus, ticks carrying Lyme disease, or untreated water infested with cryptosporidia—all of which pose bigger threats to you than large predators.

Keep yourself safe by respecting animals from a distance and being diligent in not attracting them to camp. Do not approach or feed any wild animal, and store your food (and other good-smelling stuff) so they cannot get it (see more on storing food on page 178).

The Golden Rule applies to most large predators in the Americas. Bears and cougars can be dangerous, but the power to avoid attacks and other dangerous situations is usually in human hands. Give large predators the same respect and distance you would want from them, and they'll respect you in return (if only mosquitoes lived by the same rule). Predators can also be unpredictable and dangerous. The

More About Wildlife

- *The Lost Grizzlies*, by Rick Bass (Maritime Books)
- *The Grizzly Years*, by Doug Peacock (Henry Holt)
- *Mountain Lion: An Unnatural History of Pumas and People*, by Chris Bolgiano (Stackpole Books)
- *Crossing Paths: Uncommon Encounters with Animals in the Wild*, by Craig Childs (Sasquatch Books)

following information should help decrease your chances of a dangerous wildlife encounter, although nothing can guarantee safety.

Bears

Black bears (*Ursus americanus*) can be found throughout much of the lower 48. They are slowly repopulating some of their former ranges, in the Southeast, for example, where they had been previously hunted out. In general, black bears will run from humans. They can attack if they're surprised, after your food (or protecting their own), or protecting cubs. Black bears come in a variety of colors, from mocha to cinnamon to jet black.

Brown bears and grizzlies (*Ursus arctos horribilis*; grizzlies are a subspecies) are significantly larger and fiercer than blackies. Brown bears used to live throughout North America. Now they live only in Canada and Alaska, with isolated populations in the northern reaches of Western states, especially in the northern Rocky Mountains around Yellowstone and Glacier national parks. Before hiking in these areas, check with local rangers for updates on bear activity, trail closures, etc.

Although California has a brown bear on its state flag, the last known brown bear in the Golden State was killed in 1922. If you see a bear in California, it's a black bear, no matter what color it is.

Polar bears (*Ursus maritimus*, or "sea bear") live along the fringes of northern ice, from Siberia through Alaska and across Canada. If you're planning a trip that far north, you'll need skills and equipment far beyond the scope in this book. Dress warm and inquire with local officials about how to prepare for polar bear encounters.

The largest land predators in North America, brown and black bears are naturally wary of humans (polar bears, however, are cu-rious). They are also unpredictable. On average, grizzlies kill two people and black bears kill one person each year in North America. Between five and 15 people are seriously injured annually. The following precautions can greatly reduce your risk of a dangerous bear encounter:

➤ Don't hike alone. Safety comes in numbers.

➤ Make noise. Let bears know you're coming. The most common reasons bears attack humans are sudden encounters. Avoid mutual surprise and subsequent carnage by making noise as you hike through bear country. Clap your hands or shout occasionally, or sing, talk loud, and bang stuff.

➤ Be alert. Scan your surroundings as far as you can see. Try to see bears before you are too close. Watch for signs—scats, tracks, and clawed up tree trunks. Use extra caution when poor visibility or loud, ambient sounds from wind or water prevent you and the bear from seeing or hearing each other. Pay attention to the wind; if it's at your back, animals ahead of you already know you're coming; if you're hiking into the wind, be careful, because they haven't smelled you yet. If you find a fresh kill, leave the area immediately.

➤ Don't smell like food. Bears have an excellent sense of smell, exemplified by the following saying: "If a pine needle falls in the forest, the eagle will see it, the deer will hear it, and the bear will smell it." Bears are more aggressive when they smell something good. When hiking in bear country, especially grizzly country, try hard not to smell like food by following these tips:

➤ Do not strap large fresh salmon to the outside of your pack.

➤ Do not wear perfume, cosmetics, deodorant, or any scented lotions or creams.

➤ Do not leave food out, wipe your hands on your clothes after eating, or go to sleep in clothes soaked in smoke from dinner.

➤ Prepare and eat all food at least 100 feet downwind from your tent.

➤ Wash your hands and face well after meals.

➤ Don't walk away with food still out, even for a few moments.

➤ Hang or canister everything that might smell good, including food, toiletries, sunscreen, etc. Hang smelly clothes in a garbage bag in the same area.

➤ Avoid traveling at dawn and dusk. Although you can encounter a bear anytime, they are most active at dawn and dusk.

➤ Keep children close. We forget often, but we're part of the food chain; large predators know who's on top, and your kids are tempting morsels. Keep them close at all times.

➤ Leave dogs at home. They're natural enemies, and the bear might chase your dog right to you.

➤ Pack out all garbage. Leave nothing to entice the bear to visit that campsite again.

➤ Carry pepper spray in grizzly country. Use spray designed for bears, not that small bottle on your key chain. Keep it handy on your belt; practice until you can get it off and spray it within a second or two. Spray range is not more than 10 feet (less in head- or crosswinds). You get one shot, so wait until the bear is almost on you. Statistics say you have a 75 to 85 percent chance at survival (versus a 50 percent survival rate with guns) using pepper spray. Pepper spray repels charging bears, but the spray residue attracts them. Do not spray your camp and gear to keep them away—it must smell like salsa.

➤ Guns. Bad idea. Many bears have continued attacking and killing everyone in the party for minutes after they've been shot through the head and/or heart. And that's after a good shot; a bad shot will just make it angry. Guns give you a false sense of security. Humility, respect, distance, and pepper spray are more reliable.

Learn More About Bears

➤ www.bears.org: A website dedicated to providing accurate information about bears.

➤ www.beartrust.org: Information about bears in and around Glacier and Yellowstone national parks.

➤ www.ursusinternational.org: The website of the Ursus International Conservation Institute, which is dedicated to protecting bears and their habitat, partly by helping people understand how to live with bears.

If you encounter a bear:

➤ Don't run. Black bears can run up to 30 miles per hour; grizzlies have been clocked at 42 miles per hour. You cannot outrun them (not even downhill—it's a myth). Running will only trigger their predatory instinct to chase and kill. When facing black bears, act large, yell, bang pots, and throw stuff. When facing grizzlies, be much more respectful. They are political creatures. If one's not already charging, you might be able to negotiate with it if you're not already too close; stop, avert your eyes while still facing it, back off slowly and reassure it with a respectful, calming tone. It might be scared, too. After all, we kill far more of them than the other way around. Make sure it has an escape route.

➤ Respect them from a distance. The farther away you are from the bear when you first see it, the better your chances of safety. You're asking for trouble if you approach a bear to get a better look or take a picture. As you've heard many times before, don't get anywhere near a mom and her cub(s).

➤ For added safety, always choose hiking partners who run slower than you. This is a good way to lose hiking partners, though, and it's not recommended.

➤ If attacked by a blackie, fight, kick, and scream as hard as you can, punch it in the nose—you have a chance. The experts are split about how to react to a grizzly attack. Some say roll into a ball, leave your pack on to protect your back and neck, lock your fingers behind your neck, pull your knees to your chest, and remain silent. Do this until several minutes after you're sure the bear has left. Other experts recommend fighting back by punching the nose and poking the eyes.

Cougars

Next to humans, cougars (*Felis concolor*; also called mountain lions, puma, painters, and catamounts) have the most extensive range of any land mammal in the Americas—from the Arctic to Patagonia, sea level to above 11,000 feet. Loss of habitat and other conflicts with humans have limited mountain lion range to places where there is still large, wild country for them to roam. There's also a small, struggling population in Florida. Human-cougar encounters are rare, but they do happen on trails and in backyards and neighborhoods wherever wild country meets civilization across the West. Attacks are rarer, but they can happen.

While bears survive through size and brute force, cougars specialize in stealth—stalking their prey in silence, then attacking from behind. Their teeth are designed to slip between vertebrae and slice spinal cords with surgical precision, allowing them to take elk and deer many times their size. Sightings are rare and attacks far rarer. On average since 1991, cougars attack six people each year in the US and Canada, with one fatality a year.

Increase your chances of safety by following these precautions:

➤ Hike in numbers. Lone people are more likely to be attacked; groups, almost never. In groups, the person far ahead of the group and the lone straggler are most at risk of an attack.

➤ Keep kids close. Smaller, more helpless people attract cats with the promise of an easy meal. Don't tempt them.

➤ Watch your back, especially, if you're alone at isolated springs or other water sources in the wilderness.

If you encounter a cougar:

➤ Keep your distance. Most cougars want to avoid confrontation. Give them room to escape.

➤ Do not turn away or run. Keep eye contact. Running triggers their instinct to chase. Cougars seem to be drawn to mountain bikers and runners cruising along isolated trails. Remember, they attack from behind. Face it and stand it down. Never turn your back.

➤ Act large and make noise. Open your jacket, wave your arms, shout, and throw stuff. Pick up your children to make them look larger.

➤ If attacked, fight back aggressively and scream; protect your head and neck; try to keep standing.

Wolves

Although *Canis lupus* was once more widespread across North America, wolves are now relegated to the northern lower 48, Canada, and Alaska. Attacks on humans have been extremely rare (only 28 recorded attacks since 1900, and most of those involved wolves that were either captive, accustomed to humans, wolf-dog hybrids, or wolves that were fighting with domestic dogs). If you're itching to see wolves or hear them howl, your chances are best at Yellowstone National Park, the Boundary Waters Canoe Area Wilderness, and Isle Royale National Park.

Coyotes

The coyote is one of the few predator species that has increased its range thanks to humans, because they're so adaptable. Bigger than foxes, smaller than large dogs, *Canis latrans* are nearly ubiquitous across North America. Their yips and howls add ambiance to lonely landscapes. Although normally weary of humans, coyotes used to human food have been known to bite people. Although commonly thought of as scavengers, they will hunt alone or in packs. They have been known to take dogs, cats, and small children.

Healthy, wild coyotes unaccustomed to human food will keep their distance. If a coyote seems unusually brave, chase it off by making noise, throwing stuff, etc.

Skunks

About the size of house cats, these relatives of weasels, martens, and badgers are nocturnal. It's likely they'll prowl through camp while you sleep, looking for insects, mice, rats, lizards, or scraps leftover from dinner. They're not aggressive, but they are confident, because they know that no creature in the forest with a lick of sense wants to mess with them. Be aware as you're walking through camp at night. It's far more likely your dog—curious to a fault—will be on the receiving end of a skunk's perfume.

If you get sprayed in the eyes, rinse with water until the pain and blindness subsides—about 15 minutes. For whomever gets sprayed, a tomato-juice bath will work, but the following solution works much better to wash away the stench:

- 1 quart hydrogen peroxide (3%)
- ¼ cup baking soda (sodium bicarbonate)
- 1 teaspoon liquid dish soap (one that cuts oils and grease well, like Dawn)

Apply with a washcloth or brush, rinse well, repeat until you can bear the smell.

Rodents

"Aaaw, ain't he cute!" might be the response you most often hear from people watching a chipmunk, squirrel, or mouse nibble on nuts and seeds on a fallen log in camp. Feelings of affection fade quickly once rodents chew through your backpack to get at food, or eat your shoulder straps because they like the salty taste of your sweat. And just because you've returned to the trailhead after your trip, your troubles might still be waiting; backpackers in the Sierra Nevada have discovered that marmots enjoy chewing on hoses and belts in car engines.

If chewed-through straps, a hole in your backpack, or missing engine parts are your worst consequences from encounters with

Cute, yes, but she's plotting to get your food.

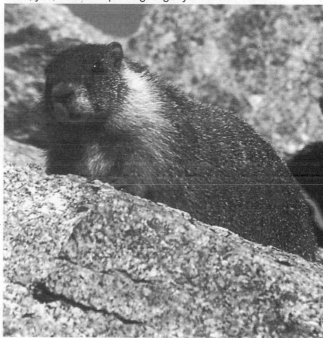

rodents, then count your blessings. Rodents can also pass on painful and deadly diseases.

All wild animals, even the smallest and cutest can be deadly. Bites from many rodents, or their fleas, can carry disease. How can you avoid such dangers in the wilderness, and how can you recognize and treat sickness you might get from these cute little balls of fur? Read on.

Bubonic Plague

Plague is a bacterium spread by the fleas of infected rodents, such as rats, ground squirrels, rabbits, and chipmunks. Although it affects only 10 to 15 people each year in the US, plague killed millions of people in Europe in the Middle Ages. Today, plague is most common in the Four Corners region of the Southwest, and in the northern Sierra Nevada, northwestern Nevada, and southern Oregon.

Within a few days of exposure to plague, victims feel fever-like symptoms, leading to swollen, painful lymph nodes. Eventually, plague spreads to the lungs, where it can pass to other people through coughing. Isolation and antibiotics are the treatment for victims and for anyone who's been around the victim in the later, coughing stage.

Rabies

In 2000, there were 7369 cases of animal rabies reported in the US and Puerto Rico. No human cases were reported. Although it is extremely unlikely you will become infected, rabies is such a nasty virus, it's best to arm yourself with the facts to prevent becoming that one truly unlucky person.

Ninety-three percent of the cases listed above were wild animals; the remaining cases were domestic animals. Raccoons and skunks were the prime culprits, followed by bats, foxes, and rabbits. Although coyotes are prime candidates, they rarely seem to get it. Infected animals can transmit the disease to pets or humans through saliva or contact through open sores or mucus membranes in mouth, nose, or eyes.

After an incubation period that lasts between several weeks and many months, rabies victims come down with flu-like symptoms that include fever, headaches, and general malaise. As the virus reaches the central nervous system and brain, confusion, anxiety, partial paralysis, hallucinations, insomnia, hypersalivation, fear of water, agitation, and delirium set in. Death occurs only days after the onset of symptoms.

Unfortunately, by the time rabies symptoms appear, the disease has progressed too far to treat. The crucial time to catch the disease is immediately after the bite.

If you are bitten by a neighborhood pet or wild animal, immediately wash the wound with soap and water. This can be an effective way to keep from getting rabies. If the bite is from a cat, wash any scratches from the cat as well; although they don't spread rabies, the scratches can be particularly septic and infection is common. Then seek medical attention as quickly as possible.

If it's possible and safe to do so, capture the animal so it can be tested by specialists. Rabies is contagious only in its final stages, after symptoms appear. Often the animal can be quarantined and observed to see if symptoms are present.

Rabies treatment usually consists of a series of injections over a 28-day period. No one has ever contracted rabies after prompt treatment following an infected bite. The best way to prevent rabies is to avoid contact with the disease and its carriers.

Hantavirus Pulmonary Syndrome

Although hantavirus is extremely rare, it is devastating to those who get it. Carriers of the disease are primarily mice. Humans get it by breathing in the virus during contact with infected mouse droppings, saliva, and urine. Hantavirus is not known to be contagious.

The disease was discovered in 1993. Since then, 313 cases have been reported, 37 percent of which have been fatal. Although it was first identified in the Four Corners region of the American Southwest, it has now been reported in 31 states (mostly west of the Mississippi River) and overseas.

Doctors are still unsure about the incubation period of hantavirus. Generally, the first flu-like symptoms appear one to five weeks after initial infection. Fever, headaches, muscle aches, nausea, and dizziness lead to coughing and breathing difficulty as the disease reaches the lungs. There is no vaccine for hantavirus, and antibiotics do not work. However, those who catch the disease early respond to oxygen and intravenous support.

from being harassed by your pet. Before backpacking with your dog, talk to your vet about a prophylactic that will prevent infection from fleas and ticks.

➤ Before backpacking, contact rangers or state or county health officials in the area about the prevalence of animal- and insect-borne diseases.

➤ Avoid areas with lots of mouse turds. Stirring up dust in the area can stir up the virus, which can infect you when you breathe them in.

➤ For more information on animal- and insect-borne diseases, check out the Centers for Disease Control and Prevention website at www.cdc.gov.

Keeping Critters Away

You can effectively prevent a majority of potentially dangerous encounters with animals by taking the following precautions while backpacking:

➤ Separate yourself from anything that might attract animals, such as food, toothpaste, candy wrappers, garbage, and other scented products.

➤ Do not leave food or garbage out. Hang these out of reach (see food storage tips on page 178).

➤ Use only unscented soaps, lotions, and toilet paper.

➤ Never approach or feed any wild animal, or let it approach you. If an animal approaches you, it's either diseased or accustomed to humans, in which case it can be dangerous as it pursues the meal it expects from you. Animals often must be killed after becoming too aggressive.

➤ Control your pets. Not only will this help them avoid the bites and fleas from infected animals, it will also protect wild animals

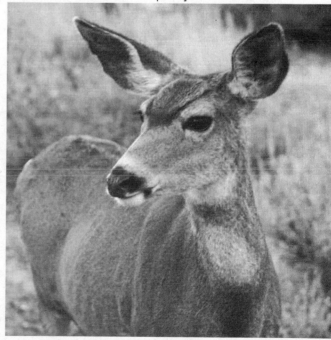
Some wild creatures are completely harmless.

This chapter offers suggestions for treatment of common minor backcountry injuries. It also offers a few general principles for identifying and managing more serious injuries. However, proper first aid protocol is far beyond the scope of this book. I strongly suggest learning first aid skills and reading the books listed later in this chapter. If you're in doubt about assessing or treating injuries and illnesses in the backcountry, seek medical attention immediately.

Administering First Aid in the Backcountry

Medical emergencies are challenging under the best of circumstances. In the backcountry, the challenges are even greater. The more training and experience you have administering first aid, the better prepared you will be to offer the best care possible for your patients. When confronted by a wilderness medical emergency, avoid making the situation worse—don't become a victim yourself; avoid making your patient's condition worse; be aware that all medications have potential adverse side effects; and always seek professional medical care immediately if you suspect serious injuries, internal injuries, severe sickness, or infection.

If you need to take any medications while in the wilderness, consult your doctor before you go. Make sure you understand the potential consequences and side effects of medications you carry before you need them in the backcountry. Although it might be helpful to share medications with hiking partners, it can also be dangerous and it's not recommended. If you feel you must give someone else medications, ask them about possible allergies, medical conditions, or other prescriptions that might create a bad reaction. Children, pregnant wom-

WILDERNESS WISDOM

The Value of a Good Bedside Manner

The mind is powerful, and the power of suggestion can do a lot to improve, or worsen, your situation. Numerous studies show that people heal more quickly when they're optimistic and happy. You can help your patient and other hiking partners by nurturing that optimism in them—healing can start as soon as you approach your patient. Calm, nurturing confidence will tell your patient that everything's OK. Skeptical, scared, or hopeless comments can actually worsen the situation. You might even say something like, "You just went through something pretty tough. But starting now, everything is going to get better."

en, nursing mothers, or anyone already taking prescribed medications for another medical condition should consult a physician before taking medication. Carefully read instructions, and use only recommended doses.

Do not take pain relievers if you're going to seek medical attention within the next few hours; pain killers can mask symptoms, which interferes with a doctor's ability to diagnose accurately. Your doctor needs to assess you in all your painful glory, so she can diagnose your situation and prescribe the best course of action.

Common Minor Injuries

In addition to blisters, sunburn, insect bites, and hypothermia, the injuries discussed here—sprained/twisted ankles, cuts, burns, and head and abdominal injuries—are the most common injuries that take place in the backcountry. As always, the best cure is prevention; use caution to avoid unnecessary missteps from becoming emergencies. But when the inevitable accident occurs, this section gives a brief introduction to these injuries and how to treat them. For a more comprehensive discussion of these and other backcountry injuries, take a wilderness first aid class or consult one of the books listed at the end of this chapter.

Sprained/Twisted Ankles

It's easy to twist an ankle, especially when walking downhill on a rocky trail. Without an x-ray, however, it's difficult to tell the difference between a sprained, strained, or broken ankle. Luckily, the treatment is the same regardless. All you need to do is think about RICE:

Rest. Stay off the injured leg, which can be tough to do if you have a long hike out. Healing will not start until you rest the injury. Walking on it can worsen the injury. Several days of rest are required at minimum; full recovery often takes six weeks or longer.

Ice. Cold packs on the injured limb will help reduce swelling and speed recovery, especially if applied in the first 24 hours after injury. Place a shirt or other material between ice and skin to avoid risk of frostbite.

Compression. Wrapping a bandage around or splinting the injured ankle snugly helps prevent further injury from movement, while helping speed recovery. Don't wrap it too tight. Make sure you can feel a pulse below the wrap. If bandage becomes uncomfortable, or if the foot starts to throb or tingle, loosen the bandage and try again—this time not as tight.

Elevation. Raising the injured part higher than the level of the heart allows for easier circulation and speedier healing.

Also check motor function and sensation in the foot by pinching the patient's toes and asking her to wiggle her toes. If there is any tingling, numbness, lack of sensation, or inability to move the extremity, seek medical care immediately. If those skills are fine, combine RICE with a non-steroidal, anti-inflammatory pain killer like ibuprofen or aspirin to reduce swelling and ease the pain.

Sore Muscles

The axiom "no pain, no gain" underscores the fact that in order to make your muscles stronger, you must first break them down. Luckily, the two types of muscle pain described here—acute muscle soreness and delayed-onset muscle soreness—aren't necessarily signs of serious injury, although they can hurt like the dickens.

Acute muscle soreness is the pain your sadistic personal trainer is referring to when she urges you to "feel the burn!" when you're working out, pushing your muscles hard. During an aggressive weights workout, or while huffing up a steep trail under a heavy pack, you are actually tearing individual muscle fibers.

Hard-working muscles also produce chemical wastes, such as hydrogen ions and lactic acid, faster than your circulatory system can flush them away. With proper care after your workout—rest, nutrition, and stretching—muscle fibers grow back in greater numbers, circulation increases, and muscles become more resistant to abuse. Acute muscle soreness is easy to identify because it fades quickly after the workout is over. If your muscles are burning while you're hiking, stop and rest until the pain subsides.

Another type of acute muscle soreness is muscle strain—the sudden tearing of muscle fibers that occurs when muscles are overworked or pushed beyond their natural range of motion. Strain pain is sudden and does not fade like the pain of burning muscles. Minor strains can be treated with the RICE protocol. More significant strains might require professional medical attention.

Delayed-onset muscles soreness (also called DOMS) can be debilitating, at least for a while. You'll know you have it the day after a big hike, when you can barely walk because your muscles are sore. The burn of working muscles fades quickly, but with DOMS, your muscles are still reeling for days. Microscopic tears in your muscle fibers are being repaired, accumulated wastes in your muscles are still being flushed out, and swelling has occurred from the damage.

Doctors believe DOMS is most significant after eccentric muscle movement. This doesn't mean you look funny when you hike (you might, but it's not contributing to DOMS). Rather, it means your muscles are contracting and expanding at the same time. Your thigh muscles (quadriceps) do this when you walk downhill; your thighs and buttocks work eccentrically when you sit down in a chair.

The best way to avoid DOMS is to train your muscles in the weeks before that big backpacking trip. Also choose trails that are well-suited to your fitness level, and be sure to warm up your muscles before heavy exertion. It's a good idea to start each day of hiking at an easy pace to let your muscles get used to the work.

After you get to camp, or back to the car, an easy walk with your pack off will help you cool down and help your blood circulate, providing fresh oxygen to, and clearing wastes from, your muscles. Next, stretch your muscles. It will help extend their range of motion (preventing tightness the next day) and flush out lactic acid and other toxins, which contribute to soreness.

If your muscles are still sore, give them a rub. Massage increases circulation to your muscles, helping to clear out toxins and speed muscle recovery. Use the heel of your hands, and push firmly along the length of sore muscles. Massage toward the heart to speed the circulatory flushing of toxins in your muscles.

Finally, replenish your system. Drink water—lots of it. Proper hydration leads to efficient circulation, which flushes out wastes and speeds healing. Eat well. Proper nutrition can replace lost electrolytes and provide good building blocks to repair damaged muscles and build stronger muscles. Doctors and sports nutritionists often recommend diets high in protein to speed the recovery of injured tissues; anti-oxidants (vitamins C and E, for example) can help repair damage that occurs to overworked muscles.

Non-steroidal, anti-inflammatory medications, such as aspirin and ibuprofen, can also help reduce swelling and speed recovery. They ease pain, too, which is a big plus. Extract from the arnica plant (available in creams or pills at many natural food and health stores), is also helpful in reducing swelling, easing pain, and speeding recovery.

Cuts

Too much blood loss can be a life-threatening emergency—without enough blood volume, the body cannot transport oxygen to cells. Luckily, most bleeding incidents don't involve enough blood loss to be dangerous; they just look scary. The bigger risk with cuts is infection. Here's how to treat all cuts to prevent both excess blood loss and infection:

➤ **Wear protective gloves.** The first rule in first aid is: Don't become a victim. The second rule: Don't make the situation worse. By wearing latex (or another synthetic, such as Nitrile, for those with latex allergies) gloves, you can protect yourself from your patient's possible blood-borne diseases, and you can prevent infecting your patient with the germs that are all over your hands.

➤ **Stop the bleeding.** Place a non-adhering, sterile dressing directly on the wound, then press firmly with your hand. Depending on the type of cut, it can take up to 30 minutes for bleeding to stop. For serious bleeds, add another dressing on top of the first (never remove dressings; doing so can tear apart the clot that's trying to form), and continue to apply direct pressure to the cut. Elevate the cut above the heart to help stem bleeding. If you need your hands free, ask the patient to apply the pressure, or stack a pile of 4-by-4-inch sterile pads directly on the wound, then wrap an elastic bandage tightly around the wound until bleeding stops. If bleeding continues, it may require more serious treatment. If your patient is in danger of bleeding to death, you may need to apply a tourniquet, a skill that is beyond the scope of this book. Learn more first aid skills from one of the sources listed on page 231.

➤ **Clean the wound.** Infection is often a bigger risk than the original injury. If bleeding has stopped and the wound is dirty, find the cleanest water you can (have someone boil water if necessary) to flush dirt from the wound. Pick rocks and other debris from the wound with tweezers.

➤ **Disinfect.** Use a sterile alcohol wipe or hydrogen peroxide on a sterile gauze pad to kills germs on the wound. For small scrapes and abrasions, apply aloe vera gel or an antibiotic ointment such as Polysporin to minimize infection and speed healing.

➤ **Cover the wound.** For small cuts, Elmo, Barbie, and superhero Band-Aids help kids and adults forget about the injury. For larger wounds, wrap the area snugly with gauze conforming wrap or other bandage material. Do not wrap so tightly that it stops circulation. If the patient experiences tingling, throbbing, numbness, or swelling below the injury, loosen the bandage and rewrap.

➤ **Treat for pain.** Give the recommended dose of non-steroidal, anti-inflammatory medication such as aspirin, ibuprofen (Advil, etc.), or acetaminophen (Tylenol, etc.) to ease pain, reduce swelling, and speed healing.

➤ **Change dressings daily.** Air can help wounds heal. It can also invite infection into the wound. Find a balance between the two. After 24 hours (hopefully enough time for a decent scab to form), unwrap the dressings, clean and disinfect the wound again, then apply fresh dressings.

➤ **Watch for signs of infection.** Redness, swelling, throbbing, pus, and fever are all signs of infection. Seek medical attention immediately if these occur. Untreated, infection can lead to amputation or even death.

➤ **Get a tetanus shot.** Tetanus bacteria are present everywhere in the soil, and it can lead to severe nerve damage and even death if untreated. Tetanus vaccinations are recommended every 10 years. When was the last time you had one?

Burns

Too-close encounters with camp stoves, the sun, cigarettes, and campfires make burns a common ailment in the backcountry. Luckily, they're pretty easy to treat. Burns are divided into three categories, depending on severity:

First degree. These burns are superficial, involving only the outermost layers of skin. Mild sunburns and burns from spilled coffee are first-degree burns.

Second degree. These burns involve deeper layers of the skin. Blisters are often present.

Third degree. These burns involve deeper tissues, such as muscles, nerves, and blood vessels. They require immediate medical attention.

To treat burns, follow these steps:

➤ Apply cool, sterile water to stop the burn. Many burns continue burning long after direct contact with the burn source has ended.

➤ Remove clothing or debris from the burn.

➤ Do *not* apply butter. Sorry to break it to you, but your grandmother was wrong. The salt in butter pulls precious water from your tissues, and unsalted butter invites bacteria into the wound.

➤ For sunburns, apply aloe vera gel to the burn to speed healing. Honey also helps speed healing, reduce infection, and minimize the formation of scars.

➤ Dress with non-adhering sterile bandage. Change dressing daily.

➤ Treat for pain with non-steroidal, anti-inflammatory medication.

➤ Seek medical attention if the burn involves deeper tissues or affects a large part of the body.

Minor Head Injuries

We all get knocked on the noggin every once in a while. Most of the time, the injuries are minor (lucky our heads are so hard), but sometimes they're serious injuries. Here's how to treat minor bumps and recognize more serious injuries:

➤ Treat open wounds as you would any cut.

➤ Apply ice for 15 to 20 minutes to reduce swelling.

➤ Treat for pain with non-steroidal, anti-inflammatory medication, according to recommended dosage, to ease pain and speed healing.

➤ Seek medical attention immediately if any of these warning signs appear:

• Bruising around the eyes (raccoon eyes) and/or behind the ears.

• Clear or pinkish fluid or blood draining from ears, nose, or back of throat.

• Mismatched pupil sizes.

• Any loss or change in consciousness (confusion, dizziness, loss of memory, etc.). Changes in consciousness can be particularly significant if they take place over hours or days. After a head injury, keep a close eye on the mental state of the patient. Don't be afraid to ask simple questions like, "When is your birthday?" or "Can you remember how the accident happened?" Changes in consciousness indicate trouble in the cranium. For example, with bleeding injuries in the head, the blood has nowhere to go within the skull cavity; the increasing pressure on the brain affects brain function. Prompt, professional medical attention is urgently required. Seek it immediately.

Abdominal Pain

Pain in the abdomen can be caused by a variety of conditions—gas, constipation, infection, ulcers, bowel obstruction, pneumonia, heart attack, urinary tract or pelvic infection, ruptured appendix, kidney stones, or internal injuries. In the backcountry, it can be hard to tell the difference between harmless pain and a serious condition requiring evacuation.

Seek medical attention if abdominal pain lasts longer than six hours, if the person experienced a serious fall or blow to the abdomen, or if it's accompanied by projectile vomiting, fever, or diarrhea that has blood or mucous in the stool.

If you're pretty sure you just have a minor stomach flu, food poisoning, or perhaps some amoebic diarrhea from drinking bad water, you can treat these non-life-threatening conditions with Imodium, Pepto-Bismol, or Kaopectate. All vomiting and diarrhea sufferers are at risk of dehydration because fluids are leaving faster than they can be absorbed (or the patient just can't keep anything down). Replace fluids and electrolytes. Create your own electrolyte-replacement potion by adding the following to a liter of water: 1 teaspoon table salt, 4 tablespoons sugar, 4 teaspoons cream of tartar, and ½ teaspoon baking soda.

For more serious cases, antibiotic treatment might be necessary to combat the bugs that are causing your abdominal stress. See a doctor quickly.

More Serious Injuries

Those who explore the backcountry with attentive awareness and caution enjoy minimal risk of serious medical emergencies, but no amount of care can eliminate all risks—after all, accidents can happen. In the unfortunate event of a medical emergency, you will need to focus every mental and physical resource you and your campmates have on getting professional medical attention fast.

Serious medical emergencies in the wilderness can tax the abilities of even the most experienced and prepared medical and rescue personnel, and a discussion of proper treatment and evacuation procedures is far beyond the scope of this book. This section, however, should help you recognize when these situations occur so you can begin the process of evacuation or rescue. Most important, this discussion should convince you to get first aid training so you can manage the basics of first aid care with confidence.

Broken Bones

It takes a doctor with an x-ray to diagnose broken bones. However, the following signs and symptoms can give pretty big clues:

➤ Inability to use limb. If your patient simply cannot walk on the leg, grip with her hand, or move an extremity without pain, the bone may be broken.

➤ Point tenderness. Touch near the break, and the patient doesn't complain so much. Touch it directly (gently!), and he hits the ceiling.

➤ Deformity. Compare the injured limb with the uninjured one, looking for differences in position, rotation, length, angulation, bones that bend where they shouldn't, or unusual bumps.

➤ Rapid bruising and swelling.

➤ Grinding sounds. Crepitus is the sound of bone ends grinding together.

If one or more of the signs above alert you to the possibility of a fracture, treat with the following steps:

➤ Avoid moving the injured body part.

➤ Gently remove clothing from the injury (cut away clothing if necessary) and evaluate the injured area by palpating (feeling for crepitus, point tenderness, and deformity) and checking the area for swelling, bleeding, and any other signs of injury.

➤ Stop bleeding according to the steps listed for cuts on page 221.

➤ Check circulation, sensation, and ability to move below the injured extremity. Feel for a pulse, or squeeze a fingernail or toenail,

The ABCS of Serious Medical Emergencies

You're enjoying a beautiful day on the trail. Suddenly, you hear a scream. You run to the sound and find a fellow hiker lying unconscious. What do you do? With every medical emergency, you can use your ABCS to guide you in treating the most important injuries first:

Airway. Without air, the brain dies in three to four minutes. Broken bones, bleeding, and other injuries won't matter if your patient isn't breathing. If a person is awake, alert, and breathing well, you can move on with your examination.

Conscious patients who are having trouble breathing are likely choking on a piece of food or other material. If they're coughing, they should be encouraged to continue. If they cannot breathe, food and other obstructions can be removed successfully. However, proper procedures are updated often and are beyond the scope of this book. Luckily, a one-day CPR class will teach you the latest techniques on how to save someone's life in these situations.

Non-choking patients with breathing difficulty might be suffering from a traumatic injury, such as a blow to the neck or throat, or from an allergic reaction to a bee sting or food.

With unconscious patients, first look at the chest: Listen and feel for breath against your cheek. Sometimes, repositioning the patient will open the airway (be gentle to avoid damage to the spine—more on that to come), allowing the patient to begin breathing on her own. If so, great! Your job now is to keep her breathing and treat other injuries.

Breathing. If the patient still isn't breathing, you will need to perform rescue breathing, which can often jump-start a patient to breathing on her own. If air won't go in, the airway could be blocked and you will need to try to clear it using first aid techniques that are beyond the scope of this book.

Circulation. If the patient still isn't breathing, you will need to perform rescue breathing and perform cardio-pulmonary resuscitation (CPR) to help circulate that oxygen to the brain and other vital organs. Another important part of circulation is to stop wounds from bleeding, because it's hard to circulate oxygenated blood if there's a hole in the plumbing (learn more about managing cuts on page 221).

Shock. As I explain in more detail on page 227, shock can kill patients even when the injuries that allow shock to occur are not fatal, so it's vitally important that you do everything you can to prevent it. Always insulate your victim from the cold of the ground by placing sleeping pads and other insulators under her; cover her with blankets to keep her warm; and raise her feet above the level of her heart to encourage maximum blood flow to the core organs that are essential to life (don't make injuries worse by moving the patient to treat for shock). There's also a psychological aspect to shock, so do everything you can to quell panic by offering a reassuring, confident, comforting, and optimistic bedside manner.

Note: Rescue breathing, airway management, and CPR are beyond the scope of this book. However, your local Red Cross chapter or community college offer one-day classes to teach these life-saving skills, and they're often free of charge! Sources for first aid training are listed at the end of this chapter.

then watch how quickly pink returns to the nail bed (if it remains white, circulation is poor). Look for a blue tint to the skin or other discoloration—a sign of poor circulation. Without proper circulation, limbs and other tissues can only survive six to eight hours.

To check sensation, gently prick the foot or hand below the injury with a safety pin, then do the same to uninjured limb. If there is less reaction on the injured limb, or if it displays tingling or numbness, there might be nerve injury.

Finally, ask the patient to grip your hand or wiggle her toes. If she cannot, or if she has impaired circulation or sensation, she may have nerve damage, which requires immediate medical attention.

➤ Splint the limb. The goal is to minimize movement of the injury, which will prevent further injury, speed healing, and make evacuation easier. It's best to immobilize joints above and below the injury. If the injury is at the joint, splint the bones above and below the joint. Splint the injury in place if possible. Use the patient's comfort as a guide.

➤ Severely deformed limbs can impair circulation and prevent splinting and might need to be aligned to normal anatomical position. This is not advised unless absolutely necessary, and instructions on how to do this effectively are beyond the scope of this book. If you try this, and the patient does not tolerate it, improvise a splint that fits the injury as found.

➤ Elevate and ice the injury.

➤ Treat for pain, using aspirin or ibuprofen according to recommended dosage.

➤ Seek medical attention immediately.

Spine Injuries

If your patient has suffered a fall, or a blow to the back, head, or neck, bones in the spine could be fractured. If so, even small movements can move those broken bones and sever the spinal cord, killing or permanently

WILDERNESS WISDOM

As you evaluate an injured patient, collect signs and symptoms that will give you clues to the nature and severity of the injury (and help you relay information to the doctor when necessary). A sign is something an observer can notice about a patient—pulse, respiration, blood pressure, redness, swelling, altered mental states, etc. A symptom is something the patient experiences and must describe—pain, nausea, dizziness, etc.

You can provide useful information to doctors if you note whether signs or symptoms (breathing rate or pulse, for example) change over time. When you think you are dealing with a serious injury, and you're still hours from professional medical care, mark the time and write down the patient's breathing rate, pulse, temperature, and blood pressure. Record them frequently. When you get to professional medical care, the doctor will be able to tell a lot from your notes, which could make a difference in her diagnosis and treatment.

crippling your patient. You can avoid this by managing your patient according to tips that follow. Proper spine management takes training and practice, but the following guidelines are better than total ignorance.

Symptoms of spine injuries include numbness, tingling, or paralysis of extremities below the injury. The mechanism of injury might also hint at a spinal injury—was there a serious fall or impact? Did you find the patient in an awkward body position? If any of the above signs or symptoms occur, use extreme caution.

Do not move the patient. "Can you move it?" is never a good question to ask someone who is complaining about a neck, back, or spine injury. Even the smallest movement can

WILDERNESS WISDOM

Never step over your patient. An accidental trip or fall could seriously complicate your patient's condition (remember the second rule of first aid—don't make the situation worse). Walking around your patient will also protect her from dirt or other debris that might fall off your feet when you step over.

cause broken bones to slip and sever the spinal cord. If the patient is responsive, ask her not to move and to answer your questions verbally—no nods or shakes of the head. If the patient is not responsive, check the airway, breathing, and circulation before anything else (see the discussion of ABCS on page 224).

Weather and other dangerous conditions might force you to move someone, even if you're confident there's a spinal injury. If you must move a patient, make every effort to keep the spine in line (that is, keep the head, shoulders, and hips in the same line), and to move the body as a single unit. For example, pull a victim from danger by supporting the head and shoulders and pulling in line with the body; roll a victim over by rolling neck, shoulders, and hips together as a single unit; use several helpers to roll or lift a person all at the same time to move the victim into safety. If possible, get help from experienced rescuers before attempting to move the patient yourself. If you must move the patient before the cavalry arrives, and you have time, practice with your fellow victim-movers; the person at the head is always the lead and calls the shots; practice on someone who's uninjured before you attempt to move the patient.

If someone has a spinal injury, you should be prepared to treat for shock (more on this next). Keep the patient warm. Normally, if someone is in shock, you would elevate the feet; do not attempt this with someone who has a spinal injury until the patient is secured to a backboard.

Get help. Ideal management of spinal injuries requires well-prepared and knowledgeable medical professionals with a backboard, straps, and pads to secure the injured person so the spine doesn't move during evacuation. Several rescuers are necessary to secure the patient on the backboard and begin evacuation. If you're alone and it's possible, keep the victim warm and comfortable in camp, and call or go for help instead of trying to evacuate the patient yourself.

Shock: The Hidden Killer

It's almost a cliché to say that someone is going into shock. Nevertheless, shock is a dangerous side effect to injury, and it's important to be vigilant in treating shock.

Shock is the body's inability to circulate life-giving blood (and hence oxygen) to the brain, heart, and other organs and tissues. It's often caused by other injuries, and it can be fatal, even when those other injuries are not. Shock is much easier to prevent than to reverse once it's started, so it's important for you to understand how it begins and what you can do to keep it at bay.

There are several types of shock, depending on the injury or condition that creates it:

Cardiogenic. This occurs when your heart fails to pump enough blood and oxygen to the rest of the body. Blood volume is normal, but it's not moving oxygen from the lungs to the rest of the body.

Hypovolemic. Picture your circulatory system (your heart, arteries, capillaries, and veins) as a giant container. When there's not enough blood and/or fluid to fill the container, there's not enough to circulate oxygen through your body. Causes can be serious internal or external bleeding, severe dehydration, vomiting, diarrhea, or burns.

Neurogenic. This happens when damage to the spinal cord (usually in the upper spine or neck) causes widespread blood-vessel dilation. Signs and symptoms include slow pulse, low blood pressure, signs of neck injury, and, often, no sweating (commonly, shock victims have pale, clammy skin).

Respiratory Insufficiency. When a chest injury or breathing obstruction prevents someone from breathing well, the blood isn't getting enough oxygen for the body, even though it may be circulating well.

Psychogenic. Also known as fainting, this type of shock is an example of the power of the mind. When someone faces an unpleasant situation (the sight of blood might be enough), blood vessels dilate, blood drains from the brain, and the person faints. Although the person often recovers once on the ground and blood returns to the brain, cuts, bruises, or other injuries are possible on the way down.

Fear and panic during a medical emergency can also send a patient or onlookers into psychogenic shock, creating increased agitation, altered blood pressure, and rapid pulse, which can make existing injuries worse. For this reason, it's important for you to be the calm, cool, and collected one during medical emergencies, even if you're scared on the inside.

Septic. Severe and prolonged infections or toxins can lead to damage of the vessel walls, which, in turn, become leaky and unable to effectively contract. This lowers blood pressure and damages tissues and organ function. This type of shock is often the result of very serious illness, injury, or surgery. Luckily, it's most common after long stays in the hospital, not on the trail while backpacking.

Anaphylactic. A severe allergic reaction (to a bee sting or some foods, for instance) can sometimes develop in seconds and lead to anaphylactic shock. Symptoms range from mild itching to burning skin, vascular dilation, edema, profound coma, and rapid death. Although it's called shock because it can happen so suddenly, *anaphylaxis* is a different medical condition than the other shocks discussed here, and it requires different medical care—often an injection of epinephrine and treatment with antihistamines.

Depending on the type of shock, patients may present very differently. Hypovolemic shock and respiratory insufficiency, for instance, present with pale, cool, clammy skin; rapid, weak pulse; rapid, shallow, irregular breathing; confused, restless, or combative level of consciousness; low blood pressure (hard to find a pulse at the wrist).

Those in cardiogenic shock may have chest pains, irregular and/or weak pulse, pale skin, and anxiety. Those with neurogenic shock display slow pulse, low blood pressure, and often an absence of sweating.

Psychogenic shock is characterized by rapid pulse and fainting. Patients with septic shock present with warm skin, rapid pulse, and low blood pressure.

The best way to treat shock is to prevent it. If serious injuries occur, expect shock

---

WILDERNESS WISDOM

When assisting a patient, abide by the two primary rules of first aid: Don't become a victim, and do no further harm. Rushing into dangerous situations to rescue other people can create more victims and fewer rescuers. It's sad but true—sometimes people can't be saved. Think twice before rushing in to help someone in trouble. If you should decide to help, don't do anything that will make injuries worse. Your patient's comfort is often the best guide to doing the right thing, although with injuries, comfort might be a relative term.

to happen and treat it in advance with the following steps:

➤ Keep the victim lying down, insulated from the ground, and covered to keep him warm.

➤ Elevate the legs (unless the patient suffered a spinal injury, in which case you need to immobilize the spine first by securing the victim to a backboard) to improve circulation to the brain, heart, lungs, and other vital organs.

With heart attacks and head injuries (unless the patient is also suffering from a spinal injury), keep the victim in a comfortable, reclined sitting position and raise the legs—pretend he's in a reclining chair. The position of greatest comfort for the patient is a good guide to follow.

➤ Seek medical help immediately.

A Few Thoughts on Pain

Some pain while hiking—the burn of working muscles, for example—isn't dangerous. Other pain can indicate serious medical situations. Here are a few thoughts on how to distinguish good versus bad pain:

➤ Pain that comes on suddenly and lingers after the pain of sore muscles fades away indicates a more serious injury.

➤ Joint pain is a sign that ligaments, tendons, and cartilage have been damaged. These tissues, which attach bone to bone, bones to muscles, or cushion bones from friction and impact, are more brittle and less flexible than muscle. Avoid this by not pushing too hard during hikes and other workouts. Pushing yourself past your fitness level means pushing

Secondary Survey

After a serious accident, your patient might have multiple injuries. The most obvious injury isn't always the most serious. Don't let blood, screams, and other distractions prevent you from noticing other injuries that might also be serious but less obvious. Use the following tips to examine your patient fully, so you can discover the full extent of injury. Always stabilize the airway, breathing, and circulation (including bleeding) first and be alert to the possibility of shock.

Once you have treated the ABCS, ask the patient if you can look over the entire body, just to make sure there isn't anything you're missing. Getting permission to treat someone is an important part of treatment; not only is it respectful, but if the person is conscious and doesn't want to be treated, he has the right to be left alone—if your patient is unconscious, don't wait for permission, just start treating him.

➤ Wear gloves to protect yourself from the patient's bodily fluids and to protect the patient from the possibility of infection.

➤ Start with the head (check bones, as well as pupil size in eyes, and look for bleeding, fluids, or bruising in mouth, nose, and in and behind ears), then move down the body to the toes. Press each area gently (be respectful with certain areas of the body—you know the ones). Check the chest, ribs, abdomen, and pelvis. For arms and legs, use both hands to encircle the limb and squeeze gently. Inspect each limb separately, and ask the patient to push and pull her feet against your hand and to grasp your hands with her hands to make sure she has equal strength in all limbs. Carefully run your hand down the patient's spine, gently pressing on each vertebra to inspect for pain or bleeding.

➤ Ask your patient if any other places hurt, not just the obvious injury.

closer to the breaking point of these fragile tissues.

Joint pain can also be a sign that your body is out of balance—that one muscle group is stronger, and working harder, than another, which can pinch, fray, and bruise the tendons in the joint.

Rest, ice, proper posture and technique, and an effort to strengthen weaker muscles around a joint are the ways to relieve this pain. Ignore it, and you're asking for injury and surgery to repair the damage.

➤ If you feel pain that comes on with activity but isn't present at rest, you might have a stress fracture. Such injuries are common in lower legs after many miles of pounding, which is common in long-distance runners and hikers. Rest, ice, and non-steroidal, anti-inflammatory pain relievers can help this pain go away over time.

➤ If you feel chest pain with activity—while hiking along a trail, for example—it's a sign you're stressing your heart. Stop and rest. After the pain resides, have someone carry your pack, walk slowly back to the trailhead (or wait for rescue if the pain was scary or doesn't subside), and drive straight to the doctor. Heart conditions can be life-threatening.

➤ Any pain that confuses you about its origin, or that does not go away after several hours or intensifies over time, deserves prompt medical treatment. See your doctor immediately.

Pain Relievers and Other Medications

There are several types of over-the-counter pain relievers. Each has its advantages and risks, and everybody responds differently to each. Consult your doctor before taking any medications. Consider bringing an assortment of the following:

Aspirin. Best for: Pain, fever, inflammation, blood thinner, arthritis. Recommended dose: Up to 650 milligrams every four hours, up to six times a day. Warnings: Hard on the stomach. Not advised for children, people with ulcers or liver or kidney disease, hemophiliacs, pregnant women, people undergoing surgery within a week, and anyone allergic to non-steroidal, anti-inflammatory drugs. Brands: Bayer, Anacin, Bufferin, Excedrin.

Acetaminophen. Best for: Pain and fever relief; best for kids. Recommended dose: Up to 1000 milligrams every four to six hours; for kids, give 7 milligrams per pound, once every four to six hours, not to exceed five doses in 24 hours. Warnings: Hard on the liver if taken in overdose. Not good for inflammation. Not advised for heavy drinkers or people with liver disease. Brands: Tylenol, Midol, and other "aspirin-free" medications.

Ibuprofen. Best for: Pain, fever, long-term swelling. Recommended dose: 400 to 800 milligrams every eight hours with food. Do not exceed 3200 milligrams in 24 hours. Considered safe for children over 1 year old in doses of 2 to 4 milligrams per pound every six to eight hours. Warnings: May cause upset stomach or heartburn (take with food to avoid), may be hard on the kidneys, not recommended if you have gastritis, ulcers, kidney disease, if you're prone to bleeding, or if you're taking blood-thinner medications. Avoid if you're allergic to non-steroidal, anti-inflammatory drugs. Brands: Advil, Nuprin, Motrin-IB.

Arnica extract. Also called leopard's bane, extracts from this plant, applied as a cream or ingested in tablet form, can help ease the pain and swelling and speed healing of sore muscles. Not recommended for children.

Vicodin or other prescription pain medication. These prescription medications can be good additions to your first aid kit, just in case; they can help manage severe pain when you're hours or days from rescue. Caution: These can be narcotic and habit-forming. Talk to your doctor about which heavy-duty pain reliever might be best for you.

Benadryl (diphenhydramine). This antihistamine can help relieve the watery eyes, runny nose, and scratchy throat from hay fever and colds. Also works on itching and swelling from other allergic reactions.

Epinephrine. People who develop serious allergic reactions to food or bee stings can die within hours without medical treatment, which is usually an injection of epinephrine (adrenaline). On the trail, the best treatment is the EpiPen, a one-shot, spring-loaded, and pre-measured epinephrine dose, designed for quick, easy administration in emergencies. If you're allergic, or if you'll be leading a large group into the wild, talk to your doctor about a prescription, so you'll be prepared to save a life with this easy treatment.

Pepto-Bismol. For relief of upset stomach, nausea, and diarrhea.

Imodium. To help control diarrhea and cramping associated with abdominal infections.

Polysporin. An antibiotic for cuts and abrasions, and for temporary relief of rashes from poison oak, poison ivy, and other irritants.

Insect sting treatment. StingEze, After Bite, and calamine lotion are reasonably effective over-the-counter treatments for insect bites. Homemade treatments can be made from meat tenderizer or baking soda; carry some in a small plastic vial.

First Aid Kit

It's not a question of if someone in your party will get hurt, but when. Your challenge is to be prepared for whatever emergencies come your way in the wilderness, because there might not be medical staff out there to help you. Your favorite outdoor store will carry several types of pre-assembled first aid kits; there should be one to fit your group size and activity. You can also assemble your own. A list of items to include in your first aid kid is in Appendix I (see page 254). Consider the following questions before packing your first aid kit or heading into the wilderness:

➤ How many people are in your group? How fit are they?

➤ How far will you hike, and how many days will you be out?

Small first aid kits handle most minor injuries.

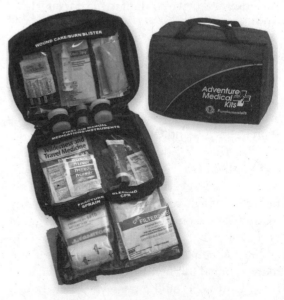

A compact survival kit

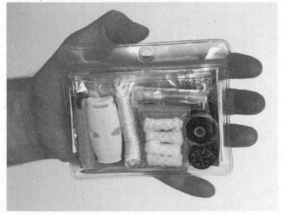

➤ What risks or hazards might you face on the trail? If it's rugged, rocky terrain, you'll need to prepare for twisted ankles; in rattlesnake country in summer, you might want to bring a snakebite kit.

➤ Do you or any of your hiking partners have medical conditions for which you should prepare ahead of time, just in case?

A first aid kit isn't enough. It's also important to know how to use it. Take this opportunity to learn first aid skills before you need them. Guaranteed, they'll come in handy sometime in the future. You'll feel more confident, less panicky, and thankful you prepared, when you have the skills to manage medical emergencies in the wilderness. The following are a few resources for first aid education:

➤ Call your local Red Cross chapter for a listing of classes near you. You can find your local chapter by calling: 202-303-4498 or logging onto www.redcross.org.

➤ Your local community college or school district might offer first aid classes through their adult-education or continuing-education programs.

First Aid Field Guides and Textbooks

➤ *Wilderness 911*, by Eric Weiss (The Mountaineers Books)

➤ *Medicine for Mountaineering & Other Wilderness Activities*, edited by James A. Wilkerson (The Mountaineers Books)

➤ There are also numerous organizations that offer Wilderness First Responder and other outdoor-emergency courses, which vary from two days to several weeks, depending on the intensity of training. They include the National Outdoor Leadership School (866-831-9001; www.nols.edu), Wilderness Medicine Outfitters (303-688-5176; www.wildernessmedicine.com), and Remote Medical International (800-597-4911; www.remotemedical.com).

➤ Practice makes better. Keep your first aid skills fresh by practicing at least once a year, or before each big trip. You'll be glad you did when you're face to face with a bloody, panicked fellow hiker.

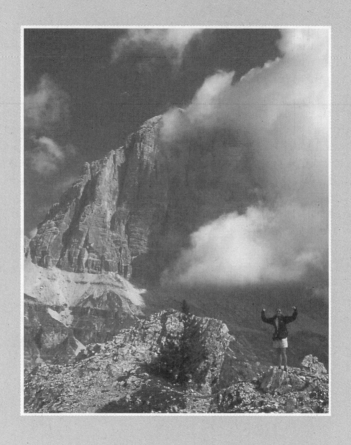

PART VII
ADVANCED BACKCOUNTRY SKILLS AND TRAVEL

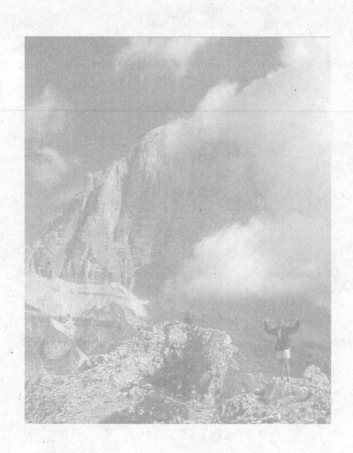

27 TRIPS FOR THE EXPERIENCED BACKPACKER

Fall in love with backpacking, and your expeditions will take you into more challenging terrain and weather for longer periods of time. This section introduces a few advanced skills you will need out there. Of course, no book can teach everything about backpacking We must all hike our own trails, make our own mistakes, and learn our own lessons—that's what makes backpacking such a wonderful adventure. Enjoy the trail!

Long-Distance Packing

If a weekend backpack trip just isn't long enough, you might be a candidate thruhiker. Most people who start out on long-distance hikes don't complete them; for example, only about 10 percent of those who plan to hike the entire Appalachian Trail (AT) make it to the other side. Long-distance hiking is more than weekend backpacking—you must be better prepared to confront the challenges of spending weeks and months on the trail, covering hundreds or even thousands of miles.

The US has numerous long-distance trails from which to choose, some of which are discussed on page 17. But these are only a few. The possibilities for a thru-hiking adventure are limited only by your creativity, ambition, and determination.

While you're first planning to begin a long-distance hike, don't think only of the sunny days and magical highlights; think also of, and prepare for, the bad things—blisters, sun, cold, rain, excruciating body odor, bugs beyond belief, tedium, and (depending on where you hike) the added risk of being days from help if you get hurt. These challenges shouldn't dissuade you from pursuing your epic trip, but the proper attitude will help you when your trip is not a picture postcard every day for weeks or months.

And although it's important to consider gear very carefully—you certainly don't want to carry too much, or the wrong equipment—the equipment isn't going to move you along the trail. How far you hike and how successful and enjoyable it is depends more on your attitude, fitness, and determination.

Pack weight is an important consideration when planning for a thru-hike. The last thing you want is 10 to 15 extra pounds on your back for hundreds of miles. Just because you'll be on the trail for a long time doesn't mean you will need a 7000-cubic-inch backpack loaded to the gills. On a long-distance hike, you will find that you can quickly pare down your needs to only the few most important items. Read the lightweight backpacking section on page 48, then carefully consider every ounce you will be carrying. More important than capacity are the comfort and durability of your pack, because you and it are going to encounter wear and tear during your trip.

A tent or shelter is highly recommended, even when hiking on a trail like the AT, which offers shelters for hikers. Shelters are crowded in the best of conditions, and they might come too soon or too late when it's time to settle in for the night. A tent or shelter can give you the freedom to camp where you want, and the freedom to avoid uncomfortable encounters with snoring, mice, crowded conditions, and bad attitudes.

Additional Sources for Long-Distance Hikers

A great way to better understand and prepare for a long-distance hike is to read the adventures and advice of those who have taken them. Here are a few great sources:

- ➤ *The Thru-Hiker's Handbook*, by Dan Bruce (Appalachian Trail Conference)
- ➤ *The Man Who Walked Through Time: The Story of the First Trip Afoot Through the Grand Canyon*, by Colin Fletcher (Vintage Books)
- ➤ *The Thousand-Mile Summer*, by Colin Fletcher (Vintage Books)
- ➤ *A Walk in the Woods: Rediscovering America on the Appalachian Trail*, by Bill Bryson (Anchor Books)
- ➤ *The Pacific Crest Trail Hiker's Handbook: Innovative Techniques and Trail Tested Instruction for the Long Distance Hiker*, by Ray Jardine (Adventurelore Press)
- ➤ *Pacific Crest Trail Data Book*, by Benedict Go (Wilderness Press)
- ➤ www.pcta.org: The website of the Pacific Crest Trail Association.
- ➤ www.aldha.org: The website of the Appalachian Long Distance Hikers Association. Also see the website for the ALDHA's sister organization at www.aldhawest.org.

Veteran thru-hiker Jim Owen offers exceptional advice on the "perspectives" section of his website, www.aldhawest.org: "The more you carry, the more you will enjoy your camping. The less you carry, the more you will enjoy your hiking. If you are going to finish a 2000-mile trail, you damn well better enjoy your hiking."

Whether you plan to hike alone or with partners, thru-hiking can be a very social activity, especially on popular trails like the AT. You will hike with, pass, and keep bumping into others. You will share shelters, eat together, and have the opportunity to join in a lot of camaraderie. Be prepared to encounter the worst humans have to offer as well as the best. The best way to deal with other hikers is to set some ground rules about your trip. The Golden Rule is a good place to start; treat others as you expect them to treat you, and tolerate all behavior, no matter how distasteful, especially if it does no harm to other people or the environment.

Although health, fitness, money, and equipment all play roles in determining the success of your long-distance hike, your attitude will be most important. How you decide to react to weather, insects, tedious days, injuries, less-than-gourmet food, and other people will play a bigger part in determining whether you complete your hike than any other single factor. Of course, there will be times when you're bored with the tedium, downright depressed with the weather, or homesick for the food, friends, family, and other comforts of civilization, but if you can find happiness and peace in the calm of resting after a long day's hike, in the glorious light of early morning or late afternoon, or in a smooth pace. And if you can find a way to flow with the challenges and the trail rather than trying to conquer them, you just might find the mindset to complete your hike of a lifetime.

Resupply

At most, you can carry enough food in your pack for a week to 10 days. If you're planning a longer trip, you will need to get new supplies along the way. If hiking through remote country, where you can't pop back into town to shop once a week, here are a few ways to get the goods so you can keep hiking:

Loop back to your car. Once a week, load up on supplies, then head back out.

Mail. If there's a town near one of the trailheads along your route, you can mail yourself a box of rations, or have a friend mail it to the specified address at a particular date: Address it to yourself, care of "General Delivery." Make sure the box is well-labeled and carries a date by which you will pick it up. It might be helpful to call the postmaster ahead of time and inquire about what would make delivery more reliable. You might also be able to send a box to businesses or even private residences near a trailhead if they don't mind, but check with them ahead of time to make arrangements. Offer to pay, perhaps.

Hand delivery. If a friend or family member is willing and able, have them meet you at a trailhead along the way to deliver your supplies in person. This is a great time to spend the day or night with them, and enjoy the nice meal and other civilized comforts they brought along as well. Professional guides or outfitters might be able to ride (or fly if you're somewhere remote, like deep Alaska) your supplies to a specified location when you need them.

Caches. Stashing provisions at a particular point along the way can be a good idea, just make sure caching is legal in the area. Package your cache in a weather- and critter-proof container.

A few other thoughts on resupply:

➤ Package all rations in a secure, reinforced box or other container, so it will endure everything it goes through before it gets to you.

➤ Write down all of the details regarding your resupply—where it needs to be delivered and by when. Include maps marked with the specific location of the drop-off point (including GPS coordinates, if necessary). Make a copy and share this contract with your resupplier. If it's not in the contract, don't be surprised if miscommunication thwarts your plans.

➤ Do all the work ahead of time. Don't expect your resupplier to shop for and package materials for you. Sort, bag, box, weigh, and label everything ahead of time to make it as easy as possible for your resupplier to provide the service you'll need. This way, you have a higher chance you will get what you need when you need it.

➤ Have a backup plan. What will you do if the resupply doesn't arrive when you need it? Where should your delivery person leave your goods if you don't show up on time? Communicate with your resupplier so each of you has a backup plan in case one of you doesn't show up at the scheduled time.

➤ Clean up. If you have a cache or other resupply point, make sure you clean all traces of your resupply when you leave.

Cross-Country Travel

Going into the real backcountry, where no trails lead, guarantees amazing adventures and natural beauty. Hiking cross-country can be rewarding and beautiful, but the risks are also higher. Arm yourself with well-developed navigation and survival skills to make sure you enjoy these adventures and come back safely.

Leave No Trace considerations are different when traveling cross-country. It's important not to create a trail that entices others to follow your route, thereby multiplying unnecessary impacts on the landscape. Travel on durable surfaces, such as rocks, logs, and soils that won't be irreversibly damaged by your

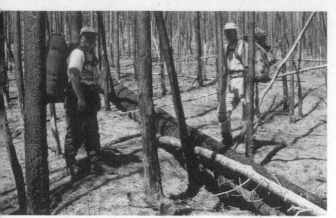

Navigation skills are important when hiking off-trail.

passing. Be particularly careful when traveling on steep slopes, which are especially sensitive to damage and erosion. If you're in a group, spread out to minimize impact on one route (in deserts, however, it's exactly the opposite; see more on desert travel on page 246). Do not create cairns, blazes, or ducks that will encourage additional traffic to your route.

When camping in pristine sites, make every effort to camp on durable surfaces, such as on bare rock or gravel. Spread out your tents, and avoid walking the same route repeatedly. Take time to naturalize your campsite before you leave; your goal is to make it look as untouched after you leave as it did when you arrived.

Navigation

Compasses and navigation techniques become essential when there is no trail, when there are no features in the landscape, when you're in winding canyons or deep forests, and when storms or fog limit visibility. Make sure you have mastered orientation, how to take a bearing, and map-compass navigation skills beginning on page 127 before you plan a cross-country trip.

When following a bearing to a desired destination (that beautiful, cool lake is waiting!), you can waste a lot of time hiking up and down over hills and other obstacles; it might be easier to walk around them. A simple way to do this is to contour by walking at a single elevation while hiking across a slope or around a hill, using your compass bearing as a general guide. Also called "sidehilling," contouring isn't always easy; it's hard on the ankles and gets old quickly. Sidehill only when necessary.

If you need to detour around an obstacle, such as a bog, cliff, or lake, but you want to keep track of your bearing, do the following:

1. When confronted by your obstacle, turn to the side that offers the shortest and easiest detour, and choose a new bearing that will take you to the side of the obstacle. Walk a straight line on this new bearing until you've cleared the obstacle. Try to walk at a constant speed, timing how long you hike off your original bearing.

2. Once you've cleared the obstacle, turn back to your original compass bearing and follow it until you have passed the obstacle.

3. To return to the line you were on before you confronted the obstacle, determine the mirror-image angle of your compass bearing from step 1. Hike at the same speed for the same amount of time as you did in step 1.

4. Re-establish your original bearing, and get on with your travels.

Careful attention to your bearing can keep you on track.

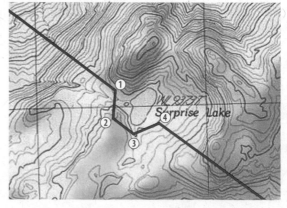

International Treks

It's a big, beautiful world, and there are too many wonderful, rewarding, and jaw-droppingly beautiful places to backpack to fit in a single book ... or life. This section aims to inspire you by mentioning a few classic destinations; learn more by asking friends, by searching the internet, and by browsing the travel section of your favorite bookstore.

Note: International backpacking does not necessarily mean hiking on trails and sleeping in tents. It's also a way to travel from town to town and see the sights, while carrying everything you need on your back (travel packs that convert from suitcase to backpack are great for this; see page 75), and while experiencing the adventure of local transportation, accommodations, and culture. In this sense, backpackers are sometimes called travelers (as opposed to tourists, who travel the world but never leave Western-style hotels, transportation, and restaurants).

Here are a few classic treks; some of which are life-list candidates:

Hut-to-hut hiking in the European Alps. Those Europeans sure know how to hike in style. Leave your stove, tent, and the bulk of your food behind and hike from hut to hut in the French or Swiss Alps, or from refugio to refugio in Italy's Dolomites. The trails are well-marked and lead through some of our planet's most stunning scenery. At regular intervals, huts and refugios are waiting with warm meals, comfortable beds, and often fine wine and beer. Learn more or sign up for tours at www.alpseurope.com.

Mt. Kilimanjaro, Tanzania. The tallest mountain in Africa is the highest in a chain of volcanoes in eastern Africa's Rift Valley. This weeklong backpack gives anyone who is decently fit the opportunity to climb to 19,340 feet without technical mountaineering skills. There are also great opportunities to enjoy African

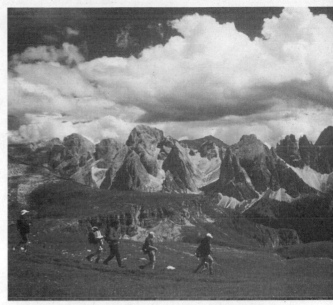

It's hard to beat hut-to-hut hiking in the Dolomites.

wildlife at nearby Ngorongoro Crater. You can get a good introduction to what this trip entails by searching "Kilimanjaro" at gorp.away.com.

Fitz Roy Grand Tour, Argentina. This 35-mile trek is considered moderate in difficulty, yet it rewards with breathtaking views of the Fitz Roy (also called Cerro Chalten by locals) group of peaks in Parque Nacionale Los Glaciares—reason enough to make the effort to get to the southern tip of South America. While you're there, you'll encounter windswept steppes, rivers of ice, and unique cultures and wildlife in one of the continent's biggest national parks. Start your research about this region at www.patagonia-argentinia.com/i/.

West Highland Way, Scotland. This 95-mile trail will lead you from the outskirts of Glasgow, past Loch Lomond, through moors, to Fort William in the Scottish Highlands. The route allows you to enjoy Scotland's natural beauty as well as her best food, hospitality, and accommodations along the way, so you don't have to carry much. Learn more by logging onto www.west-highland-way.co.uk.

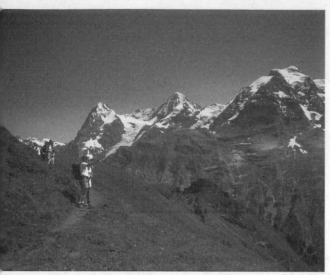

The Swiss Alps at their finest

Baltoro Glacier to K2 basecamp. This classic, monthlong trek will take you into a realm of soaring vertical spires, massive glaciers, and above 18,000 feet in the heart of the Karakoram region of the Himalayas. A Google search for "Baltoro Glacier" or "K2 basecamp" will lead you to numerous tour groups offering to lead expeditions to this spectacular region.

Milford Track. Billed as one of the finest walks of the world, this 33-mile New Zealand trek will take you over McKinnon Pass, through lush forests, past more waterfalls than you can count, and finally to Milford Sound. This trek is extremely popular, so advanced reservations are required. So is rain gear—the area receives 5 meters (yes, that's more than 16 feet) of rain each year. Begin your planning at New Zealand's Department of Conservation website at www.doc.govt.nz.

Resources for Traveling Internationally

➤ **Trail Database:** This website, www.traildatabase.org, is a great place to begin your research about international budget travel and backpacking. The quality of information on its pages varies by destination, but you're sure to find good inspiration and advice to begin planning your trip.

➤ **Passplanet:** This website, www.passplanet.com, by backpackers for backpackers (it's not sponsored by a company trying to sell you stuff), offers great destination ideas and travel advice for backpackers wanting to explore Asia and Central America.

➤ **Backpack Africa:** Although this site, www.backpackafrica.com, doesn't have the wealth of information available on Passplanet, it's a good starting point to research destinations, accommodations, and travel on the and oh-so-magical continent.

➤ **Lonely Planet guides:** Lonely Planet specializes in guidebooks for travelers and backpackers. They're good guides that focus on affordable food and accommodations, and the best cultural and natural attractions.

➤ **US State Department:** You won't find specific information on hiking destinations at this US government-sponsored site, travel.state.gov, but you'll be able to find what the US government thinks about your country of interest. You'll also learn how to get visas, and you'll find out whether travel restrictions are in place.

28 BACKPACKING IN EXTREME WEATHER AND CLIMATES

High-altitude mountaineering, winter expeditions, and high-latitude exploration (say, in the northern Arctic or Antarctica) can present explorers with extreme challenges to life and limb. Don't join any high-elevation expedition without getting your cardiovascular system into good shape (see page 145 for fitness tips). What follows is a discussion of what you'll face up there.

High Elevations

When you plan to hike at high elevations, prepare for colder weather and higher winds. Temperatures drop 3°F to 5°F for every 1000 feet you climb above sea level, which means that mountain pass 3000 feet above the trailhead might be 15 degrees colder, and windy, too.

There's also less oxygen available at altitude. Air contains about 21 percent oxygen, a constant at every elevation. However, for every 1000 feet you climb above sea level, air pressure drops by about 3 percent. Because air pressure is what pushes oxygen molecules through lung membranes into your blood, there is also 3 percent less oxygen available for your body. At 10,000 feet, about 30 percent less oxygen is available compared with sea level. At 15,000 feet, only about half the oxygen is available. Standing on the summit of Mt. Everest, at 29,035 feet, your blood, brain, and other tissues

would be forced to operate with only 30 percent of the oxygen available at sea level.

Although every body is different, everyone succumbs to the effects of altitude at some point. Although a few people feel altitude's ills lower, most people can travel to 8500 feet above sea level without incident. The few, the fit, the proud can hike strongly to 18,000 feet and beyond. How your body responds to

MY SYSTEM

High-Altitude "Guest Kit"

As a native East Coaster transplanted to Colorado, I invite my sea-level-dwelling friends to enjoy the mountains whenever they can. I make sure when we head out, I bring extra supplies to help them get along with altitude: Advil Liqui-Gels, antacids, Pepto-Bismol, an extra pair of high-quality sunglasses, strong sunblock, and energy gels that don't taste awful (usually chocolate or vanilla Gu). Oh, and one more thing: a small, pink, stuffed elephant—for when they think they have a hangover despite not having had alcohol! Pinky the Elephant is a great toy to dangle from your tent's ceiling—and a surprisingly effective distraction for a friend who needs to get his mind off how lousy the thin air is making him feel.

—**James Dziezynski**, author, *Best Summit Hikes in Colorado* (Wilderness Press)

241

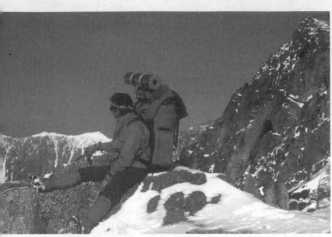
High-mountain views make all the discomfort of getting there worthwhile.

altitude depends on your fitness level and how acclimatized you are. Those who travel too high too quickly can fall victim to fluid buildup in the lungs and/or cranium, both of which can be fatal if untreated.

Fortunately, the body can compensate for this—at least to an extent—with acclimatization. The more time you spend at altitude, and the more slowly you gain elevation, the more time your blood has to produce red blood cells;

Pressure Breathing

At high elevations, you can increase the amount of oxygen available to your lungs through pressure breathing. Inhale normally. When you exhale, purse your lips so there's only a small hole for the air to escape. Then push air hard through that hole with all your breathing muscles. This simulates lower altitudes by increasing the air pressure in your lungs, which in turn pushes more oxygen over your lung threshold into your blood. It takes effort and presence of mind, but it can ease the headache, dizziness, and other symptoms of high altitude until you bag your peak and start heading back down.

the extra hemoglobin will grab what little oxygen is available. The more time you can spend at altitude before hiking, the happier you'll be. Mountaineers tackling the tallest mountains (18,000 feet and higher) spend weeks at high-elevation basecamp, getting used to the thinner air before they make their summit push.

One way to acclimatize is to hike high and camp low. If you're hiking and camping at high elevations, plan to camp lower when you can, then hike to a high point before returning to camp for the night. This simple practice helps your body prepare for your return to elevation the next day. You'll sleep and eat better lower down, too.

On that note, appetites tend to disappear at high elevations. Nonetheless, even if you're not hungry, it's important to eat anyway; your body needs the energy. Higher air, because it's colder, is also drier, which means you will dehydrate more quickly at high elevations. Drinks lots of water, then drink some more.

Altitude Sickness

You don't have to be at 18,000 feet to feel the effects of altitude. Drive quickly from your home at sea level to the trailhead at 7000 feet, then start hiking up to the pass at 10,000 feet, and you'll be lucky if you don't get a headache or nausea. While you can acclimate to higher altitude, you may still feel the effects of altitude sickness, which is affected by your speed of ascent, the altitude you reach, and how long you stay.

In addition to weakness, headaches, and nausea, high elevations can force liquid to leak from capillaries in your lungs and head, producing serious medical emergencies: High-altitude pulmonary edema (HAPE) results when your lungs fill with fluid; high-altitude cerebral edema (HACE) is the swelling of your brain. Both HACE and HAPE are extremely dangerous and can be fatal if not treated.

Luckily, the cure is simple: Descend quickly. Signs and symptoms will begin to fade quickly at lower elevations. The prescription medication acetazolamide (Diamox) can help ease the symptoms of mild altitude sickness, and it may help speed acclimatization for some people. If you do experience severe altitude sickness, seek medical care as soon as possible to avoid serious consequences.

Snow Travel

You don't have to hike in winter to face a wintery challenge. In high mountains, snow can last well into summer (late June or July in the northern hemisphere), especially on north-facing slopes. Snow can also fall on any day of the year in the mountains.

If you think you'll encounter snow and/or ice in more than a few small patches here and there, you might need extra equipment and caution to navigate with it. Snow-shoes provide extra floatation in deep snow (but in light snow with a heavy pack, expect little flotation and a lot hard work). Many models have metal teeth on the bottom to provide extra traction on ice. Ski or trekking poles provide needed stability on snow and ice.

Before traveling onto a steep, snowy, or icy slope, think first about what might happen if you slip and fall. Where will you end up? What are the potential consequences of a long, screaming tumble toward those rocks and trees, or over that cliff? Sometimes the most direct route is the most dangerous. Instead of crossing that slope, consider a detour. On icy, steep slopes, consider bringing crampons, which will help your feet gain traction on ice, and an ice ax, which you can use to self-arrest, if you know how to do it (ask a mountaineering friend to teach you, then practice on a safe part of the slope before stepping out onto high exposure). Rope together on exposed slopes,

but make sure all participants have dependable self-arrest skills.

Use caution when traveling on snow over a creek or stream. What looks like a safe route might actually be a thin snow bridge over a long drop into dangerous water. Listen to the sounds of water under the snow to alert you to the possibility of a snow bridge. Test each step with your pole before committing weight.

In spring conditions, snow tends to harden at night (if the temperature drops below freezing) and soften after a few hours in the sun. Timing can be key; depending on the particular snow conditions where you hike, snow might be easier to walk on early in the morning, or it might be easier to cross after it softens up a tad. If it warms up too much, however, you might find yourself post-holing (sinking all the way in) instead of walking on top, which is no fun with a heavy pack.

In the mountains, snow may be present, even in summer.

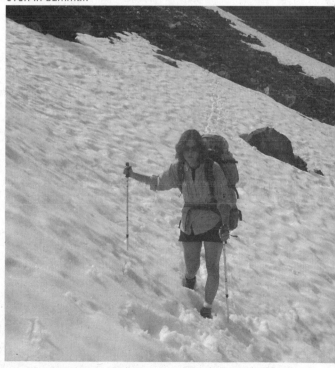

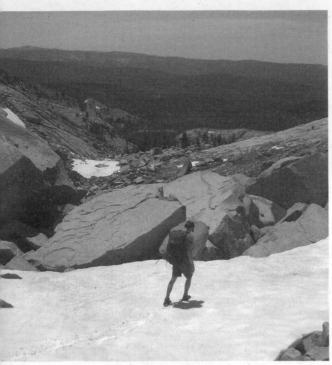

Avoid the edges of snow fields near rocks.

Use caution at the upper edges of steep snow fields, especially near rocks; in these spots, the snow may be thin, and there may be a dangerous gap between the snow and the rock or earth above it (called a bergschrund). Use caution to avoid a fall. Give a couple test kicks without committing your weight, or jab it with your pole, to make sure it's steady. When in doubt, go around.

Become Avalanche Aware

To learn more about avalanche and how to evaluate snow hazards, check out the following:

➤ *Snow Sense: A Guide to Evaluating Snow Avalanche Hazard*, by Jill Fredston and Doug Fesler (Alaska Mountain Safety Center)

➤ en.wikipedia.org/wiki/Avalanche

When traveling on glaciers in high mountains, use particular caution to avoid crevasses (deep cracks in glaciers that can kill or seriously injure anyone who falls in). Thin snow bridges can hide the mouths of crevasses. If planning a route across a glacier, advanced mountaineering skills are mandatory. All participants should be equipped with crampons and ice axes, and all should be roped together for safety. If you do not have an experienced glacier navigator in your party, hire a guide.

Traveling on snow also requires careful steps and an awareness of avalanche danger. Snow avalanches kill people on a regular basis. They can happen in winter after heavy snows, and in summer when snow layers weaken and separate from each other after months of freeze and thaw. When traveling onto large, snowy slopes or snowfields between 30 and 50 degrees steep, consider the possibility that an avalanche might occur. If mountain snow travel is in your plans, your best defense against avalanches is a knowledge of snow conditions and how to evaluate slope safety and risk. Consider taking a class to learn snow science and how to use a beacon, shovel, and probe to conduct a rescue after an avalanche.

Comfort and Nutrition

Few things are more beautiful than a snow-covered landscape in the crisp light of a clearing storm, or the profound silence that settles in the forest during soft snowfall. Backpacking in winter can be incredibly fun, but only if you keep warm and cozy, which takes a lot of equipment. This is no time to skimp on comfort. It's more difficult because you must carry more gear to stay warm, but the consequences can be fatal if you're not prepared. Keep these tips in mind to stay comfortable and safe during your travel through snow:

➤ Take off extra layers before you begin hiking, so you don't sweat from exertion, and so you don't have to stop after 15 minutes to take off your pack, remove layers, then get going again.

➤ Stop for quicker breaks and snacks throughout the day instead of long breaks that cool you off too much.

➤ Plan one-pot meals, which are quick, easy, and warming on cold days. Also bring lots of hot fluids—cocoa, soups, and stews, etc. Make sure to include extra fat with every meal. Fat has twice the calories than carbs or protein and will help keep your internal furnace stoked.

➤ Prepare to melt snow for water and meals. Water filters don't work in freezing weather. When water in the filter workings freezes, it can crack the seals, rendering your filter useless. If you're camping in snow, you may not find water to filter, anyway. Instead, you'll need to melt snow, so remember to pack the appropriate amount of fuel and consider whether your stove is effective in colder weather (see more on stoves on page 86). When you do melt snow, remember that snow melts faster when there's already some water in the pot. A hot pot without water can scald snow, which doesn't taste good.

➤ Keep your hydration pack warm. Hydration pack tubes and nozzles freeze and clog easily. Insulated tubes provide only minimal protection. If it's really cold, keep your water bottle or hydration pack (and drinking tube) in your jacket.

➤ Screw the extra weight. Bring a big, warm sleeping bag rated safely below the lowest temperatures you'll face, as well as down booties and a pair of warm, fluffy socks for night. An extra sleeping pad will insulate further again the cold ground.

➤ Tie small loops of cord to all zippers, so you can open and close them with gloves.

MY SYSTEM

Happy Hibernating

Maybe I was a Yeti in a previous life; I love winter camping! Unfortunately, my current pelt is a bit too sparse to keep me warm on chilly evenings. To get a good winter night's sleep, here's what I do: Start off by making a nice, flat surface in the snow to camp on. In my tent (or on the snow), I lay a tarp, then a closed-foam sleeping pad, and I top it off with a 1-inch-thick, inflatable, full-length Therm-a-Rest. I bring along two empty 32-ounce Nalgene bottles and fill them up with boiling water from my stove before I go to sleep. I keep one at the foot of my sleeping bag and cuddle the other one like a hard, plastic teddy bear. The heat they provide warms up my sleeping bag (saving my body the trouble) and ensures I'll have unfrozen water for the morning.

—**James Dziezynski**, author, *Best Summit Hikes in Colorado* (Wilderness Press)

Hypothermia

The life-sustaining chemical reactions that take place in core organs (heart, brain, lungs, liver, kidneys, etc.) can occur only within a few degrees of our normal 98.6°F. For example, the body begins to shiver in an attempt to warm itself when its core temperature falls to between 95°F and 98°F. With a core temperature of 94°F or below, the "umbles" take over—mumbling, fumbling, stumbling—and the brain begins to lose control over bodily functions, including the ability to understand and react to danger. Alert hiking partners should know these critical warning signs. Below 90°F, shivering stops, muscles become stiff, and the patient begins to become incoherent. Death is possible at below 80°F.

Hypothermia can occur in any cold or wet conditions, even a summer thunderstorm or sudden fall in a cold lake or stream on a warm day. The best way to treat hypothermia is to prevent it. Make every effort to stay warm in the first place. If it's too late, and you or a campmate becomes seriously cold, follow these steps quickly:

➤ Seek shelter immediately. Set up camp, get patient into dry clothes, a tent, and a sleeping bag. Have another campmate climb in the sleeping bag to help re-warm him.

➤ Re-warm the patient from the inside, using hot chocolate, soup, or other warm liquid. Do this only if the patient is conscious enough to swallow and there are no serious internal injuries.

➤ Place warm packs under the arms and against the carotid arteries on the neck (gently—you don't want to block circulation here). This warms arterial blood, which will then circulate warmth through the body. Do not worry about the arms and legs; extremities are not essential to life, and warming them first can send dangerously cold blood into the core.

➤ If your patient becomes unconscious, monitor breathing and pulse, both of which can be very slow and difficult to detect.

➤ Send or call for medical rescue.

➤ Be very gentle with the victim, because the heart is very fragile at this stage. The slightest bump can send the heart into arrest.

➤ Check the patient's pulse and breathing. Place the index and middle finger of one hand on the patient's neck, and press firmly in the notch between his windpipe and neck muscle. While doing this, place your ear and cheek close to the patient's nose and mouth. Look at the chest to see if it rises, listen for the sound of breathing, feel for breathing against your cheek, and feel for a pulse with your fingers. Do this for at least 45 seconds.

If you can detect neither pulse nor breathing, begin CPR. If you're not CPR certi-

fied, get it now; it takes less than a day and can save the life of someone you love.

➤ Do not assume your patient is dead until he is warm and dead, even if you can't detect a breath or pulse. Many people have been revived after astonishingly long periods of extreme hypothermia. However, because extremely hypothermic patients are so fragile, survival is rare without active internal rewarming and cardiac support by well-trained and well-equipped medical staff.

Desert Travel

Deserts are defined by their lack of precipitation. Because water is essential—without it, you'll die in a few days—it is the limiting factor in desert travel. Although some desert landscapes are completely devoid of water, most deserts have at least some water. Water sources may be few and far between, though. It's also heavy (8.3 pounds per gallon), so carrying more than a day's drinking supply will make your backpack really heavy.

Between the lack of water, intense sun, and crazy heat in summer, you will need to plan your trip carefully to backpack safely in the desert. Here are a few tips:

➤ Plan your itinerary around water. This is necessary in all but the wettest landscapes; make sure there's water where you plan to hike. Once you have determined where reliable water is, you might need to plan your trip around it—from spring to creek to river to spring. Carry enough water (plus some extra) to get you safely from one water source to the next.

➤ There are two ways to carry less water: Carry only the water you'll need to get to the next water source (assuming you're confident about the next water source; carry extra if it's a hot day, or if you're going to be working hard). And drink as much as you can hold. Before you leave the car, and before leaving each water source, drink as much water as you can manage, so you'll need to carry less when you're hiking.

➤ Don't trust maps. Just because your topographic map shows a spring, it doesn't mean the spring has water in it. Spring flows can change drastically from season to season and year to year. Contact local experts (rangers and other land-management officials, local hiking clubs, state wildlife biologists, etc.) to find someone who has been there recently, who can verify whether water is present. If you can't verify the presence of water, don't take chances. Carry all the water you will need, just in case.

➤ Prepare for cold. Deserts are not always hot. In winter (or cold snaps), at high latitudes, and at high elevation, deserts can be downright frigid. Once the sun goes down, heat can disappear as quickly as light. Sudden storms can also drop temperatures (and a lot of rain) quickly. Ask local experts about weather patterns and daytime versus nighttime temperatures. Always bring extra layers just in case.

➤ Avoid the hottest part of the day. On hot days, start hiking at first light. Find a cool spot to rest through the hottest part of the day, then hike again when it gets cooler. Hiking by moonlight can be a wonderful way to explore the desert.

➤ Prepare to dry camp. Water may not be available. When it is, state laws often require that you camp far away from springs and other water sources, so wildlife can access water while you're there. Dry camping means having enough water to get you through the night, and using the water you do have sparingly. With a little practice, you can learn to cook and to wash your dishes (and yourself) with only minimal amounts of water. Or you can wait to wash until there's water available. At all times, avoid infecting water sources with your own dirt, grime, and diseases.

➤ Avoid washes and narrow canyons in the rainy season. Deadly flash floods can roar through narrow canyons and fill dry washes quickly. Avoid narrow canyons and washes when thunderstorms are active. Be particularly cautious of storms you can't see that may be sending dangerous torrents toward you from a distant source far upstream.

➤ Bring a comb, tweezers, and duct tape if cacti are abundant. Combs can help remove entire segments of cholla and other cacti that "jump" onto you. Simply slide the comb between the cactus and your skin, then lift it away. Duct tape is effective at removing plentiful smaller spines.

➤ Be respectful of fragile life. Life in the desert is tough enough without you around.

Though challenging, deserts can be sublimely beautiful.

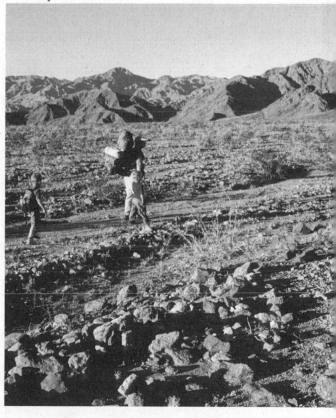

Your presence can add dangerous stress to wildlife populations; your steps can crush fragile plants. Be particularly conscious of cryptogammic (also called cryptobiotic) soils, which have a hard black or brown crust on the surface. Although these soils look barren and lifeless, the crust is actually a marriage of moss, lichen, algae, and fungi stitched together, preventing topsoil from blowing away in the wind, soaking up water during rare rainstorms, preventing the evaporation of water in the soil, and deterring invasive plant seeds from gaining a foothold. Your steps break this crust and cause all of those bad things to happen. Follow existing trails when you can. If you're a group, walk in single file.

Hyperthermia

One of the biggest challenges in hiking in hot weather is keeping your body cool. If your core temperature rises to 101°F or above, you will begin to suffer from hyperthermia, a condition that ranges from mild (heat exhaustion) to severe (heat stroke).

The signs and symptoms of heat exhaustion include weakness, dizziness, nausea, headache, dry tongue and thirst, cold, clammy skin, and a body temperature between normal and 104°F. To treat patients with heat exhaustion, have them rest in a cool, shaded spot; loosen their clothes; give them plenty of lightly salted water; and cool them with water or cold packs on neck, under arms, on chest, and in groin.

Untreated, heat exhaustion can progress to heat stroke, which occurs when your body loses the ability to keep itself cool. Heat stroke is a life-threatening condition, and your priority should be to cool the victim quickly. Signs and symptoms include high body temperature (often over 105°F), high pulse and breath rate at rest, confusion, disorientation, loss of coordination, seizure, and even coma or death. Sweating may be present or absent; the patient may have hot, dry, flushed skin if their body has lost its ability to sweat.

To treat heat stroke, cool the patient as quickly as possible. Use cool water or cover the patient with wet towels or sheets and fan aggressively. Place ice packs along side of neck, on head, under arms, on chest, and in groin. Do not give anything to eat or drink, because vomiting might occur. Treat the victim for shock by placing him on his back and raising his legs. Evacuate to professional medical care.

Backpacking is a gateway drug. Once you learn to travel fast and light, you might become addicted and want to experiment with other joys in the wild, such as mountaineering, canyoneering, river rafting and kayaking, ocean kayaking, recreational tree climbing, and bicycle touring. The best parts of these "addictions": They're good for both body and soul, and once you've invested in the necessary equipment, they're inexpensive pursuits. However, they do present unique challenges that require advanced skills to meet. Risk can be higher, too, and advanced skills are no guarantee of safety.

Canyoneering is the exploration of deep, narrow canyons, and it's the only way you will ever see the deeper secrets of the Grand Canyon, Canyonlands National Park, and any place where waterfalls in deep and steep canyons prevent access by hiking. To canyoneer properly, it's essential to have navigation and route-finding skills, as well as harnesses, ropes, helmets, and other hardware and knowledge to rappel down waterfalls. It might also be good to know how to climb up those falls with mechanical ascenders or rock-climbing skills. Knowledge of water dynamics and the threats moving water create is also good to have.

Dry bags are often necessary to protect your clothing and other gear from getting wet. Wetsuits might be necessary to protect you from hypothermia, although they might not be enough—be prepared to pursue more active warming strategies. In addition, knowledge and awareness of local weather conditions will be necessary to ensure that you don't encounter dangerous flash floods from rain in the area. To learn more about canyoneering, check out the American Canyoneering Association at www.canyoneering.net.

Llamas can make great hiking partners.

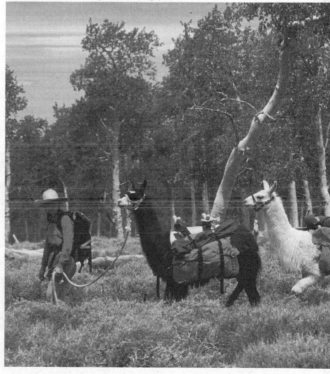

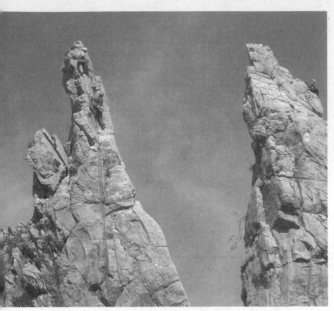
Climb to new heights in backcountry travel.

Many backpackers seek the next level of challenge in **mountaineering**, which leads to heavenly views and a wonderful sense of accomplishment. All high mountains require a level of fitness and careful efforts to acclimatize to high altitudes. Snow- and ice-covered mountains require clothing to protect you against extreme cold and storms, as well as crampons, ice axes, ropes, harnesses, and possibly skis, snow stakes, and helmets. Knowledge and experience with glaciers, steep snow and ice, altitude, rockfall, bergschrunds, seracs, and crevasses is critical. An experienced guide will help you deal with these challenges successfully as you push for the summit. Learn more about mountaineering by clicking to the following websites: www.mountaineers.org or www.traditional-mountaineering.org. You should also pick up a copy of *Mountaineering: The Freedom of the Hills* (The Mountaineers Books).

If scaling high-altitude peaks is not your thing, perhaps you should try tall trees. Who says you have to be a kid? Developments in equipment and techniques for rock climbing have opened wonderful doors (or is it branches?) for **recreational tree climbing**—exploring forests in the uppermost reaches of trees. In tropical rainforests, upper forest canopies hold secrets that ground travel will never reveal—entire plant and animal communities that are invisible from the ground. In temperate forests, you can experience amazing views and a great perspective while nestled in the arms of the oldest and wisest beings on this planet. As with rock climbing, recreational tree climbing is potentially dangerous and requires specialized equipment and skills that are well beyond tackling most neighborhood trees.

River rafting can provide both backcountry thrills and comforts.

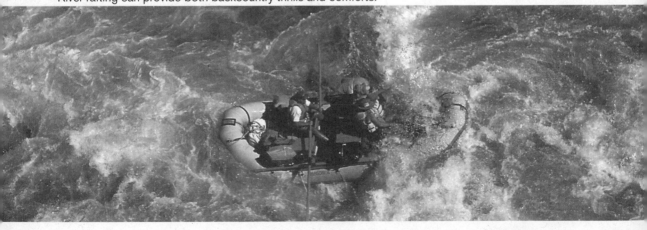

Recreational tree climbing requires the use of climbing ropes, harnesses, ascenders, and bivouac equipment (sometimes called tree boats) that allow you to hang out in trees, not just hang. Learn more at www.treeclimbing.com, www.danceswithtrees.com, www.newtribe.com, www.treeclimbingusa.com, and www.pacifictreeclimbing.com.

Yet another way to explore the wilderness is to let water lead the way. **Canoeing, river rafting, and kayaking** allow you to let water do most of the work (but certainly not all), while you watch the world drift by and hop out from time to time to camp and explore. In addition to the best watercraft to suit your needs (not all canoes and kayaks are alike), you will need specialized skills to navigate moving water safely, as well as personal floatation devices, throw ropes, knives, flotation bags, dry bags, and other equipment. Advanced swimming and water rescue techniques are also recommended. Learn more at the American Canoe Association's website, www.acanet.org; at www.paddler.net; and by reading *Whitewater Classics: Fifty North American Rivers Picked by the Continent's Leading Paddlers*, by Tyler Williams (Funhog Press) and *The Essential Whitewater Kayaker: A Complete Course*, by Jeff Bennett (Ragged Mountain Press).

Sea kayaking is a great way to explore oceans and lakes. While whitewater kayaking requires smaller, more maneuverable boats, touring kayaks are bigger, longer, and better able to track a straight line as you paddle big water. Of course, with big water come big risks. Learn more about the equipment and techniques necessary for safe and successful big water tours at www.canoekayak.com and www.seakayak.com.

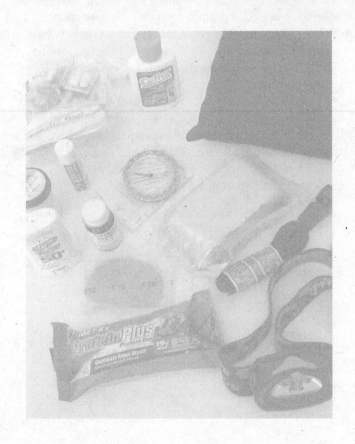

APPENDIX I
GEAR CHECKLISTS

To help you pack quickly without forgetting anything, either copy these lists or make your own. Add items you think you'll need, and take off what you don't. Keep it filed (fold it in this book), so it'll be accessible the next time you're gathering your equipment for a trip into the wilderness.

Packing

- ☐ Backpack
- ☐ Daypack or fanny pack
- ☐ Stuff sacks

Shelter

- ☐ Ground cloth
- ☐ Tent, shelter, or bivy
- ☐ Poles, stakes
- ☐ Sleeping bag
- ☐ Bag liner
- ☐ Sleeping pad(s)

Clothing

- ☐ Hiking boots/shoes and insoles
- ☐ Camp shoes/booties/sandals
- ☐ Underwear
- ☐ Base layers: synthetic long underwear (top and bottom)
- ☐ Middle layers: fleece, sweater
- ☐ Shell layers: jacket, pants

- ☐ T-shirts
- ☐ Hiking shorts
- ☐ Long pants
- ☐ Hat(s): baseball cap, beanie/warm hat, wide-brimmed sun hat
- ☐ Gloves
- ☐ Socks (one pair per day plus an extra) and liners
- ☐ Gaiters: Low/high
- ☐ Bandanna

Camp Kitchen

- ☐ Stove, with windscreen and other necessary accessories
- ☐ Fuel for _____ days
- ☐ Lighter/matches
- ☐ Cooking pots, with lids and pot grabber
- ☐ Plate/bowl
- ☐ Cup/bottle
- ☐ Utensils
- ☐ Can opener
- ☐ Pot scrubber
- ☐ Bear canister
- ☐ Dish towel and biodegradable soap

Food

- ☐ Coffee, tea, and drink mix
- ☐ Breakfast for _____ days

- ☐ Ready-to-eat trail snacks and lunch for _____ days
- ☐ Dinner for _____ days
- ☐ Spice kit
- ☐ Food for extra day(s), just in case

- ☐ Insect protection (head net, repellent)
- ☐ Straps
- ☐ Carabiners
- ☐ Trekking poles
- ☐ Pack cover

Hygiene

- ☐ Toilet paper (in a Ziploc bag, plus extra bags to pack out your tp)
- ☐ Biodegradable soap
- ☐ Hand sanitizer
- ☐ Plastic trowel (or use a stick or rock)
- ☐ Washcloth and/or towel
- ☐ Toothbrush, toothpaste
- ☐ Comb
- ☐ Deodorant
- ☐ Lip balm
- ☐ Tampons/pantyliners for women, even if not menstruating (backpacking can sometimes throw off women's cycles; pads are also great to help bandage cuts)

Ten Essentials Plus

- ☐ Water bottles, hydration bag/large water-storage bag
- ☐ Water treatment (filter and extra filters, tablets)
- ☐ Extra layers
- ☐ Headlamp/flashlight, plus extra batteries
- ☐ First aid kit
- ☐ Map and compass (guidebook/trail description; GPS optional)
- ☐ Sun protection (glasses, sunscreen, hat)
- ☐ Fire starter (matches, lighter, and/or tinder)
- ☐ Emergency whistle
- ☐ Emergency blanket
- ☐ Knife/supertool
- ☐ Plastic bags (small, medium, large)

First Aid Kit

(For augmenting, restocking, or building your own kit)

- ☐ SAM splint or other splint
- ☐ CPR shield/mask
- ☐ EMT snips, for cutting through clothing, boots, etc., without hurting patient
- ☐ Q-tips or other swabs
- ☐ Safety pins
- ☐ Notebook/pencil, in plastic bag, for recording vital signs, symptoms, etc.
- ☐ Irrigation syringe
- ☐ Antiseptic wipes or other sterilizer
- ☐ Antibiotic ointment
- ☐ Hydrocortisone
- ☐ Tweezers
- ☐ Aloe vera gel, for treating sunburn, insect bites, rashes, burns, and other skin irritations
- ☐ Protective gloves (latex, nitrile, or other material)
- ☐ Band-Aids (include fingertip and knuckle bandages)
- ☐ ¼- by 4-inch wound closure strips, for closing wounds
- ☐ Spenco 2nd Skin or other liquid bandage
- ☐ Non-adhering sterile dressings
- ☐ Gauze roller bandages
- ☐ Ace-type elastic bandage
- ☐ Moleskin and Molefoam
- ☐ Athletic/medical tape
- ☐ Medications
- ☐ Aspirin
- ☐ Ibuprofen

- [ ] Acetaminophen
- [ ] Arnica ointment or tablets
- [ ] Benadryl for allergies
- [ ] Antacid tablets
- [ ] Anti-diarrhea medication
- [ ] Activated charcoal (to take if you ingest poison/eat the wrong plant)

Repair Kit

- [ ] Duct tape
- [ ] Bailing wire
- [ ] Needle and thread
- [ ] Safety pins
- [ ] Super Glue or hot-glue stick
- [ ] Stove-repair kit
- [ ] Nylon-repair tape
- [ ] Water-filter repair kit
- [ ] Sleeping-pad repair kit
- [ ] Parachute cord or other cord, for hanging food and other uses
- [ ] Tent-pole splint

Contingency

- [ ] Money and credit card
- [ ] Personal identification
- [ ] Car keys
- [ ] Cell phone, satellite phone, or personal locator beacon (PLB)

Luxuries

- [ ] Book
- [ ] Nature guides
- [ ] Playing cards
- [ ] Camp chair
- [ ] Pillow
- [ ] Binoculars or close-up lens
- [ ] Camera, film, tripod
- [ ] Journal and pen/pencil
- [ ] Umbrella

Optional Items

Take the following, depending on your destination and hiking partners:
- [ ] Sawyer Extractor, for snakebites
- [ ] Acetazolamide (Diamox), a prescription medication for altitude sickness
- [ ] Glutose paste, for diabetic reactions and hypothermia
- [ ] EpiPen, a prescription epinephrine injector for anaphylactic shock
- [ ] Vicodin, Percocet, or other prescription pain killer for serious pain management when you're days from rescue

Other Items

- [ ] _____
- [ ] _____
- [ ] _____
- [ ] _____
- [ ] _____
- [ ] _____
- [ ] _____
- [ ] _____
- [ ] _____
- [ ] _____
- [ ] _____
- [ ] _____
- [ ] _____
- [ ] _____
- [ ] _____
- [ ] _____
- [ ] _____
- [ ] _____
- [ ] _____
- [ ] _____
- [ ] _____

APPENDIX II
BACKPACKING AND HIKING ORGANIZATIONS AND RESOURCES

Adirondack Mountain Club:
www.adk.org; 518-668-4447

Alabama Trails Association:
www.alabamatrailsasso.org

American Hiking Society:
www.americanhiking.org; 301-565-6704

Appalachian Mountain Club:
www.outdoors.org; 617-523-0636

Appalachian Trail Conservancy:
www.appalachiantrail.org; 304-535-6331

Audubon Society:
www.audubon.org; 212-979-3000

Backpacker magazine:
www.backpacker.com

Bureau of Land Management:
www.blm.gov; 202-452-5125

Calgary Outdoor Recreation Enthusiasts:
corehike.org

Colorado Fourteeners:
www.coloradofourteeners.org; 303-278-7525

Continental Divide Trail Alliance:
www.cdtrail.org; 888-909-CDTA

Desert Survivors:
www.desert-survivors.org

Gorp.com:
gorp.away.com

Mazamas:
www.mazamas.org; 503-227-2345

National Park Conservation Association:
www.npca.org; 800-628-7275

National Park Service:
www.nps.gov; 202-208-6843

North Country Trail Association:
www.northcountrytrail.org; 866-445-3628

Ozark Society:
www.ozarksociety.net

Pacific Crest Trail Association:
www.pcta.org; 916-349-2109

Pacific Northwest Trail Association:
www.pnt.org; 877-854-9415

Sierra Club:
www.sierraclub.org; 415-977-5500

Southern Arizona Hiking Club:
www.sahcinfo.org

Tahoe Rim Trail Association:
www.tahoerimtrail.org; 775-298-0012

The Wilderness Society:
www.wilderness.org; 800-843-9453

APPENDIX III
MANUFACTURER CONTACT INFORMATION

Adventure Medical Kits:
www.adventuremedicalkits.com;
510-261-7414

Aquaseal:
www.aquaseal.com; 360-794-8250

Arc'Teryx:
www.arcteryx.com; 604-960-3001

ArchCrafters:
www.archcrafters.com; 800-707-9928

BakePacker:
www.bakepacker.com; 866-576-0642

Big Agnes:
www.bigagnes.com; 877-554-8975

Black Diamond:
www.blackdiamondequipment.com;
801-278-5552

Bridgedale:
www.bridgedale.com; 802-658-8322

Campsuds:
www.sierradawn.com; 707-535-0172

Cascade Designs:
www.cascadedesigns.com; 800-531-9531

Cocoon:
www.designsalt.com; 800-254-7258

Coghlan's:
www.coghlans.com; 877-264-4526

Coleman:
www.coleman.com; 800-835-3278

Crazy Creek:
www.crazycreek.com; 800-331-0304

Dana Design:
www.danadesign.com; 888-357-3262

Dr. Bronner's:
www.drbronner.com; 877-786-3469

Dr. Scholl's:
www.drscholls.com;

Esbit:
www.esbit.de

ExOfficio:
www.exofficio.com; 800-644-7303

Exped:
www.exped.com

Fox River:
www.foxsox.com

GoLite:
www.golite.com; 888-546-5483

Gore-Tex:
www.gore.com; 888-914-4673

Granger's:
www.grangersusa.com; 800-577-2700

Granite Gear:
www.granitegear.com; 218-834-6157

Gregory Mountain Products:
www.gregorypacks.com; 800-477-3420

Injinji Socks:
www.injinji.com; 888-465-4654

Integral Designs:
www.integraldesigns.com; 403-640-1445

Katadyn:
www.katadyn.com; 800-755-6701

Kelty:
www.kelty.com; 800-423-2320

Leatherman:
www.leatherman.com; 800-847-8665

Leki:
www.leki.com; 800-255-9982

Marmot:
www.marmot.com; 888-357-3262

McNett Corporation (Seam Grip):
www.mcnett.com; 360-671-2227

Merrell:
www.merrellboot.com; 616-866-5500

Montrail:
www.montrail.com; 503-985-4000

Mountain Equipment Co-op:
www.mec.ca; 888-847-0770

Mountain Hardwear:
www.mountainhardwear.com; 800-953-8375

Mountain Safety Research (MSR):
www.msrcorp.com; 800-531-9531

Mountainsmith:
www.mountainsmith.com; 800-551-5889

Nalgene:
www.nalgene-outdoor.com; 800-625-4327

Nikwax:
www.nikwax.com; 800-563-3057

Optimus:
www.optimus.se

Orikaso:
www.orikaso.com; 800-577-2700

Outback Oven:
www.backpackerspantry.com; 303-581-0518

Outdoor Research:
www.orgear.com; 888-467-4327

Pacific Outdoor Equipment (Insul Mat):
www.pacoutdoor.com; 406-586-5258

Patagonia:
www.patagonia.com; 800-638-6464

Petzl:
www.petzl.com; 801-926-1500

Polar Equipment (Polar Pure):
www.polarequipment.com; 408-867-4576

Potable Aqua:
www.potableaqua.com; 800-568-6614

Primus:
www.primusstoves.com

Princeton Tec:
www.princetontec.com; 609-298-9331

Quantum Health:
www.quantumhealth.com; 800-448-1448

Quixote:
www.quixotedesign.com; 206-545-9555

REI:
www.rei.com; 800-426-4840

Ruffwear:
www.ruffwear.com; 888-783-3932

Sea to Summit:
www.seatosummit.com; 303-440-8977

Shock Doctor:
www.shockdoc.com; 800-233-6956

Sierra Designs:
www.sierradesigns.com; 800-635-0461

SmartWool:
www.smartwool.com; 800-550-9665

Snow Peak:
www.snowpeak.com; 503-697-3330

Spenco Medical Corporation:
www.spenco.com; 800-877-3626

Sportif USA:
www.sportif.com; 775-359-6400

Superfeet:
www.superfeet.com; 800-634-6618

Suunto:
www.suunto.com

Teko:
www.tekosocks.com; 800-450-5784

Tender Corporation:
www.tendercorp.com; 800-258-4696

The North Face:
www.thenorthface.com; 866-715-3223

Therm-a-Rest:
www.thermarest.com; 800-531-9531

Thorlo:
www.thorlo.com; 888-846-7567

Vargo:
www.vargooutdoors.com; 877-932-8546

Vasque:
www.vasque.com; 800-224-4453

Western Mountaineering:
www.westernmountaineering.com;
408-287-8944

Wigwam:
www.wigwam.com; 800-558-7760

Wolf Packs: www.wolfpacks.com; 541-482-7669

APPENDIX IV
BIBLIOGRAPHY

Anger, Bradford. *Basic Wilderness Survival Skills.* Guilford, CT: The Lyons Press, 2002.

Auerbach, Paul. *Medicine for the Outdoors: The Essential Guide to Emergency Medical Procedures and First Aid.* New York: The Lyons Press, 1999.

Barnes, Scottie et al. *The Ultimate Guide to Wilderness Navigation.* Guilford, CT: The Lyons Press, 2002.

Bennett, Jeff. *The Essential Whitewater Kayaker: A Complete Course.* Camden, ME: Ragged Mountain Press, 1999.

Bennett, Steve and Ruth. *365 Outdoor Activities You Can Do With Your Child.* Holbrook, MA: Bob Adams, Inc., 1993.

Berger, Karen. *Everyday Wisdom: 1001 Expert Tips for Hikers.* Seattle, WA: The Mountaineers Books, 1997.

Bruce, Dan. *The Thru-Hiker's Handbook.* Appalachian Trail Conference, 1997.

Bryson, Bill. *A Walk in the Woods: Rediscovering America on the Appalachian Trail.* New York: Anchor Books, 2006.

Cassidy, John. *The Klutz Book of Knots.* Palo Alto, CA: Klutz, 1985.

Connors, Tim and Christine. *Lipsmakin' Backpackin': Lightweight, Trail-Tested Recipes for Backcountry Trips.* Guilford, CT: Globe Pequot Press, 2000.

Cornell, Joseph. *Sharing Nature with Children.* Nevada City, CA: Dawn Publications, 1998.

Crouch, Gregory. *Route Finding: Navigating with Map and Compass.* Helena, MT: Falcon Books, 1999.

Fleming, June. *The Well-Fed Backpacker.* New York: Vintage Books, 1986.

Fletcher, Colin. *The Man Who Walked Through Time: The Story of the First Trip Afoot Through the Grand Canyon.* New York: Vintage Books, 1989.

Fletcher, Colin. *The Thousand Mile Summer.* New York: Vintage Books, 1989.

Fredston, Jill, and Fesler, Doug. *Snow Sense: A Guide to Evaluating Snow Avalanche Hazard.* Anchorage, AK: Alaska Mountain Safety Center, 1999.

Ganci, Dave. *Desert Hiking.* Berkeley, CA: Wilderness Press, 1996.

Go, Benedict. *Pacific Crest Trail Data Book.* Berkeley, CA: Wilderness Press, 2005.

Gookin, John, ed. *NOLS Wilderness Wisdom: Quotes for Inspiration Exploration.* Mechanicsburg, PA: Stackpole Books, 2003.

Graham, John. *Outdoor Leadership: Technique, Common Sense & Self Confidence.* Seattle, WA: The Mountaineers Books, 1997.

Graham, Scott. *Extreme Kids: How to Connect with your Children Through Today's Extreme (And Not So Extreme) Outdoor Sports*. Berkeley, CA: Wilderness Press, 2006.

Grubbs, Bruce. *Desert Sense: Camping, Hiking and Biking in Hot, Dry Climates*. Seattle, WA: The Mountaineers Books, 2004.

Hampton, Bruce, and Cole, David. *Soft Paths*. Mechanicsburg, PA: Stackpole Books, 2003.

Hostetter, Kristen. *Don't Forget Duct Tape: Tips and Tricks for Repairing Outdoor Gear*. Seattle, WA: The Mountaineers Books, 2003.

Howe, Steve, et al. *Making Camp: A Complete Guide for Hikers, Mountain Bikers, Paddlers & Skiers*. Seattle, WA: The Mountaineers Books, 1997.

Jacobson, Cliff. *Knots for the Outdoors*. Guilford, CT: Globe Pequot Press, 1999.

Jardine, Ray. *Beyond Backpacking: Ray Jardine's Guide to Lightweight Hiking*. Arizona City, AZ: Adventurelore Press, 1992.

Jardine, Ray. *The Pacific Crest Trail Hiker's Handbook: Innovative Techniques and Trail Tested Instruction for the Long Distance Hiker*. Arizona City, AZ: Adventurelore Press, 1996.

Kesselheim, Alan. *Trail Food: Drying and Cooking Food for Backpackers and Paddlers*. Camden, ME: Ragged Mountain Press, 1998.

Louv, Richard. *Last Child in the Woods: Saving our Children from Nature Deficit Disorder*. Chapel Hill, NC: Algonquin Books, 2005.

Meyer, Kathleen. *How to Shit in the Woods*. Berkeley, CA: Ten Speed Press, 1994.

Mountaineers, The. *Mountaineering: The Freedom of the Hills*. Seattle, WA: The Mountaineers Books, 2003.

Musnick, David, and Pierce, Mark. *Conditioning for Outdoor Fitness*. Seattle, WA: The Mountaineers Books, 1999.

National Outdoor Leadership School. *Wilderness Ethics: Valuing and Managing Wild Places*. Mechanicsburg, PA: Stackpole Books, 2006.

O'Bannon, Allen, and Clelland, Mike. *Allen and Mike's Really Cool Backpackin' Book: Traveling and Camping Skills for a Wilderness Environment!* Helena, MT: Falcon Books, 2001.

Pearson, Claudia. *NOLS Cookery*. Mechanicsburg, PA: Stackpole Books, 2004.

Renner, Jeff. *Mountain Weather: Backcountry Forecasting and Weather Safety for Hikers, Campers, Climbers, Skiers, and Snowboarders*. Seattle, WA: The Mountaineers Books, 2005.

Ross, Cindy, and Gladfelter, Todd. *Kids in the Wild: A Family Guide to Outdoor Recreation*. Seattle, WA: The Mountaineers, 1995.

Seidman, David. *The Essential Wilderness Navigator*. Camden, ME: Ragged Mountain Press, 1995.

Silverman, Goldie Gendler. *Camping with Kids: The Complete Guide to Car, Tent, and RV Camping*. Berkeley, CA: Wilderness Press, 2006.

Sloan, Jim. *Staying Fit Over 50: Conditioning for Outdoor Activities*. Seattle, WA: The Mountaineers Books, 1999.

Stock, Gregory. *The Book of Questions*. New York: Workman Publishing, 1987.

Tawrell, Paul. *Camping & Wilderness Survival: The Ultimate Outdoors Book*. Shelburne, VT: Paul Tawrell, 1996.

Tilton, Buck, and Bennett, Rick. *Don't Get Sick: The Hidden Dangers of Camping and Hiking*. Seattle, WA: The Mountaineers Books, 2002.

Tilton, Buck. *Tent and Car Camper's Handbook: Advice for Families and First-Timers*. Seattle, WA: The Mountaineers Books, 2006.

Weiss, Eric. *Wilderness 911: A Step-By-Step Guide for Medical Emergencies and Improvised Care in the Backcountry*. Seattle, WA: The Mountaineers Books, 1998.

Weiss, Hal. *Secrets of Warmth: For Comfort and Survival*. Seattle, WA: The Mountaineers Books, 1992.

Williams, Tyler. *Whitewater Classics: Fifty North American Rivers Picked by the Continent's Leading Paddlers*. Flagstaff, AZ: Funhog Press, 2004.

Wood, Robert: *The 2 Oz. Backpacker: A Problem Solving Manual for Use in the Wilds*. Berkeley, CA: Ten Speed Press, 1982.

INDEX

A

adiabatic lapse rate 195, 241
affordable backpacking 46
air pressure, weather 195
altitude
    hiking at 241
    sickness 242–243
American Hiking Society 14
anaphylactic shock 207, 227, 230
Animatedknots.com 142
anti-oxidants 107–108
Appalachian Mountain Club 15
Appalachian Trail 17
Atkins diet 106
Attention Deficit Hyperactivity
  Disorder (ADHD) 3, 24
attitude 218, 235, 236
Audubon Society 15
autism 3
avalanches, snow 244

B

Backpacker magazine 13, 14, 45,
  93
backpacking
    why it's great 1–3
backpacks 72–75
    capacity, explanation of
      73–74
    daypacks and travel packs
      75
    external frame 73

finding the right pack
    72–75
how to put on and adjust
    161–162
internal frame 73
kids packs 28
lightweight 73
proper fit 75
bacteria 181–182
BakePacker oven 93
barometric pressure 195
bears 212–214
biodegradable soaps 94, 96, 139,
  182
bivy sacks 79
blisters 165–166
bonking, prevention 168
boots. *See* footwear
Brower, David 47
Bullas, Roslyn 95
Bureau of Land Management 18

C

caffeine 104
cairns, rock 170
calories 103
camp chairs 55, 56
camp kitchen 86–96
Camping Life magazine 45
campsites
    breaking down 187
    choosing and setting up
      172–175
canoeing 251

canyoneering 249
car camping 39, 154–155
carbohydrates 105
cardiopulmonary resuscitation
  (CPR) 224
CD-rom maps 128
cell phones 54
Centers for Disease Control and
  Prevention 204, 208, 217
Chambers, Mary 33
checklists 152–153, 253–255
    camp kitchen 253
    clothing 253
    contingency 255
    first aid kit 254–255
    food 253–254
    hygiene 254
    luxuries 255
    optional items 255
    other items 255
    packing 253
    repair kit 255
    shelter 253
    ten essentials plus 254
children, backpacking with
  24–39
    activities for the trail 35–39
    clothing and gear 27–30
    fishing 31
    infants 25
    rules for kids 30–31
    when to start 24–25
    where to go 26–27
chlorine dioxide 90–91
chocolate 55

ABOUT THE AUTHOR

Some of Brian Beffort's favorite moments have taken place while exploring the American West and other parts of the world while carrying everything he needs on his back. He is also the author of *Afoot & Afield Las Vegas & Southern Nevada: A Comprehensive Hiking Guide.* He currently lives in Reno, Nevada, with his wife, son, and dog, and he works as the Associate Director of Friends of Nevada Wilderness.

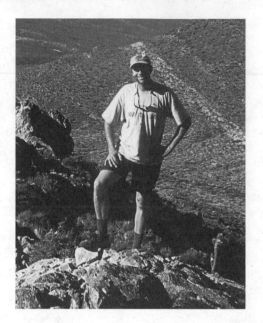